HEALTH CARE AS A RIGHT OF CITIZENSHIP

Health Care as a Right of Citizenship

THE CONTINUING EVOLUTION OF REFORM

Gunnar Almgren

Columbia University Press
New York

Columbia University Press
Publishers Since 1893
New York   Chichester, West Sussex
cup.columbia.edu
Copyright © 2017 Columbia University Press

Library of Congress Cataloging-in-Publication Data

Names: Almgren, Gunnar Robert, 1951– author.
Title: Health care as a right of citizenship : the continuing evolution
of reform / Gunnar Almgren.
Description: New York : Columbia University Press, [2017] |
Includes bibliographical references and index.
Identifiers: LCCN 2016026234| ISBN 9780231170123 (cloth : alk. paper) |
ISBN 9780231170130 (paperback : alk. paper) | ISBN 9780231543316 (e-book)
Subjects: | MESH: United States. Patient Protection and Affordable Care Act. |
Health Care Reform | Civil Rights | Social Justice | Social Security | United States
Classification: LCC RA412.2 | NLM WA 540 AA1 | DDC 368.38/200973—dc23
LC record available at https://lccn.loc.gov/2016026234

Columbia University Press books are printed on permanent and durable acid-free paper.
Printed in the United States of America

Cover design: Mary Ann Smith

Cover images: Statue of Liberty © Homestudio/Shutterstock;
Caduccus © Hurst Photo/Shutterstock

Dedicated to the memory of Edgar Borgatta (1924–2016)

Professor emeritus of sociology, University of Washington

Immigrant, World War II veteran, eminent sociologist, teacher, and mentor to generations of social scientists

CONTENTS

PREFACE

As history contemplates the 2010 Affordable Care Act (ACA), there are two plausible narratives of its meaning and significance that might emerge. The first narrative, capturing the despair of its proponents in the wake of the November 2016 elections, will define the ACA as a poorly conceived and ultimately failed expansion of the welfare state akin to mainstream history's appraisal of the Johnson administration's Great Society and War on Poverty social experiments of the 1960s. The second narrative, which this book advances as by far the most likely, is that the ACA's historical significance will not be in its largely successful expansion of health-care entitlements and insurance subsidies to millions of Americans but in its affirmation by act of Congress, for the first time in the nation's history, the idea that comprehensive health care must be available to all as a social right of citizenship. While previous acts of Congress sought to incrementally expand public and private health-care insurance to the aged, poor, and the disabled, the ACA is unique in its embracement of universal health insurance coverage to all citizens as an explicit policy aim.

Although the conservative Congresses that followed the 2010 passage of the ACA have since endeavored to repeal the ACA and the hard right results of the 2016 elections might seem to guarantee it, what matters is that the mainstream American public now views access to affordable health care as crucial function of just and effective governance, and any proposed alternative to the ACA must be reconciled with that expectation. However the ACA might be redefined, repackaged, or even diminished, neither the key health-care industry stakeholders (in particular the pharmaceutical, health insurance, and hospital industries) nor the American public will tolerate a return to the pre-ACA regime of a failing employment-based insurance system, 49.6 million uninsured Americans, and an epidemic of safety-net hospital closures. Political rhetoric is one thing; economic and political reality is another. While this book illuminates other reasons for the ACA's survival in fundamental and functional terms (if not in name), the penultimate argument is the absence of a coherent conservative alternative that will not propel the nation toward the next catastrophic health insurance coverage crisis—a health-care financing crisis that could result in the truly radical health-care reform anathema to conservatism, namely universal social insurance for health care. It is this thought that keeps health insurance industry executives and investors awake at night, as well it should.

While this book does not share the view of many that the 2016 political resurgence of the GOP is synonymous with the demise of the ACA's core provisions to expand insurance coverage to millions of poor Americans and make comprehensive health insurance more affordable to millions more of low- and middle-income families, it also does not regard the basic approach of the ACA as anything more than a politically pragmatic and necessary step toward the evolution of a social right to health care for all Americans. In its critique, the book will illuminate the ways in which the basic policy strategy and structure of the ACA are substantially inadequate to such a task, both because of its inability to achieve universal health insurance coverage and because its substantive health-care provisions fall short of the equity and equality of opportunity requisites of political democracy. Instead, an alternative national health-care policy approach is needed, and the justification and illumination of that alternative approach are ultimately what this book is about.

I make no assumptions about the health-care policy background of the readers of this book, except that they perhaps share a keen interest in the problem of creating a health-care system that is both financially sustainable and capable of making health care accessible, adequate, and affordable to all Americans irrespective of their place in the hierarchy of advantage in American society or their individual health needs. So the book begins with two chapters devoted to a journey into the origins of American exceptionalism in health care: how we managed to create a health-care system that is the most expensive in the world, the most exclusionary among modern democracies, and among the least effective in promoting the overall health of the national population, and the emergence of the most recent era of health-care reform that has the ACA as its signature achievement. In chapter 3, I interrogate the justifications for a social right to healthcare, and then, based on a synthesis of T. H. Marshall and John Rawls on the social citizenship requisites of political democracy, I advance a set of principles that address the substantive aspects of such a right. In chapter 4, I then translate these principles to a set of core health-care policy aims, which in turn provide the framework for a critical appraisal of the ACA's accomplishments and deficits, ending with the book's central argument that the ACA is but an evolutionary step toward what must inevitably be more radical and fundamental health-care reform.

The remainder of the book is devoted to what more radical and fundamental health-care reform should look like. In chapters 5 and 6, I provide the specifics of a fundamentally restructured health-care system that would realize the core health-care policy aims imperative to health system reform, thus fulfilling the substantive requisites to a social right to health care identified in chapter 3. Whether any health-care system achieves or at least makes progress toward its core policy aims is of course an empirical question, so in chapter 7, I provide the specific criterion and measures optimal to evaluating the performance of the redesigned health-care system, based on both established and emergent approaches to the analysis of health-care system performance. In chapter 8, I explore the special issues and considerations that all nations must grapple with as they seek to provide a sustainable social right to health care: the health-care needs and claims of noncitizens, the limits and boundaries of a social right to health care for all citizens, and the special entitlements to health care that might legitimately be claimed by some groups of citizens. This book is founded on the view of health-care reform as an evolutionary process, that a democratic society will inexorably move toward the collective and inclusive realization of those social rights to health care that are essential to not only the well-being of individuals but also the political voices and pathways to opportunity that define democratic citizenship. The particular approaches to evolutionary health-care reform that are advanced in the following chapters may or may not be close to what is ultimately realized, but they represent the desirable and achievable in light of the healthcare requisites of political democracy and the unique context of American exceptionalism in health care. They also represent the direction toward which the nation turned when in 2010 Congress legislated, for the first time in the history of the republic, an irrevocable acknowledgement of health care as a social right subject to claim by all Americans.

ACKNOWLEDGMENTS

First and foremost, I express my incredible gratitude to my wife and life partner, Linda, for all the ways she made this work possible and inspired its purpose. Few books that are worth publishing rise to that level in the absence of great editorial wisdom, a refined editorial eye, and, within academia, a deep knowledge of the author's field. In this regard, I have been extraordinarily fortunate to have as my primary editor Jennifer Perillo, Senior Executive Editor at Columbia University Press. The anonymous referees Jennifer recruited on behalf of the faculty and editorial board of Columbia University Press also provided invaluable critiques, which ultimately enabled me to write a better book. The manuscript was also adeptly shepherded through the editorial review process with the skillful oversight of Associate Editor Stephen Wesley at Columbia University Press, and in final production, it benefited from the meticulous proofing work performed by Erin Davis and the staff at Westchester Publishing Services.

HEALTH CARE AS A RIGHT OF CITIZENSHIP

Chapter One

STATEMENT OF THE PROBLEM

American Exceptionalism in Health Care and the Emergence of the Great Unsustainable Compromise

THE PARADOX OF AMERICAN EXCEPTIONALISM IN HEALTH CARE

There are two contrasting notions of American exceptionalism. The first, known to most elementary school children, speaks to the deeply entrenched ideology in national culture and politics that the American experiment in democracy is both unique in history and uncontested in its achievement of individualism, civic consciousness, respect for human rights, equality of opportunity, collective prosperity, and political democracy (Ross, 1991). The other version, prevalent among scholars of social policy, defines American exceptionalism in terms of its deficits in achieving equality of opportunity and collective prosperity—pointing to such features as the nation's meager social safety net and its rising levels of income inequality (Garfinkel et al., 2010). American exceptionalism in health care is in many respects a hybrid of both of these polarized perspectives. On one hand, the nation invests the most out of all modern democracies in the health care of its citizens— in fact, well over twice as much on a per-capita basis than the average of all other developed democracies (Organization for Economic Cooperation and Development [OECD], 2013c). On the other hand, the United States is one of the very few advanced democracies (along with only Turkey, Mexico, and Chile) that does not provide access to at least basic health care as a universal right of citizenship (OECD, 2012). Even should the Affordable

Care Act (ACA) ultimately achieve its central policy goals that pertain to the expansion of private and public health insurance coverage (a dubious prospect), a significant share of Americans will remain uninsured—in fact, some 23 million men, women, and children (Centers for Medicare and Medicaid Services [CMS], 2010).[1] This is the first dimension of the paradox of American exceptionalism in health care—in essence, spending the most to achieve the least.

A second dimension of the paradox of American exceptionalism in health care is represented by the fact that, contrary to the nation's political history of rejecting legislation that would extend basic health insurance coverage to all Americans as a right of citizenship, Americans have long embraced health care for all as an important national goal (Blendon, Benson, et al., 1994). Moreover, surveys of American attitudes that have been conducted over the past forty years reveal a stable conviction among the far majority of Americans (80 percent) that the assurance of affordable health care for the sick is a legitimate and important function of government (National Opinion Research Center, 2016).[2] In this vein, it is also worth noting that Barack Obama was elected twice to the U.S. presidency by a wide margin on a campaign platform that highlighted universal insurance coverage as a social and political goal of just and inclusive governance.

The third and final dimension to the paradox of American exceptionalism is that while there has long been a consensus among the primary stakeholders in the American health-care system (defined here as consumers, providers, and payers) that the system is broken and dysfunctional, there is precious little consensus on what specific reforms are needed or in the nation's best interests (Fuchs & Emmanuel, 2005). While this particular conundrum can be attributed in large part to the conflicting interests of consumers, providers, and payers of health care in any particular solution, as the proportion of the gross domestic product (GDP) expended on health care approaches 20 percent and the Medicare Hospital Insurance Trust Fund approaches collapse, it is self-evident that retention of the status quo is the worst of all possible options.

As essential context for this book's central purpose, which is to provide the basic outline of a proposed long-term solution to the paradox of American exceptionalism in health care, this chapter provides a narrative of the complex origins of American exceptionalism in health care and the main impediments to the realization of health care as a social right afforded to all Americans.

THE PATH TO THE "GREAT UNSUSTAINABLE COMPROMISE" IN AMERICAN HEALTH-CARE FINANCING

One way to think about the evolvement of the American health-care system is that it is the result of a century-long quest to reconcile the principles of political liberalism, particularly the idea that democratic citizenship requires some substantive provisions essential to fair equality of opportunity, with libertarian notions of full self-ownership, the sanctity of private property, and the pernicious nature of government. This result is described here as the "Great Unsustainable Compromise," that is, a fragmented mixed-public and private system of health-care finance and delivery that has been built around a subsidized employment-based insurance system with selective entitlements to health care for the poor and aged.

Embedded in this system are two contradictions that have led to it being unsustainable. The first is its inherently inflationary tendencies due to, among other things, its historic and continued accommodations to the interests of politically powerful stakeholder groups. The second contradiction has to do with inconsistency between selective entitlement to health care as a social right on the basis of factors such as age, social class, and race and the substantive requirements of political democracy that are crucial to political citizenship and the preservation of a permeable class structure.

Current estimates by the trustees of the Medicare Hospital Insurance Trust Fund predict that this fund will have exhausted its assets by 2030, even under the optimistic assumption that the ACA's Medicare program cost-savings measures will be implemented and as effective as anticipated. Prior to the ACA becoming law in 2010, the Medicare Hospital Insurance Trust Fund was projected to be exhausted by 2017 (Board of Trustees Medicare Hospital Insurance Trust Fund, 2014; CMS, 2009).

While it is conceded that the dominant accounts of the evolution of the American health-care system that are based on the political economy perspective are both empirically grounded and compelling (see in particular Quadagno 2004, 2005; Starr, 1982), in the narrative offered here, the origins of American exceptionalism in health care that reside within the conflicts between the libertarian and liberalist traditions in American political thought also are emphasized—in particular, their derivatives in the public attitudes toward the nature and proper role of government as a force in the life chances of individuals. Where the political economy perspective is most useful (and in fact essential) is in understanding how the particular policy compromises that have been crafted to reconcile the liberal–libertarian streams in American political consciousness have served the interests of powerful stakeholder groups, each representing the advantaged segments of American society during different periods in the history of the American health-care system. Apart from this interplay between the dominant ideologies in American political thought and political economy of health-care system stakeholders, the narrative that follows also incorporates (like other accounts of the evolvement of the U.S. health-care system) the phenomenon of path dependence in social policy—in essence, the tendency of yesterday's policy solutions to become so institutionalized as to shape the parameters of the possible in today's policy options.

While the interplay between the liberal–libertarian divide in American politics and the political economy of health care has been a constant determinant of health-care policy both before and subsequent to the immediate post–World War II years, it was the pivotal five-year period between 1945 and 1949 that set the nation on its course toward exceptionalism in health-care policy. The following analysis of this crucial period is divided into two parts to properly illuminate the two distinct but complementary roots of American exceptionalism in health care: one originating from the power of the American Medical Association (AMA) to shape national health care policy in ways that served the interests of the medical profession and the other originating from the dynamics of path dependence in social policy.

THE TRIUMPH OF THE MEDICAL PROFESSION IN POST-WORLD WAR II AMERICA (1945-1949)

At the close of World War II in 1945, a broad movement had emerged among the allied Western democracies that had triumphed over Nazi Germany and Imperial Japan to both make major investments in their health-care systems and to ultimately make health care a universal entitlement of citizenship.

Although their pace of achievement was uneven, within a generation of the war's ending, each of these democracies (with the sole exception of the United States) had ultimately created a system of universal coverage for comprehensive health care. In France, the Social Security Ordinance of 1945 expanded the heretofore very limited national insurance program to all salaried workers in industry and commerce, marking the beginning of a gradual path toward universal coverage that France ultimately achieved by 1978 (Rodwin & Sandier, 2008). In the United Kingdom, the Labour government passed the National Health Service Act of 1946, which established the National Health Service (1948), thus setting the blueprint for the single-payer public health-care system approach to universal health care. In Canada, the march toward universal health-care coverage began in 1944 with the province of Saskatchewan's universal hospital insurance coverage, which by 1958 had been extended to all Canadian provinces—although universal access to comprehensive health-care services was not fully realized until the Canadian Health Act of 1984 established Canadian Medicare (Irvine et al., 2005). In Australia, the beginnings of a national health insurance plan can be traced to the Labour government's introduction of a national prepaid hospital system in 1946. However, similar to Canada, the realization of a universal right to health care in Australia required nearly three decades—its national plan for comprehensive health insurance coverage (also referred to as Medicare) was not achieved until 1984 (Gray, 2013).

In the United States at the close of World War II, it also seemed highly likely that a plan of national social insurance for health care would be realized in the immediate postwar years. Like his counterparts in the postwar leaders of the United Kingdom, Canada, Australia, and France, President Harry Truman had also embraced a plan of national health insurance as national domestic priority. In fact, the federal investments in public health, hospital construction, and a national health insurance plan that would provide universal coverage for all Americans were Truman's signature postwar policy initiatives. In a nutshell, the Truman plan called for a compulsory social insurance system that would cover expenditures for medical, hospital, nursing, laboratory services, and dental care—while at the same time preserving the existing system of private physicians and voluntary hospitals.

When Truman announced his plan in a formal memorandum to the Congress in November 1945, he took pains to directly point out that his plan for national health insurance was not "socialized medicine," as had long been the oppositional battle cry of the AMA:

The American people are the most insurance-minded people in the world. They will not be frightened off from health insurance because some people have misnamed it "socialized medicine." I repeat—what I am recommending is not socialized medicine.

Socialized medicine means that all doctors work as employees of government. The American people want no such system. No such system is here proposed.

Under the plan I suggest, our people would continue to get medical and hospital services just as they do now—on the basis of their own voluntary decisions and choices. Our doctors and hospitals would continue to deal with disease with the same professional freedom as now. There would, however, be this all-important difference: whether or not patients get the services they need would not depend on how much they can afford to pay at the time.[3]

At the time that Truman proposed his national health insurance plan, 75 percent of Americans supported national health insurance, and it could readily be claimed that he had every reason to expect that comprehensive health insurance for all Americans would be a legacy of his presidency. However, by the end of his first term in office four years later, only 21 percent of the public favored his plan—thus setting the nation off on its divergent course toward the most expensive and exclusionary health-care system in the world (Quadagno, 2005). How was it possible that such a dramatic reversal in the public's support for a social insurance approach to universal health care occurred in such a short time?

To begin with, it must be acknowledged that the public consensus that a national plan of compulsory health insurance coverage was acceptable (or even necessary) was a fragile one. At the time that Truman proposed his plan, by his own admission (acknowledged in his November 1945 message to Congress proposing a plan of national health insurance), only 3 to 4 percent of Americans were enrolled in comprehensive health insurance plans available from private insurance, although it is clear that many more had the means to afford the very modestly priced private health insurance premiums available at the time. Second, as a reflection of the strong stream of libertarianism in American politics, shortly after Truman's message to Congress advocating a national plan of health insurance, the nation's political preferences took a sharp turn toward the right, resulting in the Republicans gaining control of both chambers of Congress in the 1946 midterm elections.[4] Third, support for national health insurance by American labor was itself operating on a delicate accord that a government insurance plan was preferable to benefits realized through collective bargaining—an accord that quickly fell apart as collective bargaining rights and pro-labor ideology became a primary target of the new Republican majority in Congress eager to roll back the large gains that labor had made during the New Deal administration of Franklin Roosevelt. With the successful passage of the Taft-Hartley Act of 1947 (famously denounced by

President Truman as "a slave-labor" bill), not only were unions deprived of some of their most essential organizing and collective bargaining rights, but under one provision unions were also required to ban and even purge their communist members (Cockburn, 2004; Quadagno, 2005). This provision, which in the rhetoric of the McCarthy era made socialism synonymous with communism, caused unions to both expel their more radical members and eschew support of any national legislation that might be tagged with the label of "creeping communism"—including, in particular, social insurance for comprehensive health care.

The main story of this debacle, though, resides in the medical profession's power to shape public beliefs and to employ the mechanisms of political power to its own interests, as manifested through the ideological foundations and strategic triumphs of the AMA. At each juncture over the past century, whenever and wherever the nation was engaged in a debate over the assurance of affordable health care for all Americans, the AMA was a formidable and ultimately successful opponent of publicly funded comprehensive universal health insurance. In recent decades, the health insurance industry has eclipsed the AMA as the dominant opponent to publicly sponsored health care. However, the health insurance industry is beholden in its more recent policy successes to the strategic themes and imagery employed by the AMA that are tied to (1) Americans' general distrust of government and special distrust of social programs that are tied to expansions of the welfare state and (2) the resilient belief among most Americans in the benign authority of the medical profession as a whole (and their own physicians in particular) in all matters related to personal health and well-being (Quadagno, 2004; Starr, 1982).

While the former theme is tied to the deeply embedded strain of libertarianism in American culture and politics that became manifest during the nation's early colonial history, the latter theme emerged during the late nineteenth and early twentieth centuries as a distinctive strategic accomplishment of a heretofore fairly disreputable profession eager to advance its status, power, and capacity to shape a national health-care system toward its own ends (Starr, 1982).

Even a greatly condensed version of the authoritative narrative of this accomplishment by the medical profession, Paul Starr's landmark book *Social Transformation of American Medicine* (1982), cannot be done justice in this brief chapter. I will instead highlight the main argument of Starr's analysis of the rise of the American medical profession to dominance over the public interest—that is, the medical profession's achievement of what Starr refers to as *cultural authority*. In contrast to other forms of authority, which extend primarily to the capacity to compel obedience, cultural authority possesses the capacity to define reality (pp. 13–14). The crucial reality defined by the medical profession (as embodied in the AMA) during the early twentieth century and continuously reinforced thereafter is the enduring conviction by a large share of the American public that their own best interests are synonymous with those of their personal physician and, by extension, the medical profession as a whole (Starr, 1982).

The convergence of these two strategic themes has been at the heart of the AMA's popular media campaigns against publicly funded health care over much of the past century. While this dual-message strategy was first successfully employed in the halls of the U.S. Congress in the AMA's opposition to the renewal of the Sheppard-Towner maternal and infant public health-care legislation in 1927,[5] its pivotal triumph is represented in the demolition of the public support for the comprehensive approach to social insurance for health care advocated by the Truman administration that occurred between 1945 and 1949. Arguably, the most effective component of the AMA's public opinion strategy was the grassroots and media campaign that employed as their centerpiece a compelling nineteenth-century tableau: Sir Luke Fildes's 1891 portrait of a physician in practice, aptly titled *The Doctor* (figure 1.1).

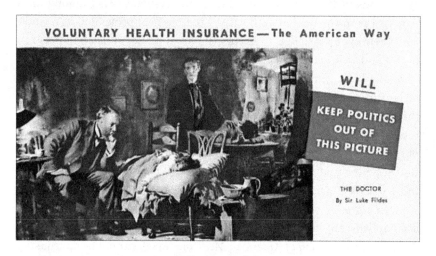

FIGURE 1.1. Sir Luke Fildes's *The Doctor* (1891), adapted by the American Medical Association.

Source: Courtesy of the American Medical Association Archives.

The viewer of *The Doctor* is drawn into the struggle and quiet heroism captured by the artist. As the doctor gazes at his gravely ill patient and ponders his next therapeutic action, we find ourselves hoping that the doctor's competence and wisdom will triumph over suffering and death—the compassion itself is self-evident. Our hopes, fears, and questions are mirrored in the face of the physician's assistant who gazes at the doctor; we all wait in subordinate silence for the doctor to exercise his authoritative and ever benevolent powers of comfort and healing.

However, in contrast to the original version of *The Doctor* displayed for the Royal Academy in London, the AMA's adaptation of Fildes's tableau (the version replicated in this book) is embellished with two political messages that not only represent the convergence of the AMA's two strategic themes but also promote voluntary health insurance as being both acceptable to your doctor and in keeping with what it is to be American. Embedded in this message is not only the blatant point that government involvement in health care is a dangerous obstacle to the practice of medicine and an impediment to the doctor–patient relationship but also the idea that to act against the interests of one's physician (however defined by the AMA) is both a betrayal of doctor–patient trust and contrary to one's own best interests. It is this secondary message that, when joined with notions of free enterprise and professional autonomy rooted in populist libertarianism, enabled the medical profession to shape the organization and financing of health care in ways that privileged the interests of the medical profession over a social right to health care. That is, we witness in the politicized version of *The Doctor* the AMA's successful bid to extend and transform American medicine's cultural authority into what Starr refers to as *professional sovereignty*—defined as the capacity of a profession to extend and transform its authority into social privilege, economic power, and political influence (Starr, 1982, p. 5).

As noted by medical historian John Harley Warner in his *Lancet* essay, "The Doctor in Early Cold War America," *The Doctor* appeared as an official 1947 U.S. postage stamp (sans the blatant political text) and, in its AMA-politicized version, was widely disseminated in pamphlets available in doctors' clinics, in advertisements in popular magazines, and even on banners at medical conventions (Warner, 2013, p. 1452). For the patient, the AMA version of *The Doctor* effectively conveyed the AMA's version of who to trust (your doctor) and who not to trust (President Truman and the government as a whole). For the medical community, *The Doctor* embodied all that would be lost if socialized medicine were allowed to triumph over medical free enterprise.

As brilliant as the selection of *The Doctor* was as the centerpiece of the AMA's strategy to sway public opinion toward the national embracement of medical free enterprise and voluntary health insurance, to achieve its full potential as a symbolic weapon, *The Doctor* required an equally brilliant campaign strategy to advance its message. For this, the AMA relied on the husband-and-wife public relations firm of Williams and Baxter, the architects of the California Medical Association's defeat of a state health insurance plan sponsored by then Governor (and later Supreme Court justice) Earl Warren (Quadagno, 2005).

Launched in 1948, the Williams and Baxter campaign to defeat the Truman plan can be characterized as having an inside and outside strategy. Within the AMA, the campaign characterized the fight against national health insurance as a fundamental struggle against government domination not only of medicine but also of individualism and liberty (Quadagno, 2005, p. 35). Doctors were fighting for not only medical free enterprise and the doctor–patient relationship but also democracy and the American way of life. The outside strategy, made possible with the inspired commitment of an energetic AMA rank and file, enlisted local medical societies throughout the country in a grassroots public information blitzkrieg against the Truman plan that included text for speeches at local clubs and interviews and op-eds for local papers, pamphlets to fill the racks of doctors' waiting rooms, and even office posters depicting the AMA's ever ubiquitous politicized version of *The Doctor*. An additional key asset to the AMA's grassroots campaign was the wives of physicians acting through their local medical society auxiliary organizations (Quadagno, 2005; Warner, 2013). As with the AMA's national-level campaign, claims of comprehensive entitlement to health care as part and partial of a communist conspiracy (consistent with the politics of Cold War–era McCarthyism), massive expansions of government bureaucracy, and the imagery of assembly-line medicine were key to the rhetoric of these local campaigns. While the AMA led the political opposition to the Truman plan and crafted its public messaging strategy, it also coordinated its campaign with both ideological and economic allies.

Ideologically, the AMA was aligned with the U.S. Chamber of Commerce and its local chapters as well as with conservative organizations as the American Legion. Ultimately, even the American Bar Association and most of the national press favored the notion of *voluntary* health insurance over a compulsory national plan (Starr, 1982). The AMA could also count on its economic bedfellows in the insurance industry committed to the preservation and expansion of the nascent voluntary health insurance market, including the not-for-profit Blue Cross health insurance associations and the Insurance Economic Society (Quadagno, 2005). On the other hand, the hospital industry found itself in the difficult position of being economically and ideologically sympathetic to the idea of universal health hospital insurance while being beholden to the goodwill and, in many communities, subject to complete de facto administrative control of the local medical societies. No community hospital administrator could publicly embrace anything but voluntary insurance for hospital care without provoking the collective ire of their medical staffs or their local hospital board.

It was thus inevitable that the powerful American Hospital Association, composed largely of professional hospital administrators, chose to oppose the Truman plan and instead favored government subsidies for the purchase of private health insurance (Starr, 1982). In summary, by the end of the 1940s, the Truman plan had lost both its broad public support and the support of the hospital industry.

Still, to ultimately triumph over the notion of universal social insurance for health care and thereby set the nation on a divergent path from other Western democracies, the AMA required that the Truman plan be co-opted by some form of a publicly funded safety net for the millions of Americans who would never be in a position to have even very basic health insurance coverage for catastrophic hospital costs. Thus, the AMA's victory was ensured by a seemingly progressive piece of legislation that, over the decades, poured billions of federal dollars into expansion of the American hospital industry in the absence of any meaningful federal oversight over where and how those public dollars were invested, or any congressional questioning of whose ends would be ultimately served.

THE HILL-BURTON ACT, WAGE CONTROLS, AND THE EMERGENCE OF PATH DEPENDENCE IN AMERICAN HEALTH-CARE POLICY (1945-1949)

The Hill-Burton Act and Its Inflationary Legacies

There were two components to Truman's postwar vision for a national plan of health care. One was universal social insurance for health care, and the other entailed massive federal investments in the national health-care infrastructure—in particular, the nation's already antiquated and altogether inadequate hospital system. Until the mid-nineteenth century, the government's role in the funding of hospital construction was largely limited to the public health hospitals created to serve the maritime industry, hospitals for soldiers and veterans, and, at the state level, asylums for the mentally ill. The county hospital system, such as it existed, was poorly funded, antiquated, and not at all capable of absorbing the millions of Americans in need of hospital care who, with the greater availability of health insurance, would be able to afford it. In response to the crisis, in 1942 the American Hospital Association organized the National Commission on Hospital Care, which recommended that the nation invest $1.8 billion into the building of an additional 195,000 hospital beds (Starr, 1982). In 1946, Congress passed the Hill-Burton Hospital Survey and Construction Act, which Truman then signed into law—apparently not anticipating the ways in which key provisions of the Hill-Burton Act would then advance the AMA's political agenda in opposition to national health insurance by (1) providing the nation with a morally acceptable alternative to denying hospital care to those unable to afford voluntary health insurance and (2) creating for physicians a publicly subsidized private practice revenue stream in the provision of hospital care in the absence of any government impediments to medical free enterprise.

With respect to the first benefit of the Hill-Burton Act to the medical profession, the $3.7 billion allocated between 1947 and 1971 for local hospital construction in effect were treated as long-term loans, to be paid back to the public over the course of many years through the provision of charity care to poor and uninsured patients (Clark et al., 1980). The availability of so-called Hill-Burton charity care funds as a part of a community hospital's annual budget thus provided both the moral rationale and the public subsidies essential to a national system of hospital care predicated on private voluntary health insurance—at least for the crucial postwar decades when other Western democracies and World War II allies (Great Britain, France, Canada, and Australia) developed more universalistic publicly funded approaches to health insurance coverage.

The secondary benefit of the Hill-Burton Act to the medical profession was to provide, for physicians in private practice, a publicly funded venue for the very lucrative fee-based hospital medical and surgical care for their private patients. That is, while Congress intended that Hill-Burton funds would place a priority on the expansion of hospital bed capacity in lower-income communities, in reality, the Hill-Burton funds were disproportionately allocated to middle- and high-income communities—those suburbs and counties that were best situated to support medical free enterprise (Hochban et al., 1981).[6] In addition, from its implementation in 1947 until 1963, the Hill-Burton Act permitted the use of its funds to construct racially segregated facilities for African American patients and also disproportionately allocated hospital construction funds to white suburbs over inner-city African American communities (Quadagno, 2005; Starr, 1982).

However, the real damage that the Hill-Burton Act did for the prospects of universal health insurance was more long term and far more profound than its immediate effects on undermining the case for the Truman plan. This damage stems from its fostering of health-care cost inflation through both its emphasis on investments in hospital care over primary care outpatient infrastructure and its creation of the spatial context for capital-based competition between hospitals competing for the same pool of insured patients in overlapping service areas. That is, while the Hill-Burton Act was designed to build hospital capacity in accordance with local needs, it is well established that the act played a pivotal role in the rapid growth of U.S. health expenditures for decades after its initial investments in hospital care had been distributed (Chung et al., 2012).

In large part, this particular inflationary effect had to do with a phenomenon called "Roemer's law" (named for UCLA health economist Milton Roemer), which in its essence holds that supply tends to induce its own demand when a third party guarantees reimbursement of use (Roemer, 1961). Or, to rework the famous line from the beloved American baseball movie *Field of Dreams*, "Build the beds and they will come." This in fact was precisely the situation of American hospitals from 1960 to 1980, when health-care expenditures and inflation bypassed that of other modern democracies. Through massive infusion of federal dollars initially via the Hill-Burton hospital construction program and then later through Medicare program provisions (which allowed hospitals to finance their capital investments as a part of the cost of care for Medicare patients), hospitals were positioned to expand their bed capacities with the assurance that they could (through the recruitment of the right mix of medical specialties on their medical staffs) create the demand essential to fill their beds with insured patients. This inflationary juggernaut was only possible because the Hill-Burton Act, over a period of two decades, provided billions in federal hospital construction funds to politically and economically well-positioned communities—in the absence of any systematic way of allocating those funds in accordance with federal criteria for the determination of local area health-care infrastructure needs ("The Hill-Burton Act," 1979).

The second inflationary component to the Hill-Burton Act, again stemming from the lack of any federal oversight of determining local area needs for hospital construction investments, is the role that the act played in creating the geography of capital-based competition between hospitals. In essence, capital-based competition takes place when two hospitals vie for the same pool of insured patients seeking competitive advantage, not through price or quality of care but through more attractive physical facilities and/or the latest innovations in sophisticated health-care technologies (Almgren, 2007). That is, hospitals engage in a kind of medical arms race that blurs the distinction between quality of care (as measured in patient care outcomes) and the appeal of state-of-the-art physical facilities and cutting-edge medical technologies. To cite a specific example, should Hospital A serving the same community as Hospital B acquire the latest version of a multimillion dollar magnetic resonance imaging (MRI) facility, Hospital B would then be compelled to invest millions to acquire its own such technology, even though the hospitals in question are within minutes of travel of each other and could share the same MRI facility without detriment to the population health of the community they both serve. This is one reason why there are 34.5 MRI machines per million persons in the United States, while there are only 8.7 MRI machines per million persons in France with no discernable disadvantage in population health benefits (OECD, 2013d).

The significance of all these inflationary aspects of the Hill-Burton Act to the prospects for the realization of a national plan for universal health care is profound. In essence, to the extent that the Hill-Burton Act is implicated in the growth in health-care expenditures in excess of the baseline inflationary rate for the economy as a whole (and thereby consuming an ever larger share of the nation's GDP), the notion of expanding access to health care to the nation's millions of uninsured has become less viable—both politically and fiscally. Over the decades since the act, we have heard many in Congress decrying the unaffordable burden of entitlement programs on the national economy and the American taxpayer, lending an economic basis to what historically has been an ideological argument against universal health care. While evidence from other nations has long suggested that universal health insurance coverage through a single-payer fund would likely stem the tide of health-care inflation in the United States (Evans, 1990), the reality is that the Hill-Burton Act, in combination with later developments in both the employment-based insurance market and the Medicare program, created a hospital-based political economy of health care that has become institutionally entrenched, thus providing the first crucial root of *path dependence* in American health-care policy. The second root was the subsidized employment-based health insurance approach to financing health care.

Wage Controls, Subsidized Employment-Based Health Insurance, and Path Dependence in Health-Care Policy

As used in this book, *path dependence* refers to the phenomenon that, through the selection of particular policy choices, both social and political constituencies and complementary institutions are created that both entrench these policy choices and constrain future policy alternatives (Page, 2005). While it has been shown how the Hill-Burton Act fostered one form of path dependence in American health-care policy by providing the foundations of an inherently inflationary hospital-based health-care system, conceivably the system could still have been transitioned to a publicly financed system of health insurance that would have included all Americans. That it did not had far more to do with the development of a powerful private health insurance industry, aided and abetted by the largely unintended consequences of federal wage controls imposed both during and after World War II, than any solidified ideological barrier to social insurance for health care among the broad public. As it happens, these federal labor market policies also played perfectly into the AMA's agenda to push the nation toward a commitment to voluntary private-sector health insurance as an alternative to social insurance for health care as a social right of American citizenship.

As concisely summarized in Quadagno's (2005) authoritative narrative of the emergence of employment-based health insurance, the nation's central vehicle for health-care financing, four federal labor market policies enacted during the World War II era propelled the nation toward this preference—three of them made by unelected officials on federal boards charged with the task of restraining the growth of wages as a mechanism to counter inflation. The first was the Revenue Act of 1942, which limited the allowable wartime profits by corporations and thus created incentives for corporations to funnel their excess wartime profits into group insurance plans and health insurance as an allowable business expense (p. 51). This fueled the growth of the private insurance industry and reinforced the role of the employer as the provider of health security for workers and their families (J. Klein, 2005). Then in 1943, the National War Labor Board, charged with the task of controlling the growth of wages in a time of extreme labor shortage, ruled that employer contributions to benefits (including health benefits) would not be counted as wages, thus both incentivizing unions to turn their bargaining power toward the acquisition of health insurance benefits and adding crucial momentum to the insurance industry's rapid development of what had been an heretofore neglected employment-based group health insurance market (J. Klein, 2005).

Finally, during the critical immediate postwar years of 1946 to 1949, when the Truman administration's plan for national health insurance hung in the balance, the last two nails in the plan's coffin were driven in by two pivotal labor market policy decisions. The first was a decision by the National Labor Relations Board in 1948 that ruled (in contrast to more restrictive interpretations of the 1947 Taft-Hartley Act) that fringe benefits were subject to collective bargaining; the second was a 1949 decision by the Wage Stabilization Board that held that fringe benefits (in contrast to wages) were noninflationary (Quadagno, 2005, p. 52). Taken together, these two decisions pushed the then powerful labor movement to abandon any of its heretofore lukewarm support for a national plan of health insurance in favor of securing health insurance benefits at the bargaining table. In a related development, health insurance benefits for workers and their dependents were subsequently ruled by both the Internal Revenue Service (IRS) and the National War Labor Board to be a nontaxable form of employment compensation—thus furthering the rapid expansion of the employment-based health insurance market and ultimately the demise of the New Deal vision of an all-inclusive national plan of social insurance for health insurance (Helms, 2008).

To get a sense of the pace and magnitude of the growth of employment-based insurance, figure 1.2 shows the trend in the percentage of the national population covered by hospital insurance and surgical insurance (covering physician services) for the two postwar decades that set the course for American exceptionalism in health care. While employment-based hospital insurance had been in existence with the development of the first Blue Cross

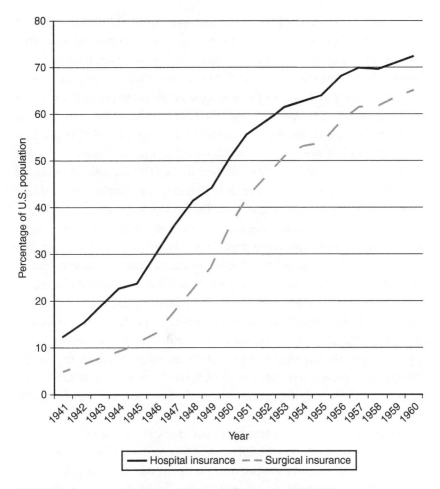

FIGURE 1.2. Percentage of the U.S. population covered by insurance, 1940–1960.

Source: Historical Statistics of the United States: Colonial Times to 1970: Series B 401–412 (Washington, D.C.: U.S. Census Bureau, 1975).

plan in 1929,[7] in 1941, just 12.4 percent of Americans were covered by either group or individual health insurance policies for hospital care. By 1950, that figure had swelled to 50 percent, and by 1961, nearly three of four Americans were covered by at least hospital insurance (U.S. Census Bureau, 1975).

Nothing illustrates the phenomenon of path dependence in social policy with more clarity than postwar expansion of the employment-based insurance industry and the emergence of subsidized employment-based insurance as the preferred mechanism for the financing of health care. Use of the term *subsidized employment-based insurance* highlights the fact that the voluntary employment-based health insurance approach advocated by the AMA entails a significant infusion of tax subsidies, both in dollar value of health insurance benefits that are a part of the compensation package for workers and also in the nontaxed employer share of the costs of health insurance benefits. Although the relative value of tax subsidies was fairly modest during the first two decades following the end of World War II, by the end of the 1970s (as health-care cost inflation began to exceed 10 percent of the GDP), the tax subsidies for health insurance skyrocketed from the 2015 dollar equivalent of \$13 billion in 1969 to \$120 by the mid-1990s to \$300 billion by 2009 (Congressional Budget Office, 1994; Helms, 2008).

Thus, the institution that became the penultimate impediment to social insurance for health care is the employment-based insurance industry. The fact that the employment-based health insurance industry has been dominated by the traditionally not-for-profit Blue Cross and Blue Shield organizations has been irrelevant to the health insurance industry's role as the most formidable post–World War II opponent to publicly financed health care. The organization that represents the health insurance industry in its opposition to the expansion of publicly financed health care, the Health Insurance Association of America (HIAA, now known as America's Health Insurance Plans [AHIP]), represents both the profit and not-for-profit health sectors of the industry.

As noted by Quadagno (2005, pp. 206–207), since the mid-1960s, the HIAA has completely superseded the AMA as the key player in opposition to national health insurance, not only via its considerable funds for lobbying, political contributions, and media campaigns but also via its capacity to mobilize other powerful stakeholders against health-care reform (e.g., the National Federation of Independent Businesses). In an example of the health insurance industry's clout (to be delved into further at a later point), the defeat of the Clinton administration's Health Security Act can in large part be attributed to the \$100 million the HIAA was able to raise in opposition (Goldsteen et al., 2001).

MEDICARE, MEDICAID, AND THE ESTABLISHMENT OF THE GREAT UNSUSTAINABLE COMPROMISE (1965-1974)

Since the 1950s, the AMA's power to shape national health-care policy in accordance to its interests has lessened as the power of the health insurance industry has grown. However, in its final major exercise of its waning influence during the mid-1960s, the AMA did manage to effect (in concert with organized labor and the health insurance industry) a reluctant compromise that sustained the continued viability of the employment-based insurance model as an alternative to social insurance for health care. This compromise involved three essential bargains between (1) the AMA's historically vehement opposition to any form of government financing of health care and pragmatists who recognized the failures of the voluntary insurance market, (2) employers, their health insurance carriers, and the hospital industry, and (3) liberals and conservatives in Congress divided over the role of government as a provider of health insurance.

What made this compromise ultimately unsustainable were the inflationary elements already built into the American health system and the ways in which these inflationary elements were aided and abetted by the structure of new federal health-care entitlements that were the policy outcomes of this great three-part compromise. I refer in particular to the 1965 amendments to the Social Security Act that define Medicare and Medicaid health-care entitlement programs.

The AMA and the Medicare/Medicaid Bargain

The AMA had for decades steadfastly and vociferously opposed any financing alternative to voluntary health insurance, but by the early 1960s, it was clear that two populations could not access health care through the voluntary health insurance market sustained by employment-based insurance: those unable to work or find work and their dependents, and retired workers and their dependent spouses. With respect to the first population, while the AMA had a long history of opposing public financing of health care, the organization eventually conceded the necessity of some form of means-based health insurance subsidy for the poor administered by local and state authorities (Fleming, 1971). Medicaid was thus distasteful to the AMA but not viewed as a threat to its core commitment to medical free enterprise sustained by voluntary health insurance. Medicare, on the other hand, was social insurance for health care. Although confined to adults aged sixty-five years and older, Medicare represented a large and dangerous step toward what the AMA defined as socialized medicine—an all-inclusive social insurance fund for health care as intended by the Truman administration two decades before. This, in fact, was precisely the hope and intent of the liberal wing of the congressional Democrats representing the aspirations of their aging New Dealer political mentors.

Although the AMA pulled out all stops to oppose Medicare, it was ultimately unable to overcome the political realities of a Democratic sweep in 1964 of both chambers of Congress, the grassroots campaign by a coalition of the National Council of Senior Citizens and the AFL-CIO (the latter viewing government health insurance for retired workers as ultimately consistent with the employment-based insurance model and collective bargaining power), and the defection of the health insurance industry as a political ally against Medicare (Marmor, 2000; Quadagno, 2005). The Medicare program was structured to provide for a large supplementary health insurance market, and furthermore, many health insurance industry experts questioned the viability of a voluntary health insurance product line for comprehensive care that would be affordable to the elderly (Quadagno, 2005; Social Security Administration, 2014a; Starr, 1982).

However, in the very close fight to have Medicare get through Congress, the AMA did win two crucial and extremely inflationary concessions pertaining to that part of Medicare (Medicare Part B) covering physicians' services: (1) physicians would be allowed to charge patients more for services that Medicare would pay, preserving the AMA's traditional medical free enterprise ethos, whereby doctors could maximize their income by charging patients in accordance with what they could afford and (2) fee schedules for Medicare reimbursement to physicians would be based on "usual, customary, reasonable" charges for physician services (Marmor, 2000; Schroeder, 2011). As noted by Starr (1982), as soon as physicians learned they could collectively raise the Medicare fee payments schedule for physicians by hiking the fees in their private practices for all patients, the medical profession embraced the Medicare program.

While this compromise with the AMA helped to secure victory for Medicare's proponents, it fueled inflationary trends in physicians' fees for all insured patients for decades to come. When joined with other even more inflationary elements of the Medicare program (to be highlighted in later discussion), it was in important respects a pyrrhic political victory in the sense that the rampant inflation in health-care entitlement programs that was built into the Medicare/Medicaid legislation in subsequent years became a major economic and political obstacle to the achievement of universal health care as a social right of citizenship.

The Bargained Covenant Between Hospitals, Employers, and Health Insurance Carriers on Uncompensated Care

After the Medicaid and Medicare programs were created in 1965, there remained a residual population of the uninsured who were not poor enough for Medicaid, old enough for Medicare, or with sufficient personal resources to pay for their hospital care. Although the Hill-Burton Act's charity care obligations were an important resource for these patients, the typical hospital's annual allocation of Hill-Burton charity care funds was in fact never sufficient to cover the total burden of bad debt accrued from uninsured patients. Instead, in a widespread industry practice known as cost shifting, hospitals balanced their books by building their bad debt losses into their schedule of inpatient and outpatient care fees charged to insured patients. Health insurance carriers for their part then simply passed these "uncompensated care" costs onto employers via proportionally higher costs for insurance premiums.

During this era, health insurance premiums were typically based on a community rating system, through which insurance risks were based on a defined geographic area (typically counties) rather than the health insurance risks specific to individuals or their employers. This meant that every employer that sponsored health insurance for their employees paid an equal price for an equivalent insurance plan and absorbed an equal share of the burden of the costs of care for uninsured patients. For the most part, this arrangement existed in communities all across the nation as an unwritten cost-shifting covenant between employers, insurance carriers, and hospitals—sustained by a kind of collective goodwill, overlapping interests in the preservation of the employment-based insurance approach to the financing of health care, and the relatively low costs of health insurance benefits as a proportion of overall labor costs (Scofea, 1994). The cost-shifting covenant, which had evolved with the growth of employment-based health insurance during the 1950s, began to unravel in the 1970s as the inflationary seeds sown by the Hill-Burton Act, the payment mechanisms of the Medicare program, and the subsidized employment-based health insurance model took root together and blossomed.

The Bargain Between Liberals and Conservatives Over the Role of Government in Health Care

Starr (1982, p. 369) aptly describes the 1965 Medicare and Medicaid entitlement legislation as a kind of three-layer cake representing the different layers of a complex political accommodation to the ideological priorities of both Democrats and Republicans, although the three-layer cake metaphor seems to have originated with Wilbur Cohen, the leading architect of the Social Security Act's social insurance programs and the Johnson administration's Great Society programs (Marmor, 2000). The first layer, the Democratic approach, was represented in the social insurance fund for Medicare Part A (hospital) benefits. The second layer, Medicare Part B, incorporated the subsidized voluntary insurance approach advocated by Republicans. The third layer, Medicaid, served as the means-tested program of medical care assistance for the poor that incorporated the concerns of both political parties. For Democrats, Medicaid represented a massive expansion of the federal role in financing health care for the poor. For Republicans, Medicaid was a means-tested entitlement that at least retained a significant role for the states in determining the extent of their investments into health care for the poor and the administration of Medicaid eligibility determination and benefits.

Thus emerged the "Era of the Great Unstainable Compromise," represented by a vibrant employment-based insurance structure that was expanding its coverage and benefits, the expansion of Medicare and Medicaid enrollments to capture an ever larger share of the heretofore uninsured, the ability of hospitals to provide care to the uninsured through cost shifting, and major investments in hospital construction and technology financed through a cost-based payment system that was written into the Medicare program rules and replicated in the health insurance industry (Garrison & Wilensky, 1986).

THE UNRAVELING OF THE GREAT UNSUSTAINABLE COMPROMISE: THE DEMISE OF THE UNCOMPENSATED CARE COVENANT (1974–1992)

The Decline of the Employment-Based Insurance Subsidies for High-Risk and Uninsured Patients

By the early 1970s, as the costs of health care were approaching 8 percent of the GDP, the proportion of labor costs attributable to health insurance benefits had nearly doubled over what it had been in 1965 (Burtless & Milusheva, 2013). Employers, who year by year saw their health insurance premiums going up in lock-step with the unrelenting pace of national health-care costs, began to control the growth of their health insurance benefits costs through a combination of three strategies that spelled the end to one key component of "the great unsustainable compromise"—the tacit agreement between employers, insurance companies, and hospitals that had allowed hospitals to recover their uncompensated care costs through higher fees to insurance patients. The first strategy was for employers to abandon health insurance plans that were based on the "community rating" of insurance premiums in favor of insurance plans that were based on the "experience rating" of the employer's actuarial risk, which in effect meant that larger employers and employers with healthier workforces were able to avoid the subsidy costs for higher risk populations that were embedded in plans based on the community rating. The second strategy, enabled by the Employee Retirement Income Security Act of 1974 (ERISA), was for large employers to self-insure, in essence enabling large employers to reduce their health insurance costs by paying directly for the health-care claims of their employees. The third strategy, matched with the first two, was for large employers to also negotiate lower hospital care prices for their employees and their dependents through preferred provider contracts that excluded the cost recovery charges for uninsured patients.

By the early 1980s, the preferred provider contract strategy began to transform the health insurance industry as a whole, as the hospitals, physicians' clinics, and other ancillary health-care service providers banded together to form preferred provider organizations (PPOs)—in essence, closed networks of providers that could contract with health insurance plans to offer discounted fees in return for volume. In 1982, the American Hospital Association's first survey of PPOs reported thirty-three such organizations, and by 1984, the newly formed American Association of Preferred Provider Organizations (AAPPO) counted 143 operational PPOs nationally (Gabel & Ermann, 1985). As PPOs and their discounted contracts became the dominant insurer–provider relationship in the hospital industry, the ability of hospitals to readily cost-shift their uncompensated care costs to insured patients receded into history, right along with the charity care funds that had originated with Hill-Burton obligations incurred during the boom in hospital construction in the two decades following the 1946 Hill-Burton Act. As a result, hospitals were pushed to find ways to avoid uninsured patients under the emergent threat of bankruptcy. The range of tactics employed by hospitals to make their doors less open to uninsured patients included diverting uninsured patients in need of emergency care to federally subsidized community clinics, discouraging medical staff from treating uninsured patients, and sending military veterans without health insurance to the nearest Veterans Affairs (VA) hospital. When Congress combated these tactics with the 1986 Emergency Medical Treatment and Labor Act (EMTALA), which required hospitals with emergency rooms to treat and admit patients in urgent need of hospital care irrespective of financial status, many hospitals responded by closing their emergency rooms. In low-income communities with high proportions of uninsured patients, hospital bankruptcy was often unavoidable. For example, between 1970 and 1990, more than half (53 percent) of the hospitals serving African American neighborhoods in Chicago closed, a development that contributed further to the already dramatic health disparities in the city's racially segregated communities (Almgren & Ferguson, 1999).

The Decline in Employment-Based Insurance

As larger employers and those with more educated workforces sought to contain their rising employee health insurance costs through employer-based rating plans, community rating plans went into a kind of death spiral, in that community-rated insurance plans were left with a higher proportion of high-risk subscribers as healthier workers and their dependents were siphoned off by employer-based rating plans, and in consequence, community-rated insurance plans were forced to raise their premiums even further relative to plans that were based on the employer-based risk rating.

The casualties of the shift from community-rated health insurance plans to employer-based rating plans that included two groups that to some extent were subsidized by the community rating system of health insurance pricing: individual policy holders, and the owners and employees of small businesses that represented that segment of the national economy that employed the highest share of low-wage workers. Individual health insurance policy holders include not only those who are self-employed in high-risk occupations but also older adults who have retired early due to health conditions. Low-wage workers, typically with limited education, tend to incur higher health-care expenditures consistent with the well-established socioeconomic health status gradient (Scott et al., 1989). Both groups were increasingly priced out of the health insurance market as their health insurance costs escalated over the 1980s. Among male workers with a high school education, the demographic group upon which the employment-based health insurance model was predicated, the rate of employment-based insurance coverage decline was particularly pronounced. While in 1979, 90 percent of men with a high school education held a job with health insurance, that number had declined to 75 percent by 1992 (Olson, 1995).[8]

Another crucial component of the decline in employment-based insurance was the retreat in the coverage available for the dependents of employees, again driven by unrestrained health-care cost inflation and the continued growth of health insurance coverage as a share of labor costs. During the particularly pronounced decline in employment-based health insurance that occurred between 1987 and 1996, when the employment-based insurance coverage plummeted from 70 to 65 percent of the non-elderly population, 80 percent of the decline was due to the loss of coverage for dependents. This occurred as employers placed an ever larger burden of the cost for dependent coverage on workers, at a time when wage growth for low- and middle-income workers had become stagnated (Monheit & Vistnes, 2005). When workers were compelled to make a choice between mortgage payments and health insurance, they tended to choose the certainty of a roof over their heads over insurance protection against the possibility of catastrophic health expenditures.

FAILED REFORM, FAILED INCREMENTALISM, FAILED COST CONTAINMENT, AND THE RISING TIDE OF THE UNINSURED (1992-2010)

Failed Reform

When Bill Clinton was elected president in 1992, he pledged to make the realization of affordable health care for all Americans the first achievement of his presidency. True to his campaign promise, he embarked on a plan for health-care reform that would put into place a plan of health insurance for all Americans by 1994. In 1993, it seemed that Clinton's success was all but assured; nearly all of universal health care's traditional opponents had conceded the necessity of both fundamental health reform and the need for a universal plan of compulsory health insurance—including the AMA, the HIAA, the U.S. Chamber of Commerce, and even GOP Senate Minority Leader Robert Dole. Nonetheless, by 1994, Clinton's Health Security Act was politically dead. As suggested by Starr's (1995) definitive postmortem analysis of the debacle, the Clinton reform plan was defeated by a combination of factors that included presidential political miscalculations, wasted time, policy complexity, poor public relations, contextual shifts, divisions among the pro-reform coalition, and the formidable determination and resources of the opposition, most notably the health insurance industry (Almgren, 2007; Starr, 1995).

Central to the defeat of the Clinton administration's Health Security Act was the HIAA (now known as AHIP)—in particular, its "Harry and Louise" public media campaign, which represented the Clinton plan for health-care reform as both an inept government intrusion into private choices and a threat to the quality of health insurance for everyday Americans.[9] This infamous media campaign accounted for only a small share of the estimated $100 million spent by the HIAA for media advertising and grassroots campaigning against the Clinton plan (Jaffe, 2005), and it is credited with turning public opinion from being receptive to the Clinton plan to becoming overwhelmingly unfavorable (Goldsteen et al., 2001).

The Clinton plan's vulnerability to this kind of campaign was in large part attributable to three factors. The first was the complexity of the Clinton plan, which like Obama's Affordable Care Act proposed a mixed public and private solution to health-care financing that was in essence a combination of health insurance market reform, employer insurance mandates, and the retention of the Medicare and Medicaid entitlement programs. The second was the fact that the nation's most active voters, then as now, were those individuals already covered by insurance either through employment-based insurance or Medicare. Thus, the HIAA campaign could capitalize on fear of change and loss of choice. The third factor was a libertarian strain in American politics that views government as inherently either pernicious at its worst or inept at its best. As illuminated by Goldsteen et al. (2001), the HIAA anti–Health Security Act campaign was brilliant in its exploitation of each of these points of vulnerability to public opinion manipulation.

Failed Incrementalism

Following the demise of the Clinton plan, the proponents of universal health care abandoned the vision of sweeping reform in favor of incrementalism both in health-care policy and in political strategy. In policy, it entailed the gradual expansion of the Medicaid eligibility and health insurance subsidies and incentives to shore up the employment-based insurance system. In political strategy, it emphasized the targeted expansion of Medicaid to the population that garnered the most political sympathy: low-income children. There was also an incremental political strategy that pinned its hopes on a state-by-state innovation and diffusion process whereby universal health care could be gradually achieved through a critical mass of states finding their own solutions. Examples of the latter include Hawaii's AlohaCare (1994), various state-level popular initiatives to create single-payer plans such as Health Care for All in Oregon (2002), and then finally the Massachusetts Commonwealth Care plan (2006) that was the central accomplishment of then Governor Mitt Romney (although as a candidate for the GOP party nomination in 2012, Romney appeared loath to admit it). While the successful state-level policy innovations that achieved near-universal health insurance in Hawaii and Massachusetts demonstrated the viability of a state-based approach to universal health care in states with a strong stream of progressivism, throughout the two decades after the demise of the Clinton plan, it became evident that the hoped for diffusion to other states failed to materialize.

In terms of national policy, the penultimate example of the incremental approach was the State Children's Health Initiative Program (SCHIP), passed by Congress in 1997. As a block grant program that provided an enhanced federal match to state expenditures for Medicaid and other vehicles for publicly subsidized health insurance to children in families with incomes in excess of 200 percent of the federal poverty level, SCHIP received widespread bipartisan support. For Democrats, SCHIP represented an expansion of health-care entitlements to the children of the working poor. For Republicans, it reserved for individual states both the discretion to participate in SCHIP and the power to determine income levels for eligibility standards.

Perhaps more critically, to the extent that SCHIP eligibility standards needed to move further up the family income level to reduce the numbers of uninsured children, SCHIP also represented tacit admission that the employment-based insurance approach was failing. In this regard, within five years of SCHIP's implementation, the average state eligibility threshold for states was 213 percent of the federal poverty level (Hill et al., 2005). This fact was not lost on President George W. Bush, who in 2007 vetoed legislation that would have further raised the income eligibility threshold of SCHIP over the objections of many within his own political party, including the staunchly conservative Senator Orrin Hatch (R-Utah).

Although the SCHIP program reduced the number of children without health insurance by nearly one-third (from 7.9 million to 6.1 million) during the first five years of its implementation (Rosenbach, 2007), the reality is that the combination of state-level SCHIP budget reductions, reductions in both employment and employment benefits during recession, and the exclusion of the children of undocumented immigrants from SCHIP eligibility resulted in there being 6.5 million uninsured children by the end of the decade (Alker et al., 2012). That is, there were actually more uninsured children at ten years after the passage of the bill. Moreover, the largest share of uninsured children were those who were most at risk for poor health: the children below 200 percent of the federal poverty level (Alker et al., 2012). While SCHIP can be credited for its success in somewhat restraining the growth in the numbers of uninsured children over the most recent decade, as an incremental policy measure intended to bolster the viability of the employment-based insurance approach to health-care financing, SCHIP was a policy failure.

Failed Cost Containment, or the Rise and Fall of Managed Care

One of the hallmarks of the 1990s, aside from the demise of health-care reform under the Clinton administration, was the dramatic drop in the annual increase in health-care inflation, plunging from a high of 8 percent in 1990 to an effective rate of 0 percent by 1993 (Altman & Levitt, 2002). While both the threat of health-care reform and the health insurance industry's aggressive pursuit of various forms of managed care in their insurance products each played a role in reversing the trend in health-care inflation for a time, by the end of the 1990s the annual rate of health-care inflation had once more climbed to 8 percent (Altman & Levitt, 2002). The disappearance of health-care reform from the national agenda no doubt was an important factor, but the larger cause was the extreme backlash against the aggressive managed care tactics employed by the health insurance industry by providers, special interests (such as the medical technology and pharmaceutical industries), and most of all, the middle class, who were outraged at the insurance industry's explicit rationing of health care to middle-class patients (Mechanic, 2004). By the end of the 1990s, the distrust of a larger government role in health care that had its roots in American libertarianism was eclipsed by a more significant phenomenon—the public's collective antipathy toward the powerful and by then thoroughly discredited health insurance industry, a distrust that had crucial ramifications on later prospects for health-care reform.

The Rising Tide of the Uninsured

After a brief rebound in employment-based health insurance coverage in the late 1990s in response to a booming national economy, employment-based health insurance coverage began another downward trajectory that continued unabated through the first decade of the new century (Gould, 2012). In 2011, the proportion of the national nonelderly population covered through employer-sponsored health insurance had dwindled to 56 percent and altogether, the voluntary approach to health insurance coverage had plunged to its lowest level since the early 1950s, the period when the United States had first embarked on its ill-fated pursuit of employment-based health insurance as the preferred solution to affordable health care for all Americans (Henry Kaiser Family Foundation, 2012; U.S. Census Bureau, 1975).[10] While some attribute the decline in employment-based health insurance to the "crowd-out effect" of public entitlement programs, the evidence reveals that the effects of public entitlement program expansions on the decline of employment-based insurance coverage have been quite small relative to other factors, most notably the affordability of insurance coverage and its declining availability to low-wage workers (Monheit & Vistnes, 2005). Of more relevance is the fact that in 2010—when the nation's newest experiment with health-care reform (the Affordable Care Act), was being signed into law—the population of nonelderly Americans without any form of health insurance, public or private, had swelled to 49 million (Gould, 2012).

FINAL JEOPARDY: THE IMPENDING COLLAPSE OF THE MEDICARE HOSPITAL INSURANCE TRUST FUND (2010-2026)

While the gradual failure of the employment-based insurance approach had by the 2008 presidential elections pushed the country toward just enough of a popular consensus on the need for health-care reform to yield the 2010 ACA, as later events have proved, the consensus remains a fragile one; roughly half of the American public (46 percent) remains opposed to health-care reform four years after the ACA's passage (Henry Kaiser Family Foundation, 2014a).[11] In large part, the public's divided opinion about the need for health-care reform is based on the fact that the employment-based approach to health insurance continues to work for a great share of voters (Blendon et al., 2005). That is, for the large share of middle- and upper-class voters who are at low risk of losing their health insurance, health-care reform is not viewed as either a political priority or even necessarily a good thing for the country. Conversely, the uninsured largely comprise populations that either lack voting rights or are less likely to exercise them. For fundamental health-care reform to truly become a national imperative, the health insurance coverage for a significant proportion of the voting public would need to be at risk. That is precisely the situation that exists with the Medicare Hospital Insurance Trust Fund.

In 2009, the year preceding the passage of the ACA, the Medicare Hospital Insurance Trust Fund was predicted by the Medicare Program's Board of Trustees to become insolvent by 2017. In essence, the elderly who depend on Medicare for their hospital insurance would face a catastrophic slash in their health-care benefits or the program's obligations would need to be heavily subsidized from general tax revenues (Van de Water, 2009). This would pit older adult voters against those of working age in an intergenerational Armageddon that politicians from both dominant political parties have sought for decades to prevent. Five years later, even should the ACA remain largely intact and with the heroic assumption that its cost containment provisions will be both fully implemented and as effective as envisioned, the Medicare Hospital Insurance Trust Fund is *still* predicted to become insolvent by 2030 (Board of Trustees Medicare Hospital Insurance Trust Fund, 2014). So while the ACA may have postponed intergenerational warfare by as much as ten to fourteen years, the unvarnished truth is that the modest Medicare program cost containment provisions embedded in the ACA will not by themselves prevent a collapse of the

Medicare program within the near future. The imperatives of an aging population's rising health-care needs, in combination with the deeply embedded high costs of the American health-care system, will compel radical health-care reforms that will affect health care across the complete life spans.

CONCLUDING REMARKS: TAKING THE LONG VIEW OF HEALTH-CARE REFORM, ITS PURPOSES, AND ITS PROSPECTS

The Inevitability of a New Phase of Fundamental Health-Care Reform

The American health-care system has been built upon a three-legged stool that represents what has been described as an ultimately unstainable compromise between the liberal idea that democratic citizenship requires some substantive provisions essential to fair equality of opportunity and libertarian notions of full self-ownership, the sanctity of private property, and the pernicious nature of government. The first leg of the stool, the voluntary employment-based insurance system, gradually weakened as the unrestrained rise in health-care costs drove up the cost health insurance benefits so much that they became far less accessible to lower-wage workers and their dependents. The second leg, the Medicare program for older Americans, is within a decade or so of insolvency even *with* the full implementation of the very ambitious cost control measures embedded in the ACA. The third, the Medicaid means-tested entitlement originally designed for the poor, under the ACA bears an ever greater share of the burden for the failures of the employment-based insurance system to cover low-wage workers and their dependents, with total state discretion over the extent to which it actually does. In sum, even should the ACA be wildly successful with respect to reforms and subsidies intended to restore some strength to the employment-based insurance leg of the American health-care system stool, one leg remains ultimately doomed (Medicare) and the other (Medicaid) can only be extended to the low-income uninsured at the discretion of the individual states, making a social right to health care a matter of geography as much as it had been heretofore a matter of race and social class. Since three-legged stools collapse when any one leg becomes too weak, it is inevitable that the nation must contemplate another phase of health-care reform beyond the ACA within the decade if not sooner—a phase of reform that must take on more directly the problem of determining the bases and limits of health care as a social right of citizenship. There are four reasons why this is so:

1. *The ACA is here to stay.* As will be fully argued in chapter 3's analysis of the history of health-care reform and the emergence of the ACA, in its most fundamental provisions, the ACA is here to stay. To mention just one reason among many, the ACA's health insurance market reforms that have benefited middle-class voters as well as less advantaged uninsured are politically inoculated against repeal and are well on their way to becoming institutionalized.

2. *The idea that universal health insurance coverage as a social right is here to stay.* As will be discussed in more detail in chapter 2, the ACA represents the first time in the history that Congress has passed comprehensive health-care legislation with the explicit intent of achieving de facto universal health insurance coverage for all citizens, both through federal subsidies and compulsory health insurance mandates. The previously most radical expansion of the health-care entitlements, the 1965 amendments to the Social Security Act that created Medicare and Medicaid, entailed targeted expansions of health-care coverage for the two populations left outside of the employment-based insurance system—older Americans and the poor. In contrast, the ACA expands Medicaid coverage to encompass low-income individuals, provides direct subsidies to middle-class households for private health insurance coverage, and imposes significant federal health insurance market reforms to facilitate the expansion of both individual and employment-based insurance. Thus, since the 2010 enactment of the ACA, millions of American citizens are entitled to affordable health insurance and are responsible for acquiring coverage instead of being relegated to the ambiguous category of the uninsured. Significantly, while a large share of the American public voices dissatisfaction with the ACA, four years after the law's enactment, less than a third would repeal it as opposed to either keeping the law as is or working at ways to improve it (Henry Kaiser Family Foundation, 2014a). In sum, the ACA as originally signed into law made health insurance coverage both an entitlement and a responsibility of citizenship—an idea that is supported by the majority of the American public, as evidenced not only by post-ACA polling data but more directly by the reelection of a president who has expressed and enacted a commitment to a social right to health care for all citizens as a national policy priority.

3. *The ACA is inadequate to the task of providing all Americans with a social right to health care.* When the ACA was signed into law in 2010, the CMS estimated that when fully implemented in 2019, the ACA would extend health insurance coverage to 93 percent of the U.S. population, a forecast that, when adjusted for the exclusion of undocumented immigrants, predicts that no more than 5 percent of Americans would be without health insurance, many by choice rather than by exclusion from affordable health care coverage (CMS, 2010). Aside from excluding undocumented workers and their dependents from the social right to health care afforded to citizens and legal residents under the ACA (an issue examined in chapter 8), three other fundamental flaws in the ACA approach to health-care reform preclude its ability to ensure a social right to health care (defined for the purposes of this discussion as affordable health insurance coverage). The first is the ACA's assumption that some of the populations most in need of health insurance coverage (e.g., the homeless and mentally ill) will have the motivation and capacity to navigate the Medicaid enrollment bureaucracy to acquire coverage. The second is the assumption by the architects of the ACA that the stigma long associated with Medicaid will not be a major obstacle to Medicaid enrollment among the low-income uninsured who, under the ACA, become newly eligible. Research suggests that the stigma of means-based social entitlements can be a significant barrier to enrollment (Stuber & Kronebusch, 2004). This issue may be particularly problematic in states where the political discourse equates Medicaid with "dependency" and "welfare." The third flaw (related to the second) is the ACA's inability in the wake of the U.S. Supreme Court's decision in *National Federation of Independent Business (NFIB) v. Sebelius* (U.S. Supreme Court, No. 11–393, decided June 28, 2012) to enforce the cooperation of states in its provision of expanded Medicaid eligibility to the working poor despite the availability of federal funds to do so. As a result, four years into the ACA's implementation, only twenty-seven states implemented the ACA's Medicaid expansion provision, excluding as many as 5 million otherwise eligible Americans from health insurance coverage through Medicaid (Henry Kaiser Family Foundation, 2014b).

4. *The Medicare Hospital Insurance Trust Fund is nearing an impending collapse.* As discussed in the preceding section, even with the full and successful implementation of the ACA's cost containment provisions, the Medicare Hospital Insurance Trust Fund (Medicare Part A) is projected to become insolvent by 2030 absent more radical reform, and this will force

the nation to grapple with the choice between either a catastrophic slash in the Medicare programs hospital care benefits or a massive infusion of Medicare program subsidies from general tax revenues, the latter translating to a higher tax burden on younger generations of working age. It is this choice, contextualized by the ACA symbolizing a national commitment to universal health insurance coverage as a right of citizenship, that will bring about an unprecedented national conversation on health-care cost containment, a balance of health-care entitlements between the old and the young, and a pathway to health-care reform that realizes an achievable and sustainable social right to health care.

Two Critical Dialogues in the National Conversation on the (Inevitable) Next Phase of Health-Care Reform

Shortly after the ACA being signed into law, eminent social policy historian Theda Skocpol published her analysis of the political prospects for the ACA's implementation. The central point of Skocpol's analysis is that, in the case of fundamental structural advancements in social policy, broad public acceptance and institutional adaptation take several years (Skocpol, 2010). Under the not terribly heroic or radical assumption that in its essential form the ACA is here to stay, two distinct but deeply connected health-care policy dialogues will emerge that arise from the contradictions between the ACA in its current form and its manifest goal of realizing a social right to health care. The first of these critical dialogues will pertain to the contradictions related to those aspects of the ACA that are tied to the ways the law's provisions reflect and perpetuate various forms of social stratification (or social injustice, if one is an egalitarian), such as the exclusion of undocumented workers and their dependents from health-care access subsidies, the inherent stigma attached to a means-tested entitlement to health care, the ACA's perpetuation of the linkage between educational and occupational stratification and entitlements to health care, and geographic variations in the ACA's capacity to extend health-care coverage to the uninsured (especially the poor and low-income classes) created by the federalized structure of the ACA's means-tested entitlements. The second dialogue, arising from the contradiction between the continued health-care policy hegemony of health-care industry stakeholder groups and the fiscal sustainability of the ACA's mixed public and private system of health-care financing, will interrogate the alternative values and principles that might be applied to a rational process for the determination of national health priorities. The chapters that follow lend substance primarily to that second critical dialogue.

This book's premise is that the full realization of health care as a social right of citizenship is not something that is merely desirable on humanitarian grounds or even as a matter of global economic competitiveness, but that such a social right is inexorably linked to the structural requisites of democratic citizenship and democratic political institutions. The advancement of this premise is the principal task of chapter 3, which provides the theoretical foundations for the structural requisites of democratic society and democratic citizenship based on a synthesis of the works of political philosopher John Rawls and sociologist T. H. Marshall, the two theoretical giants of twentieth-century political liberalism. As crucial context for that discussion, chapter 2 will provide an overview of history health reform efforts toward the advancement of a universal social right to health care and the emergence of the new era of health-care reform that yielded at least a symbolic affirmation of that right in the form of the ACA. The book also takes on the tasks essential to constructing a plausible future wherein the priorities for national health-care investments are determined not by the interests of powerful health-care provider and insurance industry stakeholder groups but by the extent to which particular investments in health care are essential to the realization of full democratic citizenship for the largest share of the national population and to the achievement and preservation of a permeable class structure.

Chapter Two

THE EMERGENCE OF THE NEW ERA
OF REFORM

A BRIEF HISTORY OF FUNDAMENTAL HEALTH-CARE
REFORM IN AMERICA

Up until the enactment of the Affordable Care Act in 2010, the nation's attempts to reshape its health-care system have assumed four general forms: fundamental health-care reform initiatives aimed at achieving universal health care; incremental health insurance market reforms; expansion of health care with entitlements targeted toward the eventual realization of universal health insurance coverage through employment-based insurance and means-based public programs; and reforms in pursuit of health-care cost containment.[1] The first to be considered will be the fundamental health-care reform initiatives aimed at achieving universal health care, which for reasons that will be made clear are referred to as *progressive* efforts to achieve universal health care.

Progressive efforts to achieve universal health care are distinguished by their premises that the provision of health care to all citizens is (1) a social right of citizenship, (2) in the best interests of national prosperity, and (3) a distinctive and primary responsibility of the federal government. This is in contrast to the incremental approach to the eventual realization of universal access to health care, which views the role of the federal government as facilitative of universal health care as a social good, realized primarily through the market economy and the exercise of individual preference and self-responsibility. Historically, the contrast between the two approaches has played out not as a contrast between socialism and libertarianism so much as between liberalism (and its earlier traditions in progressivism) and the conservative allies of powerful health-care industry stakeholder groups that have strategically employed populist libertarian sentiments to stave off more fundamental approaches to health-care reform.

Within the progressive definition of efforts to achieve universal health care, it can be argued that there have been seven U.S. presidents, from Theodore Roosevelt to Barack Obama, who endorsed and sought legislation to achieve universal health insurance coverage as either a social right of citizenship or a social good to be provided to all as a matter of national prosperity and political necessity.

Theodore Roosevelt (1901–1909 and 1912 Progressive Party Candidate)

Although Theodore Roosevelt is generally credited as the first U.S. president to propose a program of national health insurance for all Americans, he did so as an unsuccessful Progressive Party candidate for president in 1912 rather than during the years of his presidency (1901–1909). The Progressive Movement (1890–1919), as the forerunner of modern liberalism, sought to reform capitalism through a combination of social insurance, industrial reform, and government regulation of capital markets. As noted by Paul Starr (1982), the Progressive Movement's center was the American Association of Labor Legislation (AALL), which had a broad pro-labor class agenda that included child labor reform, unemployment insurance, workers' compensation, and ultimately health insurance—all of which became integral to the Progressive Party's 1912 campaign platform under Theodore Roosevelt. Presaging the New Deal policies of Franklin D. Roosevelt a generation later, the Progressive Party's official platform statement called for cradle-to-grave social insurance for health care, unemployment, and old age income security, described as "the protection of home life against the hazards of sickness, irregular employment and old age through the adoption of a system of social insurance adapted to American use" (Teaching American History, 2012, p. 1). Roosevelt's defeat by the Democratic Party's Woodrow Wilson spelled the end of this first effort at national health insurance, after which the Progressive Movement itself withered away as it pursued an unsuccessful state-by-state strategy to achieve social insurance for health care.

Franklin Delano Roosevelt (1933–1945)

Elected to the Oval Office in 1932, exactly twenty years after his fifth cousin Theodore Roosevelt's failed bid to rewin the White House under the banner of the Progressive Party, Franklin D. Roosevelt (FDR) dedicated his presidency to the realization of progressivism's cradle-to-grave vision of social and economic security. Coincidently, just as FDR assumed the presidency in 1933, the Committee on the Costs of Medical Care (CCMC), a privately funded coalition of economists, physicians, public health specialists, and social reformers, had released its long-awaited final recommendations for national health care infrastructure investments and financing, which called for the encouragement of publicly subsidized voluntary group insurance as an alternative to compulsory social insurance for health care (Klein, 2005). In contrast, FDR favored a comprehensive plan for social security that would encompass both income security throughout the life course and social insurance for health care. The pragmatists on his key Committee on Economic Security (most notably Secretary of Labor Francis Perkins and Harry Hopkins, administrator of the Federal Emergency Relief Agency) recognized that opposition from the AMA would doom the Social Security Act legislation to failure—thus, FDR elected to pursue social insurance for health care in later amendments to the Social Security Act of 1935 when politically feasible (Klein, 2005; Starr, 1982). Due to the nation's immersion in World War II, that opportunity did not materialize until social insurance for health care became a part of FDR's postwar domestic agenda, an agenda that became his successor's when FDR died in April 1945, just as he began his fourth presidential term (Morone, 2010).

Harry Truman (1945–1952)

As already well covered in chapter 1's discussion of the origins of American exceptionalism in health care, it was during the Truman administration's first four years (1945–1949) that the old Progressive Party vision of social insurance for health care seemed to have been well within reach, only to be squashed by the well-financed and strategically brilliant campaign orchestrated by the AMA. To recap, the so-called Truman plan that Truman introduced to Congress in November 1945 called for an expansion of the Social Security Act of 1935 that would create a social insurance fund for comprehensive health care, inclusive of physician services, hospital care, ancillary diagnostic services, and even dental care. While Truman was very specific in his point-by-point delineation of the distinction between social insurance and socialized medicine and the plan's emphasis on both the preservation of medical free enterprise and patients' voluntary choice of providers, the AMA and its allies in both the small business lobby and the insurance industry framed social insurance for health care as part and parcel of a larger communist agenda to destroy democracy—and the fight waged against national health insurance as a fundamental struggle against government domination not only of medicine but of individualism and liberty (Quadagno, 2005, p. 35). Also as pointed in chapter 1, while in 1945 an astounding 75 percent of Americans supported the idea of national health insurance, by 1949, that proportion had plummeted to 21 percent. Thus ended Truman's quest to fulfill the old Progressive Party and New Deal Democratic vision of health care as a social right of citizenship.

Lyndon Johnson (1963–1968)

Late in the night on November 22, 1963, President Lyndon Baines Johnson had at last retired to bed at the urging of his cardiologist. Less than eight hours before, Johnson had been standing next to the newly widowed Jacqueline Kennedy, still in her blood-spattered pink travel suit, as the presidential jet sat on the sweltering Dallas–Fort Worth airport tarmac, reciting the Oath of Office. Unable to sleep, Johnson summoned three of his closest aides so he could share his thoughts about the presidential responsibilities and opportunities that Kennedy's assassination had thrust upon him. As recalled by Jack Valenti, one of Johnson's top advisors, even on that terrible first day in office, Johnson had already identified a social right to health care as a key presidential priority—on par with civil rights, voting rights, and education. "Well, I'm going to tell you," said Johnson, "I'm going to pass the civil rights bill and not change a word of it. I'm not going to cavil, and I'm not going to compromise. I'm going to fix it so everyone can vote, so everyone can get all the education they can get. I'm going to pass Harry Truman's health bill."[2] Thus, the 1912 Progressive Party's vision of a national plan of health insurance for all Americans was revitalized for a second time, more than a decade since its seeming final demise at the hands of the AMA and its powerful allies in the small business and insurance industries.

Despite Johnson's commitment to the FDR/Truman vision of social insurance for comprehensive health care as the final extension of the Social

Security Act of 1935 (and his legendary capacity to exercise his will in congressional politics), a national plan of health insurance did not have the popular support and the national outrage at injustice (fueled by televised witnessing of racial violence) that had propelled his two other bedside pledges to eventual achievement—the Civil Rights Act of 1964 and the Voting Rights Act of 1965. In the early 1960s, employment-based health insurance was still expanding to cover an ever larger share of the national population, thus helping the AMA to continue to make its Cold War–era case that voluntary health insurance is "the American way." In the end, Johnson had to settle for a partial, yet major, victory over the AMA's enduring opposition to social insurance for health with the 1965 amendments to the Social Security Act that established the Medicare and Medicaid programs. Both major health-care entitlements were made politically possible because it was abundantly clear to most stakeholders in the national health-care debate (including employers, unions, hospitals, and many physicians) that employment-based voluntary health insurance was unworkable for two populations that were not a part of the labor market: the elderly and the poor.

It can be said that there are three particularly enduring legacies of the presidency of Lyndon Johnson that stand in stark contrast to his tarnished image as the original "Vietnam War president." His first two legacies, achieved in a short-lived partnership with Martin Luther King Jr. (Kotz, 2005), were the 1964 Civil Rights Act and the 1965 Voting Rights Act.

These two pieces of legislation transformed the lives and prospects of African Americans and presaged the election of the nation's first African American president some four decades later. His third enduring legacy, Title XVIII and Title XIX of the Social Security Act (known as the Medicare and Medicaid programs), provided the nation with the second and third legs of the public and private three-legged stool that characterizes the American approach to the financing of health care. Ever after the Johnson administration, most approaches to health-care reform have been defined by the preservation of the deeply institutionalized three-legged stool comprising social insurance for older adults (Medicare), means-tested health-care entitlements for low-income and poor people (Medicaid), and employment-based insurance for workers and their dependents.

Richard Nixon (1969-1974)

In contrast to the four preceding presidents who had adopted a national plan of health insurance as a political aim of their presidency (Theodore Roosevelt as a candidate for reelection to the presidency and FDR, Harry Truman, and Lyndon Johnson as presidents), Nixon's advocacy of a national plan of health insurance was not inspired by a progressivist belief in health insurance as a social right of citizenship, but rather by a combination of economic necessity and political strategy. Throughout his political career as a Republican moderate in the tradition of Dwight Eisenhower (Nixon had served as Eisenhower's vice president from 1953-1960), Nixon had been a staunch supporter of the AMA's position on the sanctity of medical free enterprise and voluntary health insurance.[3] However, during the first term of Nixon's presidency (1968-1972), rising health-care costs, a genuine concern about the plight of the uninsured born from family experience, and the possibility that political rival Senator Ted Kennedy (D-MA) might use universal health insurance to defeat Nixon in the 1972 elections forced Nixon to come up with a plan of his own (Quadagno, 2005).

As a counter to the single-payer social insurance approach advocated by Senator Kennedy and his powerful ally, House Ways and Means Committee Chair Wilbur Mills (D-AR), in March 1972, Nixon proposed his Health Insurance Partnership Act in a memo to Congress. Under Nixon's plan, the health-care coverage gap would be closed by (1) an employer mandate that would require employers to share the cost of an adequate plan of basic health insurance benefits and (2) a subsidized federal health insurance plan (the Family Health Insurance Plan or FHIP) that would be available to the unemployed and the low-income self-employed.

Medicaid for the disabled and the poor would remain in place as would Medicare for the old. Under Nixon's health reform proposal, affordability and health-care cost containment would be realized through the subsidized development of health maintenance organization (HMO) plans as the preferred mechanism for health insurance coverage (Nixon, 1972). While Nixon had involved the AMA, the health insurance industry, and the corporate business interests in drafting his plan, in introducing the HMO component favored by large employers, Nixon also took a position in direct opposition to the AMA, which despised the HMO concept only slightly less than the social insurance approach advocated by the Kennedy/

Mills approach (Quadagno, 2005). In a nutshell, Nixon was quite willing to throw the AMA under the bus in pursuit of his reelection ambitions.

While Nixon's Health Care Partnership Act failed to gain political traction in Congress and ultimately withered away after Nixon's landslide victory in 1972, in his 1974 State of the Union Address, Nixon once more introduced his intention to pursue new legislation that would "bring comprehensive, high quality health care within the reach of every American" as a major policy aim of his presidency (Nixon, 1974). As with his earlier Health Care Partnership Act, it is likely that Nixon's primary motivations for introducing a national plan for universal health insurance were more political than progressive—in this second instance as a futile diversion from the Watergate scandal that ultimately led to his resignation from the presidency in August of that same year. Tragically for the millions of Americans who remained unable to afford health care, Nixon was the last president to seriously pursue universal health insurance coverage until Democrat Bill Clinton was elected to the presidency nearly two decades later.

Bill Clinton (1992-1998)

More than any preceding president in U.S. history, with the sole exception of Harry Truman, Clinton elevated comprehensive health care for all Americans as a central aim of his presidency. Even welfare reform, for which he is (perhaps dubiously) credited, was more thrust upon him as a political necessity than embraced as a desirable presidential legacy. Akin to Nixon's health reform plan of the early 1970s, Clinton's Health Security Act (HSA) sought to expand health-care coverage and contain health-care costs through a combination of health insurance market reforms, employer mandates to provide insurance, and health insurance purchase subsidies. However, in contrast to the Nixon administration's Health Care Partnership Act, Clinton's HSA departed from the three-legged Medicare, Medicaid, and employment-based insurance stool approach that was the legacy of the Johnson administration and eliminated Medicaid for all but those receiving AFDC (Aid to Families with Dependent Children) cash assistance in favor of subsidies to low-income families for purchasing health insurance. However, under Clinton's HSA, even Medicaid recipients would have their health benefits provided through health alliances—essentially health insurance purchasing cooperatives with insurance market regulatory powers (Robbins & Robbins, 1994). Aside from reducing the costly and cumbersome state and federal Medicaid bureaucracy in favor of acquiring insurance coverage through "regional health alliances" organized by the federal government, under the goals and structure of the HSA, low-income patients would not be encumbered by the social stigma associated with being a Medicaid recipient or experience the all too typical difficulties in finding a willing Medicaid medical provider.

In essence, Clinton's HSA was a hybrid of both liberal and conservative approaches to social policy. From the liberal perspective, the HSA expanded health-care coverage to all Americans younger than sixty-five (with Medicare remaining for older Americans) through both insurance and labor market regulation and insurance purchase subsidies to low-wage employers and families. From the conservative perspective, Clinton's HSA retained the employment-based insurance model while imposing health insurance market reforms that would reduce costs through what became known as "managed competition." Under the HSA's mantra of "managed competition," all Americans not covered through the self-insurance plans of large employers would be required to purchase a standard insurance plan through a regional health alliance—in essence, a federal agency organized at the regional level that would enforce health insurance market regulations, enroll subscribers into insurance plans, collect health insurance premiums, disburse payments to health insurance plans, and serve as a clearinghouse for information about insurance plan costs and insurer/provider performance. Under the employer mandate provision of the HSA, employers would be required to pay for 80 percent of costs of health insurance premiums, with workers providing 20 percent—thus sensitizing workers to costs of more expensive health insurance plans and the relationship of health benefits as a wage substitute (Robbins & Robbins, 1994).

As discussed in chapter 1, while in 1993 it appeared that comprehensive health insurance reform that would yield universal coverage was all but inevitable (even in the eyes of health-care reform's traditional foes), by late in the summer of 1994, Clinton's HSA was political carrion. The factors in its demise included presidential political miscalculations, wasted time, policy complexity, poor public relations, contextual shifts, divisions among the pro-reform coalition, and the formidable determination and resources of the opposition—most notably the health insurance industry (Starr, 1995). While some believe that Clinton may have resurrected some version of comprehensive health reform during his second term had it not been for the squandering of political capital on his legendary personal conduct scandals, in reality, the prospects for comprehensive health-care reform with a GOP-controlled Congress were nil. Instead, Clinton opted to work with the Republican leadership on the incremental expansions of health insurance coverage that *were* politically feasible.

INCREMENTAL REFORM IN PURSUIT OF UNIVERSAL ACCESS TO HEALTH CARE

Despite the demise of the HSA in 1994 and the legacy of that major policy humiliation that Clinton has endured since, two significant health-care policy accomplishments of the Clinton administration can be credited to his progressive principles and formidable skills as a bipartisan negotiator.[4] The first is Clinton's 1995 hardline defense of the Medicaid program against the Republicans' attempt to use their newly won majority control of both houses of Congress to turn Medicaid from a federal entitlement into a block grant program—with the near-certain consequence of millions of low-income and poor people being gradually pushed out of Medicaid eligibility. Clinton's refusal to give ground on Medicaid's preservation as a federal entitlement was one of the central elements that led to the government shutdowns in late 1995 and early 1996, which ultimately resulted not only in the preservation of Medicaid but also a loss of public confidence in the Republican Party's capacity to govern. The second major health-care accomplishment was the State Children's Health Initiative Program (SCHIP), which provided a large, albeit incremental, expansion of health-care coverage for the millions of low-income children who had fallen in the ever-widening gap between Medicaid and the failing employment-based insurance system.

From the mid-1960s to Clinton's second term (1996–2000), the most significant reforms targeting increased health-care access for the poor were (1) expansions of the Medicaid program during the late 1980s and early 1990s that required states to cover all pregnant women and children younger than six up to 133 percent of the federal poverty level and allowed states to expand Medicaid coverage for young children up to 185 percent of the federal poverty level and (2) the 1986 Emergency Medical Treatment and Labor Act (EMTALA) that requires emergency departments to provide medical screenings and urgent/emergent care regardless of ability to pay (Almgren, 2007; Cutler & Gruber, 2001). Despite the pre-Clinton era expansions of Medicaid coverage to poor and low-income pregnant women and children, by the beginning of Clinton's second term, it was evident that the continued decline of employment-based insurance coverage (for women and children in particular) was outpacing small incremental expansions in Medicaid coverage (Monheit & Vistnes, 2005). In return for tax reduction provisions in the Balanced Budget Act of 1997 that were popular with the Republican-led Congress (including in particular a large reduction in the capital gains tax), SCHIP was created, which Clinton considers the crowning health-care policy achievement of his presidency and was in fact the largest expansion of federally subsidized health insurance coverage since the Johnson administration had enacted Medicare and Medicaid three decades ago (Cutler & Gruber, 2001).

From the standpoint of progressivist social policy, the SCHIP program represented two significant achievements. The first is that the SCHIP legislation provided $24 billion in block grant funds over a five-year period that would allow states to expand Medicaid eligibility to children and pregnant women up to 200 percent of the federal poverty level, with flexibility left to states to use SCHIP funds to leverage even higher-income thresholds. At the point that the SCHIP program had completed its first decade, its enrollment had climbed to 7.4 million (CMS, 2014a). The second significant achievement of the SCHIP program was that, by allowing states to extend enrollment eligibility to encompass incomes of even middle-class families unable to acquire or afford employment-based insurance, it shattered the fifty-year-old myth promulgated by conservatives that the employment-based insurance approach worked for all but the poor and unemployable. It was this aspect of SCHIP that caused George W. Bush to veto, on two occasions during his tenure as president, renewal of SCHIP legislation that would have expanded SCHIP access to the growing numbers of nonpoor families that could not access affordable employment-based health insurance (Kenney & Pelletier, 2009).

HEALTH-CARE REFORMS IN PURSUIT OF COST CONTAINMENT

Since the early 1970s, the principal structural (as opposed to political) impediment to the realization of universal health care coverage in the United States has been the nation's ever-rising health-care costs, reflected in the growth in the proportion of the gross domestic product (GDP) devoted to health care. At the point that Congress committed the country to financing the Medicare and Medicaid programs in 1965, expenditures for health care represented about 6 percent of the GDP. By 1975, health-care expenditures had mounted to 8 percent of the GDP, and the pace of health-care inflation was increasing annually as well. By way of contrast, the 8 percent GDP threshold was not reached by other modern democracies until 2000 (Almgren, 2007). While by 1970, the (seemingly) unsustainable rise in health-care expenditures and its effects on the costs of the Medicare and Medicaid programs had caught the attention of both President Nixon and Congress, efforts at cost containment both nationally and at the state level were stymied by the vigorous opposition of the AMA, the hospital industry, and the health insurance industry's reluctance to embrace cost control as a function of health insurance (Quadagno, 2005).

The 1970s: The First Efforts at Cost Control

At the time that Medicare and Medicaid were enacted in 1965, Medicare hospital payments were made on a cost-plus fee-for-service basis, thus permitting hospitals to obtain full reimbursement from the Medicare program for any patient services that could be medically justified—in essence, any and all services ordered by any physician with hospital admitting privileges. Physicians, in turn, were reimbursed on a fee-for-service basis from Medicare Part B, which rewarded the promotion of health-care utilization over clinically beneficial outcomes. These arrangements were wildly lucrative for doctors as well as hospitals, and the only restraint on costs built into the original Medicare "conditions of participation" for hospitals was the requirement that hospitals needed to have a "utilization review plan" that provided for the systemic review of hospital cases for the medical necessity of inpatient admissions, length of stay, and the professional services furnished (Social Security Administration, 2014b). However, because hospital utilization review plans required the sanction and direct involvement of hospital medical staff with vested interests in unfettered medical free enterprise and the protection of their profitable referral relationships with their medical colleagues, the Medicare utilization review requirement was wholly ineffective as a means of cost control. While President Nixon imposed direct inflationary controls on physician fees and hospital charges between 1971 and 1973, this was a temporary measure as opposed to a long-term structural solution. Meanwhile, in 1972, Congress finally acted and created amendments to the Social Security Act that entailed two provisions that were intended to control rising health-care costs.

The first of these 1972 provisions permitted Medicare beneficiaries to choose enrollment in an HMO as an alternative to traditional Medicare fee-for-service plans, while the second established professional standards review organizations (PSROs), which were panels of local physicians charged with the task of reviewing hospital care for necessity and aspects of quality. There is virtually no evidence that the 200 or so PSROs that had been established by 1974 had any impact on either cost containment or enhancing the quality of care, largely because PSROs functioned as no more than an extension of local medical societies (Brown, 1992).

However, over the objections of the AMA, Congress did pass the Health Maintenance Act of 1973, advocated by the Nixon administration, which allocated $375 million in development costs for HMOs and added a provision to the Fair Labor Standards Act that required employers to offer an HMO option in employment benefit plans. While HMOs failed to be the panacea to rising health-care costs envisioned by Nixon, the act is credited for ultimately fostering the formation of hundreds of HMOs that over time would cover nearly 60 million Americans (Galewitz, 2011).

Another avenue of cost containment undertaken by Congress in the 1970s was the Health Planning Resources and Development Act of 1974, which sought to reduce the growth of health expenditures by restraining and rationalizing hospital industry expansion and modernization. Under this legislation, local health systems agencies were funded and established, under federal guidelines, to review major investments in hospital facilities and service expansions and determine the justifications for a certificate of need (CON), which in turn would be a requirement for Medicare reimbursement. Theoretically, the authority of local health systems agencies to deny CONs representing costly and unnecessary expansions in hospital infrastructure should have been a significant restraint on rising health-care costs. In reality, the health systems agency review process often functioned as the battleground between competitive hospital systems seeking market dominance over the geography of insured patient populations. Despite federal requirements that health systems agencies must include consumer representation on their governance boards, provide avenues for public input in the CON review process, and engage in objective analysis of proposed investments in local health-care infrastructure, health systems agencies were at best a small impediment to rising health-care costs (Brown,

1992). While several individual states also endeavored to control rising health-care costs through the establishment of hospital care "rate commissions" during the latter part of the 1970s, this approach failed to gain traction nationally, and the evidence as to their effectiveness is at best mixed (Atkinson, 2009).

At the federal level, the last major cost control effort of the 1970s was President Jimmy Carter's Hospital Cost Containment Act of 1977, which sought to both calibrate the growth in hospital charges to the general inflation rate and place an annual cap on hospital capital expenditures. Carter introduced this cost control legislation as an essential platform for his ultimate plan of comprehensive health care for all Americans through insurance market reforms and a new federal insurance program for low-income individuals that would merge Medicare and Medicaid. As an alternative to the Carter plan for direct price controls, the hospital industry proposed and implemented its own voluntary cost control initiative, and congressional support for Carter's Hospital Cost Containment Act evaporated. Predictably enough, once the threat of federally mandated cost controls was removed, the hospital industry's voluntary initiative had served its political purposes and it quickly withered away (Davis & Stremikis, 2009).

The 1980s: The Emergence of Medicare's Prospective Payment System and Managed Care

In 1982, Congress passed the Tax Equity and Fiscal Responsibility Act or TEFRA, which, in addition to its direct cost control provisions limiting hospital reimbursement and expanding the incentives for Medicare HMO enrollment, contained a provision that required the Department of Health Education and Welfare (now Health and Human Services) to submit to Congress a new prospective payment system (PPS) for Medicare. The PPS approach to hospital care reimbursement was to be based on selected case characteristics that proved to be highly predictive of hospital care costs, as opposed to the unrestrained fee-for-service approach based on economically lucrative claims of medical necessity. Thus, under the PPS system, the incentives to provide unnecessary care to hospital inpatients were eliminated in favor of providing care that would yield desirable clinical outcomes at the lowest possible cost.

49

In a move that stunned all but the political insiders of the hospital industry, in 1983, Congress replaced the traditional fee-for-service hospital reimbursement system with PPS, thus forever changing the hospital industry's inflationary incentives.[5] In essence, the Medicare PPS based its reimbursement to hospitals for an individual patient's hospital stay based on that patient's assignment to a diagnosis-related group (DRG) at discharge, which in turn was determined by a range of characteristics such as age, the presence of comorbid conditions, and type of surgical interventions provided. While the PPS system was designed and intended to be fiscally neutral for hospitals during its phase-in period, over time, this system would constrain hospital price inflation by both removing the incentives for lengthy hospital stays and unnecessary care and also providing a more direct and simple way to impose payment controls.

The effect of PPS on Medicare hospital expenditures was dramatic. In the ten-year period preceding the implementation of PPS, the average cost per hospital day for a Medicare patient grew by about 14 percent per year, a rate of growth that fell to about 9 percent in the decade that followed (Scanlon, 2006). Hospital usage by Medicare patients also declined by 20 percent during this same post-PPS period. However, the PPS could not wholly counter the health-care utilization incentives built into the Medicare program, the costs associated with new technological innovations in surgery and diagnostic medicine, or the health-care demands of an aging population. In sum, while the PPS system extended the solvency of the Medicare Hospital Insurance Trust Fund for a period, other more significant structural changes in Medicare remained necessary.

As state Medicaid program administrators, business groups, and health insurance organizations observed the cost containment success of the Medicare PPS approach, various adaptations of the PPS form of reimbursement diffused throughout the health-care industry. Of equal importance were the ways in which the Medicare PPS incentives promoted the development of highly sophisticated hospital utilization management strategies and outcomes-based clinical protocols that became essential for hospitals striving to compete in the new managed care insurance environment. By the end of the 1980s, these managed care innovations were providing the foundations for the coming age in American health care, where the shared interests of the insurance industry and employers in cost containment triumphed over the heretofore sovereign rule of medical free enterprise. In 1988, traditional health insurance plans accounted for 73 percent of the employment-based insurance market, whereas by 2000, that market share had dwindled to 8 percent as most employment-based plans shifted to HMO and preferred provider organization (PPO) coverage (McQuire et al., 2011).

Incremental Cost Containment Reforms Since the 1980s

Despite the success of Medicare's PPS in at least slowing the pace of growth in Medicare program hospital expenditures, the Medicare program has remained embedded in the epidemiological paradigm that defined the state of medicine in the 1960s. That is, Medicare was designed as a system of reimbursement and provider relations that was suited to short-term clinical interventions for the treatment of acute episodes of illness, as opposed to a program designed for the management of the chronic diseases associated with the dramatic advancements in old age life expectancy that have taken place in the decades since Medicare was signed into law. Because of the fears of older adults about loss of their Medicare benefits and the power of both provider groups and the supplemental health insurance industry, Congress has remained stymied in its attempts to fundamentally reform Medicare in ways that would adapt its financing structures and provider incentives to the needs of an aging population burdened by chronic disease and disability.

In absence of the political feasibility of more fundamental reforms of Medicare, Congress has pursued the path of incremental Medicare reform through encouraging enrollment in alternatives to the traditional Medicare fee-for-service structure under Medicare Part C—known today as the Medicare Advantage program. Although Medicare Part C options to traditional fee-for-service Medicare originated with the 1982 TEFRA amendments to Medicare that permitted enrollment in HMO plans, it was not until the Balanced Budget Act of 1997 that Congress pushed hard on promoting enrollment in HMO and PPO managed care alternatives to traditional Medicare—known as Medicare "Medicare+Choice" (later renamed "Medicare Advantage" under the Medicare Modernization Act of 2003). Despite the thirty years that have elapsed since the TEFRA amendments established Medicare Part C options to traditional Medicare (including HMO plans, PPO plans, and medical savings accounts), the majority (70 percent) of Medicare beneficiaries have preferred to remain in traditional Medicare fee-for-service plans (Henry Kaiser Family Foundation, 2014b).

The reluctance of Medicare beneficiaries to embrace managed care plans as an alternative to the more costly fee-for-service coverage is in dramatic contrast to the employer-sponsored insurance market, where traditional fee-for-service plans have all but disappeared in favor of plans that pursue cost containment through managed care, preferred provider networks, or high-deductible catastrophic coverage (McQuire et al., 2011). However, as highlighted in chapter 1, after some initial dramatic success at halting the growth in health-care expenditures in the early 1990s, the aggressive managed care strategies that characterized the employment-based insurance market during the first half of the 1990s ultimately alienated both providers and health insurance beneficiaries (Mechanic, 2004). As a result, by the end of the 1990s, the health insurance industry had largely abandoned its more aggressive managed care cost containment strategies and tactics, and the annual rate of health-care inflation resurged to 8 percent (Altman & Levitt, 2002).

THE NEW ERA OF HEALTH-CARE REFORM: ITS TRIUMPHS AND ITS CONTRADICTIONS

It can be said that "the new era of health-care reform" began with a speech made by President George W. Bush in Cleveland, Ohio, on July 10, 2007. In what was intended to be a routine wide-ranging political stump speech to a friendly audience of Ohio businessmen, Bush famously claimed, "I mean, people have access to health care in America. After all, you just go to an emergency room."[6] This statement (which even had some members of Bush's own party scratching their heads) unleashed a firestorm of criticism and ridicule directed not only at Bush's personal ignorance of the plight of the nation's millions of uninsured but at the preposterous idea that care sought in desperation at a crowded and overly taxed hospital emergency room could be equated with genuine access to health care. Although he had not intended to, with a seemingly offhand remark, Bush managed to reawaken the sleeping giant of a broad-based call for national health-care reform, just at the point when the public's attention was beginning to shift toward the defining issues of the upcoming 2008 presidential primary season. In making this remark, Bush also managed to remind Americans that when it came to fundamental health-care reform, it was the Republican Party that was the defender of the health-care status quo—43 million uninsured Americans, a Medicare Hospital Insurance Trust fund that was approaching insolvency within the decade, and a middle class increasingly affected by the loss of employment-based health insurance and the specter of medical bankruptcy.

The Legislative Phase, 2008–2010

The Context of the ACA's Passage

Although the political context for the ill-fated 1992–1994 era of health-care reform was also characterized by an initial broad-based consensus in support of health-care reform that would yield some form of universal health insurance coverage (Starr, 1995), two crucial shifts in the political context of the 2008–2010 era of health-care reform legislation made the prospects for success more likely than they were in 1992.

The first contextual shift was that, in 1992–1994, the level of antipathy toward the health insurance industry had not risen to the point where it was regarded by the general public and health-care providers with the same disdain as that heretofore accorded to "big government." By the end of the 1990s, however, both the middle class and health-care providers were frustrated with the run-amok bureaucracy and health-care access barriers for which the health insurance industry had become infamous (Mechanic, 2004). This made the health insurance industry as vulnerable to media sound-bite vilification as had been, in previous reform eras, federalized health-care reform in the name of a social right to health care.

The second crucial contextual shift was the extent to which diminished access to health insurance coverage had, by 2008, become a major financial threat to the middle class, in the wake of the continued decline in the availability of affordable employment-based insurance for the families of middle-income workers (Monheit & Vistnes, 2005), the increased prevalence of high levels of debt and bankruptcies among the middle class due to uncovered catastrophic medical expenses (Doty et al., 2008), and the loss of health insurance benefits due to recession-related job losses (White & Reschovsky, 2012). Since the early 1970s, most of the middle class had supported the notion that it was an important responsibility of the government to ensure universal access to health care. However, to the extent that the opponents of health-care reform could frame such reform as a threat to health-care access for those with employment-based insurance, the proponents of reform lost the crucial middle-class vote (Blendon et al., 2005). By the end of the George W. Bush's presidency in 2008, all of this had changed. A continuation of the status quo had at last for the middle class become more frightening than the prospect of fundamental health-care reform. Social welfare historians will long ponder why the nation's first African American president was able to succeed in his quest to enact legislation that would make universal access to comprehensive health care a social right of citizenship, whereas some of the most able and determined Euro-white presidents in history had failed.

In part, Obama's success at achieving the passage of the Affordable Care Act is attributable to the two contextual shifts just highlighted, but there were other fundamental reasons as well. Among them is the fact that because Obama was elected with the largest Democratic vote since 1964 on a platform of health-care reform, he could legitimately claim that he had a mandate from the American electorate to reform the health-care system. This was in contrast to Clinton in 1992, who had won the presidency with only 43 percent of the popular vote (thanks to the third-party candidacy of Ross Perot). Most crucially, Obama also had, for his first two years in office, a party majority in both chambers of Congress *and* the lessons learned from the Clinton administration's health-care reform debacle—notable among these Clinton era lessons was the knowledge that Obama could not win against the combined strength of both the health insurance and pharmaceutical industry lobbies. Thus, in return for his pledge not to pursue legislation that would allow the federal government to exercise its purchasing power to negotiate lower drug prices (a concession that outraged the political left), Obama gained not only the support of PhRMA (the Pharmaceutical Research and Manufacturers of America) for his Affordable Care Act but also $100 million in media advertising in support of the ACA (Blumenthal, 2010). Although the ACA squeaked through the House of Representatives with a five-vote margin, at the time the ACA was signed into law in March 2010, public opinion had already shifted toward a slight majority in opposition to the legislation, in part because many on the political left objected to the Obama administration's abandonment of a provision in the original ACA for a public insurance option at the behest of both the health insurance and the for-profit hospital industries (Mogulescu, 2010). The ACA's passage was that close, but it was also a done deal.

The Essentials of the ACA

The ACA can be fairly described in a variety of ways, including that it (1) represents the largest expansion of the welfare state in the past half-century and (2) is fundamentally an extension of the 1965 compromise between the political moderates of both majority parties that created the mixed public and private health-care financing marriage of subsidized employment-based insurance with a means-tested public entitlement to health care for the poor (under the ACA, this has been extended to those of relatively low income). However, as crucially distinct from the 1965 compromise, the ACA embodied a congressional concession to the inevitability of a universal health care coverage as a social right of citizenship—albeit a reluctant one.[7]

While it is beyond the purpose of this chapter to delve deeply into the specifics of the ACA, in a nutshell, the ACA has four manifest policy aims. It seeks to (1) expand health insurance enrollment to over 90 percent of the national population, (2) increase health-care quality, (3) "bend the curve" of ever rising health-care costs, and (4) leave intact the nation's extremely complex mixed private/public model of health-care financing. Under the ACA as originally signed into law, expansion of health insurance coverage to near-universal inclusion is achieved through a combination of regulatory insurance market reforms, health insurance purchase and coverage subsidies, insurance purchase mandates for individuals and employers, and expansions of public entitlement programs—most particularly Medicaid. Health-care delivery system reforms that are intended to both increase quality and restrain the growth in health-care inflation include heavy investment in preventative health services, increased investment and payment incentives in primary care, significant investment in innovative approaches to the management of chronic disease, payment mechanisms that reward cost-effective clinical care over the promotion of health-care utilization, and identification and elimination of inflationary provider incentives (such as proprietary doctor-owned hospitals).

The most controversial provisions of the ACA include the so-called individual mandate that requires citizens and legal residents to have qualifying health coverage as an alternative to payment of a tax penalty and (as originally signed into law) a de facto requirement that states expand Medicaid coverage to most citizens and legal residents younger than sixty-five (children, pregnant women, parents, and adults without dependent children) with incomes up to 133 percent of the federal poverty level based on modified adjusted gross income.

The Implementation Phase, 2010–?

Successful social policy entails three accomplishments. First, the policy must be essentially implemented as designed. Second, the policy must achieve its basic aims. Third, the policy's unintended consequences must not be so detrimental as to outweigh its intended benefits.[8] By far the most elusive of these three requisites for successful social policy is the implementation of policy as designed, as both theory (Pressman & Wildavsky, 1984) and the early experience of the ACA's implementation will attest.

Obstacles to Implementation

While full implementation of the ACA requires that its *ninety* most significant provisions be implemented by 2018 (Henry Kaiser Family Foundation, 2014c), realistically, five critical obstacles to the ACA pertain to a small number of its core provisions and assumptions. The first critical obstacle to the ACA's implementation, in fact its very survival, entailed the constitutionality of its individual mandate—in essence, whether the federal government could require that an individual carry health insurance and thereby engage what heretofore had been a voluntary health insurance market. The second critical obstacle, also pertaining to the constitutional powers granted to the federal government, concerned the provision of the ACA that permitted the federal government to financially coerce states into participating in the ACA's Medicaid coverage expansion to individuals and families above the federal poverty level. In the summer of 2012, the U.S. Supreme Court ruled on litigation that challenged both the individual mandate and the ACA's requirement that states expand Medicaid, upholding the individual mandate but then preserving for states the authority to determine whether to accept federal funds for Medicaid expansion.[9] Taken together, these two decisions meant that the ACA's insurance market reform efforts that would both make health insurance more affordable for high-risk populations and eliminate exclusions for preexisting medical conditions could go forward, but the prospects for expanded Medicaid enrollment in politically conservative states would be poor at best. As of early 2014, half of the nation's fifty states had not accepted ACA funds for Medicaid expansion, leaving approximately 5 million low-income uninsured Americans ineligible for Medicaid that in other states would have been (Henry Kaiser Family Foundation, 2014d).

A third critical obstacle to the ACA's implementation, easily as formidable as the first two, entailed the rapid development of the state-level health insurance exchanges that were the ACA's crucial vehicle for connecting consumers and small businesses to health insurance plans that meet the ACA's requirements for comprehensive coverage and affordability—the latter achieved through both competitive pricing and the availability of federal subsidies for the purchase of health insurance. While the preferred mechanism for this part of the ACA was for states to develop their own health insurance exchanges by the health insurance enrollment startup date of October 1, 2013, the ACA also included a provision that would enroll those seeking insurance from the states that elected not to develop their own health insurance exchanges in a federal health insurance marketplace developed by the U.S. Department of Health and Human Services (HSS). In essence, in this respect, the ACA lurched toward to a kind of mixed success that by January 1, 2014, provided a just sufficient enough health insurance market infrastructure to make possible the achievement of ACA's health insurance enrollment targets. Reflecting the state-level political opposition to the ACA, only seventeen states had elected to develop their own health insurance exchanges, while the remainder either relied on a federal–state partnership in the development of their insurance exchanges (seven) or totally defaulted to the federal health insurance exchange developed by the HSS (twenty-seven) (Henry Kaiser Family Foundation, 2014e).[10]

The fourth critical obstacle to the ACA's implementation, which in the final analysis represents the ACA's true prospects for success, is the extent to which the ACA proved able to meet its health insurance enrollment targets during its first crucial open enrollment period from October 1, 2013, to March 31, 2014. Unlike the public opinion polls that measure attitudes and beliefs about health-care reform and the ACA, the extent to which the uninsured and those seeking more affordable health insurance enroll in the ACA's new health insurance options (through either the state-level health insurance exchanges or federally operated health insurance exchange) represents actual health insurance market behavior and, for that matter, the ACA's true "buy-in" by the American public. During this first crucial period, there were two pivotal enrollment targets: the overall number of Americans using the health insurance exchanges to obtain either Medicaid or private health insurance and the extent to which those acquiring health insurance coverage represented young adults between the ages of

THE EMERGENCE OF THE NEW ERA OF REFORM

eighteen and thirty-four—this being essential to balance health insurance usage risks between the relatively young and healthy and those older and typically less healthy.

With respect to the first pivotal target (in a development that surprised both the Obama administration and the ACA's opponents), by the end of the first open enrollment period on March 31, 2014, President Obama was able to triumphantly announce that the ACA health insurance exchanges had enrolled 7.1 million Americans—thus just meeting the Congressional Budget Office target enrollment benchmark of 7 million made at the point that the ACA was launched (Bergman, 2014; Office of the Press Secretary, 2014). As to the second, during the first five months of the ACA's open enrollment period, young adults comprised 25 percent of the enrollment—which fell well short of the 40 percent benchmark required to balance insurance plan expenditures and revenues (Assistant Secretary for Planning and Evaluation, 2014; Levitt et al., 2013). While it is quite feasible that the enrollment of young adults might accelerate in response to a more favorable labor market for young adults and as the idea of carrying health insurance becomes more normative, this crucial aspect of the ACA's implementation has a guarded prognosis. The fifth and penultimate obstacle to the ACA's successful implementation is purely political—in essence, the ability of Congress to either critically impede key provisions of the ACA's implementation or repeal the ACA altogether. Both are what the GOP has vowed to do since the day the ACA was signed into law on March 23, 2010. Taken at face value, the GOP's dozens of unsuccessful votes to repeal the ACA over the first four years of its implementation would be chilling for the ACA's long-term prospects—particularly given the very real possibility of a GOP resurgence in the 2016 elections that would yield the presidency and both chambers of Congress. However, some important considerations preclude the GOP's regaining political dominance as being necessarily synonymous with the demise of the ACA.

First and foremost, written into the ACA is a timeline of implementation that put into place its most politically popular provisions during its first few years: in particular, expanding mandated employment-based insurance coverage of dependent children to age twenty-six, the elimination of preexisting conditions as an obstacle to obtaining affordable health insurance and as a means of denying health insurance claims, imposing a threshold of the profits made by health insurance carriers, and the provision of health insurance purchase subsidies for middle-class families. These upfront ACA provisions are in effect a poison pill in any legislation that would actually substantially repeal the ACA. Second, repeal of the ACA's Medicaid expansion provisions would return millions of low-income Americans to the ranks of the uninsured and would quite likely be catastrophic to an already deeply strained national health-care safety net.

Third, the GOP would have to introduce a viable alternative to the ACA that would convince key stakeholder groups (including hospitals, the health insurance industry, the pharmaceutical industry, and both large and small employers) that they would be actually better off under some as yet to be proposed non-ACA alternative that is in any way different from the failing pre-ACA status quo. Finally (but not exhaustively), the GOP would have to contend with the detrimental effects of an ACA repeal on both the solvency of the Medicare Hospital Insurance Trust Fund and reductions in the federal deficit—both of which are substantially aided by the ACA (Congressional Budget Office, 2014; Congressional Research Service, 2013).

Contradictions

The take-home points from the preceding analysis of the ACA's first four years of implementation are that (1) the ACA has been mostly successful in surmounting its critical obstacles to implementation and (2) despite the sound and the fury from its most vociferous opponents, in its essentials, the ACA is here to stay as the next major phase toward the realization of a social right to health care for all Americans.

That said, the ACA falls well short of the full realization of that achievement, due to a number of inherent contradictions between the structure and scope of its health-care entitlements and the requisites of health care as a social right of citizenship as it is broadly construed. These inherent contradictions include the ACA's exclusion of undocumented workers and their dependents from eligibility, the ACA's dependence on a highly stigmatized means-tested health-care entitlement (Medicaid) as the major pathway for low-income Americans to access health care, the ACA's reliance on an employment-based health insurance system that maintains the linkages between social stratification in the labor market and social stratification in health care, geographic exclusions from a social right to health care based on the ACA's inability to transcend the constitutional limitations imposed on the powers of the federal government, and finally (and perhaps most significantly) the inherent contradiction between the continued health-care policy hegemony of health-care industry stakeholder groups and the fiscal sustainability of the ACA's mixed public and private system of health-care financing. Although these are significant points of critique, there needs to be a more comprehensive appraisal of the ACA in light of what should be the core policy principles of a national commitment to a social right to health care. These core health-care policy principles, and their basis in the social citizenship requisites of political democracy, are illuminated in the next chapter.

Chapter Three

THE THEORETICAL FOUNDATIONS FOR
HEALTH CARE AS A SOCIAL RIGHT
OF CITIZENSHIP

The perspective that undergirds this chapter, and for that matter the book as a whole, is an optimistic one that sees the nation as evolving, albeit in fits and starts, toward a more complete realization of a truly democratic society. While there are ample grounds for a skeptical view of the nation's democratic future, there are also abundant grounds for a more hopeful view, if we consider the progress of both civil rights and political rights for various groups that have been among the oppressed and excluded at different points in our national history—women; African Americans; Native Americans; the lesbian, gay, bisexual, and transgender (LGBT) community; and, as always throughout our national history, the most recent waves of immigrants (Shklar, 1991). Indeed, few of us predicted that the same generation that witnessed the racial brutality of 1965 Selma, Alabama, would, by 2012, see the nation elect for a *second* term as president the biracial child of an African immigrant and a single mother.

As I argue in this chapter, because the realization of certain kinds of democratically essential social rights (including universal access to some essential forms of health care) is intrinsically bound to the evolvement of more inclusive civil and political rights, the fulfillment of certain social rights is not only plausible but also in the end imperative to the whole process of democratic progression. In this vein, the Affordable Care Act (ACA) is seen as a large and historically unprecedented step toward the embracement of universal access to health care to what has become an *essential* social right of citizenship.

The primary task of this chapter, then, is to show why, from the standpoint of a progressive democratic political philosophy, some kinds of social rights (defined broadly as economic security provisions and human capital investments that are granted to all citizens) are *essential* to the realization of what American political philosopher John Rawls refers to as the "moral powers of citizenship" in a democratic society (Rawls, 2001, p. 20). For this primary task, I draw on not only the arguments of Rawls's original (1971) theory of justice and his later revisions but also mid-twentieth-century theoretical essays of British sociologist T. H. Marshall on the evolving nature of citizenship in democratic societies and the interdependence of social mobility and democracy. Because John Rawls transformed the social justice sentiments of early twentieth-century progressives and FDR's rationale for the social legislation of the New Deal into a coherent theory of social justice and, by extension, liberal social democracy, his arguments are of course foundational to the task of this chapter. T. H. Marshall, on the other hand, provides the lens through which we can view certain kinds of social rights as not only crucial to a socially just society but also essential to the viability of political democracy in the face of the relentless and enduring forces of social stratification.

While the arguments made in this chapter concerning the linkages between democratic citizenship and certain kinds of social rights belong solely to Rawls and Marshall, in this chapter, I weave them together into a more concise synthesis of complementary ideas. Once this primary task is accomplished, I conclude with the theory-based justifications for the essential social rights that are the institutional preconditions to the realization of democratic citizenship and social mobility, including in particular the social right to health care. However, before embarking on this ambitious intellectual journey, here are some key terms and constructs that, because they have varied meanings and interpretations, require highlighting and specification.

DEFINING CRUCIAL CONSTRUCTS

The Definition of a "Democratic Society"

There are various forms of democratic governance and also societal variations within particular forms of democratic governance. Although the two principal theorists providing the substantive arguments for this chapter, John Rawls and T. H. Marshall, shared some overlapping and complementary ideas concerning citizenship and social rights, they formulated their propositions in reference to two very different democratic societies with distinct kinds of social hierarchies and variants of democratic governance.

Rawls, an American political philosopher, formulated his ideas within the context of a society with a federalist form of democratic governance and a deeply entrenched racial hierarchy. Marshall, a British sociologist, developed his ideas in the context of a parliamentary democracy with a deeply embedded class structure. However, both the United States and Great Britain are defined within a common class of democratic societies— that is, constitutional democracies with market economies. Such societies (1) define the rights and responsibilities of citizenship explicitly through a formal social contract established through the consent of the governed and (2) produce and distribute the material resources of the society primarily through the aggregate private interactions of individuals acting in their own perceived self-interest. This general class of democratic societies (which includes such other countries as France, Japan, Sweden, Germany, and South Korea) represents the general case to which both the theories of Rawls and Marshall apply. As such, this general class will serve as the book's definition of a democratic society.

The Definition of "Citizenship"

The most basic and theoretically coherent definition of citizenship is that provided by T. H. Marshall in his seminal essay *Citizenship and Social Class*, first published in 1950: "Citizenship is a status bestowed on those who are full members of a community. All who possess this status are equal with respect to the rights and duties with which the status is bestowed" (Marshall & Bottomore, 1992, p. 18). If by *community* we mean (as Marshall did) a democratic society, it should become apparent that as simple and perhaps as intuitive as this definition is, the genuine realization of citizenship in accordance with this definition imposes formidable demands of justice on a society's political and social institutions. For example, if citizenship in a particular society includes an *equal* right to a free public education, it means that the accessibility and quality of that free public education are unaffected by gender, race, income, or place of residence. Similarly, if particular political rights (such as voting rights) are bestowed to all those to whom the term *citizen* applies, it means that there can be no barriers, inconveniences, or obstacles to voting that would make it more difficult for one citizen or category of citizens to exercise their voting rights than any other.

Aside from providing a concise and timeless definition of citizenship, Marshall's *Citizenship and Social Class* delves deeply into the complex and multidimensional nature of citizenship in democratic societies, such as it has evolved in the case of Great Britain, beginning with the *civil* dimension of citizenship in the eighteenth century, the *political* dimension of citizenship in the nineteenth century, and the *social* dimension of citizenship in the twentieth century (Marshall & Bottomore, 1992, p. 10). In fact, Marshall's illuminating essay on these three interdependent aspects of democratic citizenship and their chronology of emergence as a reflection of the evolutionary nature of democratic societies represents his major intellectual contribution to our understanding of the relationship between social rights and political rights. At a later point in this chapter, when Marshall's theory of citizenship will be considered in depth, the nature of these three dimensions of democratic citizenship and their implications for social rights will be examined in detail.

DEFINING HEALTH AND HEALTH CARE

There are many definitions of health, and any theory of particular rights to health care must begin with its chosen conceptualization of health. In this book, I adopt the perspective that health is of special significance to the moral powers of citizenship in a democratic society and embrace the definition of health advanced by political philosopher Norman Daniels. That is, health is conceptualized as the absence of pathologies that prevent or inhibit "normal human functioning" as it is understood within the context of human biology and social context (Daniels, 2008).[1] While Daniels's defense of this particular definition of health is an extensive one, for the purposes here, only some essentials that are relevant to arguments made in later chapters will be highlighted.

First, in defining health in terms of "normal human functioning," Daniels places particular emphasis on those capacities that are essential to the requirements of justice as articulated in John Rawls's theory of justice— both in Rawls's two principles of justice and in his ideas pertaining to the two moral powers of democratic citizenship (Rawls, 1971, 2001). With respect to Rawls's two principles of justice, embedded in the second principle is the idea that a democratic society (as "a fair system of cooperation") must provide those rights and resources that are essential to "fair equality of opportunity"—meaning not just a de jure "equality of opportunity" as an ideological abstraction but as a de facto opportunity structure in which factors such as class, race, and gender are independent of the genuine prospects to enjoy the full benefits of democratic citizenship.[2] As argued by Daniels (2008), health in the sense of "normal human functioning" is an essential precondition to that fair equality of opportunity.

Although there is a wide range of definitions for *health care*, in this book, health care refers to the services (procedures, methodologies, and products) that are provided to persons and populations for maintenance or restoration of health. Health services thus may be preventative, curative, or restorative (Hessler & Buchanan, 2002). *Health care rights* are defined as a *social right* of citizenship, which in the context of democratic citizenship are resources or actions on our behalf that are owed to us based on our possession of the status of "citizen."

There is somewhat of a conundrum entailed in the distinction between *health rights*, which encompass all aspects of societal structure and social resources that can be shown to affect both the overall level of population health and its distribution (as, for example, income inequality and clean air and water), and *health care* rights. Philosopher Sridhar Venkatapuram suggests that the health rights discourse can be organized into four categories: claims to disease and disability-specific responses, claims to health affecting goods and services (e.g., preventative health care, sanitation, clean water), more general kinds of human rights that are shown to affect health (as in the relationship shown between freedom of the press and famine prevention), and health rights that are derived from formal theories of justice (Venkatapuram, 2011, pp. 182–183). In this book, *health care rights* as opposed to the more encompassing *health rights* are seen as referring to the first two categories: (1) claims to disease and disability-specific responses and (2) claims to health affecting goods and services.

As considered in this book, the term *universal* as applied to health care has two crucial aspects. The first aspect refers to coverage and inclusiveness; *universal* means applied to all persons falling within the discrete category of citizen. The second aspect of *universal* as applied to health care refers to equal treatment of equal cases, meaning that whatever is regarded as *essential* health care by the definitional rules adopted is distributed in accordance with principles of equity. For example, under the meaning of universal health care adopted here and as used in subsequent chapters, persons regarded as equal with respect to the clinical need for hip replacement surgery must have equal prospects for obtaining a hip replacement surgery as an extension of their equal standing as citizens—independent of factors such as race, gender, age, social class, or place of employment. Finally, the term *essential* health care acknowledges that rights to health care, even if universal, are inherently limited by the finite nature of health-care resources. Every nation that provides universal health care must continuously grapple with what range of health services can feasibly be available to all within its particular scheme of health services. This problem, and the suggested approaches to it, will be taken up in the later chapters devoted to the setting of national health-care priorities. For now, though, we will say that *essential* health services are those that are demonstrably necessary to the requirements of democratic citizenship.

EXPLORING ALTERNATIVE JUSTIFICATIONS FOR UNIVERSAL HEALTH CARE

This book is largely devoted to the justification of a universal right to health care based on a particular synthesis of twentieth-century political philosophy and empirically grounded social theory. However compelling in its own right, this justification should be considered in light of other kinds of arguments for a universal right to health care—in particular, those alternative justifications that are particularly well represented in the contemporary public and political discourse on "the right to health care." These justifications include a universal right to health care based on popular preference, economic competitiveness, humanistic moral arguments (both secular and faith based), and a universal right to health care derived from formal theories of social justice (specifically utilitarianism, neo-Marxism, liberalism, and the capabilities approach).

Justification Based on Popular Preference

Essential to the nature of democratic governance, in contrast to monarchies and dictatorships, is the enactment, amendment, and repeal of social policies in response to popular preference (Madison, 1788b). While there are limits to this pertaining to the protection of individual liberty rights,

social policy by popular preference remains a central basis of policy justification. Perhaps the most notorious example of the enactment and then
repeal of social policy in response to popular preference was the Volstead
Act of 1919, thus beginning the era more generally known as Prohibition.
In 1933, again by popular preference, the Volstead Act was repealed and
Prohibition came to an end. By far the most dominant example of health-
care policy in response to popular preference is the Medicare program,
which, despite its status as a form of socialized medicine, is contrary to
conservative principles. However, it is considered by even the conservative
political establishment to be firmly entrenched and all but politically un-
touchable. This is because the Medicare program is highly popular among
the general public relative to most social programs, most particularly
among older adult voters, who directly benefit from Medicare entitlements
to health care.

In many respects, the ACA is itself illustrative of social policy that can
be justified on the grounds of popular preference. Notwithstanding dissent
over many of the specifics of the ACA, particularly the so-called individual mandate that requires a broad class of U.S. citizens to either carry
or purchase health insurance, there is strong evidence from decades of
national surveys that most Americans believe (1) that health care should
be available to all citizens and (2) that the assurance of health care for all is
a legitimate function of government. For example, as discussed in chapter 1,
since 1972, the General Social Survey has regularly asked a representative
sample of American adults the same question pertaining to the role of
government versus the individual in ensuring access to affordable care. Despite claims and common assumptions to the contrary, less than 20 percent
of the public believe that paying for health care is solely a matter of individual responsibility (National Opinion Research Center, 2006). In a more recent national survey jointly sponsored by National Public Radio, the Kaiser
Family Foundation, and the Harvard School of Public Health, it was shown
that 72 percent of the public favored an expansion of government-sponsored
health-care programs for low-income individuals—with nearly half of the
public (44 percent) supporting a single-payer government plan financed
through taxes (Sussman et al., 2009). Moreover, the 2008 election and then
2012 reelection of Barack Obama to the presidency on a platform that advanced universal health-care coverage for all citizens adds to the evidence
of popular support for the general idea of health care as a social right of
citizenship—despite enduring divisions over the specific means of fulfill-

ing this right. Had the majority of Americans not embraced the idea of health insurance coverage for all as an important function of government and political priority, it is unlikely that Obama would have been elected to a first term, let alone a second one.

Justification Based on Economic Competitiveness

The justification of universal access to health care on the basis of economic/ competitive necessity has two related but distinct lines of reasoning and evidence. The first line of reasoning derives from the observation that the dramatically higher costs of the mixed public and private U.S. health-care system (2:1 relative to other democratic nation-states that have universal coverage) undermine the global competitiveness of U.S. firms through the dramatically higher health-care costs imposed on U.S. exports (OECD, 2011). In essence, this line of reasoning attributes the high costs of health care in the United States to its historic and deeply entrenched treatment of health care as a market commodity as opposed to a universal social entitlement. This, in turn, supports the argument that countries that provide universal health coverage see health care as primarily a public good in the interests of collective economic advantage—thus, they also embrace a stronger government role in reducing the costs of health care.

The second line of reasoning considers more directly the beneficial human capital investments in health and other kinds of social welfare entitlements on global competitiveness. For example, it is noted that each of the four countries ranked more highly than the United States in the 2011–2012 *World Economic Forum Global Competitiveness Report* (Switzerland, Singapore, Finland, and Sweden) provides not only universal health care but also an extensive array of other social welfare benefits (Callahan & Bradley, 2012). In fact, of the ten most competitive national economies in the world, only the United States (ranked fifth) fails to provide health care as a right of citizenship (Callahan & Bradley, 2012; World Economic Forum, 2012).

Justification Based on Humanistic Moral Arguments

Although there are many definitions of humanism, as applied here, humanism refers to an ethical perspective that is grounded in beliefs about intrinsic human worth, human equality, and moral imperatives concerned with the preservation and advancement of human well-being. Two forms of humanism share a similar ethos but arise from different assumptions about the origins and bases of human worth—often referred to as *secular humanism* and *faith-based humanism*.

Secular Humanism

Secular humanism, which threads its way from the rationalism of the early Greek philosophers through the European scientists and philosophers of the Enlightenment, is characterized by its ethos of intrinsic human worth, equality, and the advancement of human well-being through the human capacities for reason, rationalism, and compassion (Bristow, 2011; Edwords, 2008). In contrast to more formal moral theories that originate from either organized religion or rational philosophies, secular humanism does not adhere to a theologically derived doctrine or a particular system of thought with a coherent set of ethical principles and moral rules. Secular humanism instead embraces a general conception of the good—that which protects and advances human dignity and well-being, including a range of human rights that in most variants of secular humanism include health care.

Perhaps the most well-known version of secular humanism that advances universal health care as a human right and ergo a social right of citizenship is the *United Nations Universal Declaration of Human Rights*, which in Article 25 states, "Everyone has the right to a standard of living adequate for the health and well-being of himself and of his family, including food, clothing, housing and medical care" (United Nations, 1948).[3] The perspective on health care as a universal right derives from secular humanism, because it accommodates a wide range of religious beliefs and political ideologies and is also reflected in the health-care policy positions statements across an array of professional associations, scientific societies, and health-care advocacy organizations that espouse health care as a universal right or a crucial societal goal. Examples include the National Association of Social Workers' (NASW) official policy statement on health care, which supports a national policy that "ensures the right to universal access to a continuum of health and mental health care throughout all stages of the life cycle" (NASW, 2011, p. 170); the Physicians for a National Health Program (PNHP) mission statement, which reads in part that the "PNHP believes that access to high-quality health care is a right of all people and should be provided equitably as a public service rather than bought and sold as a commodity" (PNHP, 2013, p. 1); and the American Public Health Association's (APHA) *Fourteen Points on Health Care Reform*, which includes among its criteria for national health reform "universal coverage for everyone in the United States" (APHA, 2009, p. 1). Secular humanism is also represented in the millions of agnostic and even otherwise apolitical Americans who support universal health care as a collective humanitarian obligation.

Faith-Based Humanism

As noted by Edwords (2008), except for the belief that a deity or spiritual force plays a role in the human condition and provides the ultimate basis for moral principles that guide human conduct, faith-based beliefs about intrinsic human worth and dignity, as well as one's obligations to protect the vulnerable and advance human well-being, are often indistinguishable from the ethos of secular humanism. That said, faith-based convictions about social justice and human rights, including rights to health care, still occupy their own powerful place among the moral frameworks that provide justifications for universal health care.

Although faith-based humanistic moral arguments in support of universal health care are not limited to monotheistic religions (the belief in one supreme deity), the monotheistic traditions of Islam, Judaism, and Christianity each share a common ethical thread that reifies care of the sick as a moral duty—specifically an act of obedience to God's will. Briefly stated, this arises from a theological ethic referred to as "theological voluntarism" or "divine command," which in essence is the belief that one's sovereign duty in life is that of obedience to either God's will or God's specific commands (Olson, 2012, p. 192). By this theological ethic, all other moral principles in life are subservient to this one. Although monotheistic faith traditions depart from each other and manifest their own internal schisms with respect to the ideas, events, and moral principles that are presumed to represent God's will, all rely on the exercise of a faith-based inference process that links sacred ideas and moral principles to the moral evaluation of particular social policies—including the question of universal entitlement to health care.

In this vein, within the reform tradition of Judaism, a universal right to health care is inferred to derive from not only a long tradition in Jewish communities to care for their sick as a communal imperative but also the conviction "that God endowed humanity with the understanding and ability to become partners with God in making a better world" (Religious Action Center of Reform, 2013, p. 1). Within Islam, scholars of the Quran point out that health care as a right derives in part from the Prophet's great emphasis on health as being only secondary to faith in God's blessings, thus conferring a duty upon Muslims to protect and promote health in themselves, their families, and their community (Al-Khayat, 2004, p. 14). In turn, Christian proponents of universal health care often attribute their moral imperative to promote a universal right to health care to both the example of Jesus's caring for those afflicted with stigmatizing illnesses as a central object lesson of his ministry and his categorical imperative (as paraphrased from the Christian New Testament, Matthew 22:37–40) that one's duty to God can be summarized by "loving God, and loving your neighbor as you would love yourself" (Olson, 2012, pp. 192–193).[4] As just one example of this moral inference among many in the Christian tradition, there is the 2009 statement by Roman Catholic bishop William Murphy, chair of the U.S. Bishops' Committee on Domestic Justice and Human Development on the criteria for just health-care reform: "Reform efforts must begin with the principle that decent health care is not a privilege, but a right and a requirement to protect the life and dignity of every person. . . . *The bishops' conference believes health care reform should be truly universal and it should be genuinely affordable.*"[5]

It should be noted that Judaism, Islam, and Christianity (in particular, the Roman Catholic Church) all have enacted their common moral imperative that care for the sick is a duty owed to God through the building of hospitals that serve all patients, regardless of ability to pay. Within the Islamic religious traditions, the hospitals and medical schools that serve all needing medical care can be traced to the founding of the city of Baghdad in the eighth century A.D. Among the largest in early Middle East history was Mansuri Hospital in Cairo (established 1248 A.D.), which had its own pharmacy, library, lecture halls, and places of worship for both Muslim and Christian patients (Dharmananda, 2004).

In the United States, most hospitals can trace their roots to either Jewish or Christian philanthropists, beneficence societies, and religious orders with an institutional mission to serve all those in need of hospital care—such as the Sisters of Providence on the West Coast that emerged in the nineteenth century (Rosenberg, 1987). The health-care financing mechanisms that were originally intended to make hospital care affordable to all (employment-based health insurance, Medicare, and Medicaid) that ultimately led to the commodification of hospital care in ostensibly not-for-profit hospitals were later developments.

Justifications for Universal Health Care Based on Theories of Social Justice

Justifications for universal health care from the standpoint of obligations that are owed to the individual as a matter of just governance arise from specific theories of social justice. While the term *social justice* itself has a variety of meanings, as applied here, social justice refers to a construct derived from a political theory or system of thought used to determine what mutual obligations flow between the individual and society. With respect specifically to health care, at least four major theories of social justice provide a moral basis for a universal entitlement to health care, including utilitarianism, neo-Marxism, liberalism, and the capabilities approach (Almgren, 2013). While it is beyond the purpose of this chapter to review these four theoretical perspectives in depth, I will summarize in brief the essential moral basis for a universal entitlement to health care from each perspective. The order of theories of justice reviewed is framed by philosopher William Talbott's thesis that the dominant theories pertaining to just governance and human rights represent different stages in the evolutionary progression of human rights, with each theory representing a "moral improvement" over the preceding one—with no particular theory representing the final penultimate statement on social justice and human rights (Talbott, 2010).

Utilitarianism

Of the four theories of social justice to be considered, the utilitarian approach is at once the most intuitive and also the most fragile as a justification for a universal right to health care. In essence, the utilitarian perspective, as applied to the just distribution of health-care resources, argues that health-care resources should be distributed in accordance with the principle of utility (also referred to as the principle of maximum utility), which holds that the optimally just distribution of scarce resources is based on *whatever scheme yields the average level of maximum good to the maximum number of people* (Rescher, 1966). In this vein, utilitarian proponents of universal health care point out the evidence from cross-national comparisons of population health that shows

that among industrialized countries, the achievement of universal entitlement to health care is correlated with the realization of higher levels of
overall population health.

However, there are two problems with this argument. The first is that
a number of other factors tend to co-occur with the achievement of
a universal entitlement to health care, such as the rise in per-capita
income, advances in population education, lower levels of income inequality, and higher levels of nutrition. The second is that under the utility principle, population health might be even further advanced by
reducing the entitlements to health care among groups who tend to incur very high health-care expenditures, with little chance of contributing to the average level of population health, and instead shifting those
health investments to those groups who would most contribute to the
average level of population health. In fact, this particular utilitarian argument provided a substantial part of the basis of renowned bioethicist
Daniel Callahan's controversial proposal that old age should be a limiting factor in individual entitlements to health care (Callahan, 1987).[6] The
logic of this utilitarian argument might also be extended to the limiting
of health-care entitlements among the severely developmentally disabled, accident victims with little hope of recovery to full health, and
any other groups or individuals who share the common trait of incurring great health-care expenditures with little added contribution to the
average level of population health.

Neo-Marxism

The term *neo-Marxism* is used here to acknowledge the fact that Marx himself did not regard his theory of societal evolution to be a theory of justice
but rather a theory of history. He left it to others to translate his ideas to
political theory and then later theories of social justice based on what are
presumed to be Marxist principles of justice. Also, like other nineteenth-
century political philosophies, Marxist theory in its original form does not
deal specifically with the just distribution of health care, except through
logical inference. That said, a universal right to health care has been, at least
in principle, the centerpiece of every regime over the past century predicated on Marxism. This emphasis on health care as a social right in Marxist regimes has its origins in at least two tenets of Marxist ethics. The first
is the collective ownership of the national system of health care for the benefit of workers, and the second is the elimination of any disparities in the

rewards for labor—including by logical inference disequities in access to health care (Peffer, 1990). Another Marxist justification for universal health care as a social right can be traced to a simple ethical maxim stated directly by Marx himself: "From each according to his ability, and to each according to his needs" (Marx, 1938, p. 10). This would infer a collective obligation to provide health care on what might be termed a humanistic ethos within Marxist thought, which is consistent with Karl Marx's particular concern with the ways in which the Industrial Revolution had destroyed the bases of human dignity in the common working man. Tragically, Marx had not anticipated the rise of entrenched Stalinism and other tyrannical versions of Marxism that were at least as dehumanizing as the extremes of the laissez-faire capitalism that had motivated and framed his analysis of modern history.

Liberalism

While the origins of political liberalism, as with libertarianism, can be traced to the Enlightenment writings of John Locke (1632–1794) on the natural rights of man and the idea of the social contract as the basis of just governance, it took the social philosophy of the American Progressive Era (1890–1920) to imagine an activist government that would balance the extremes of laissez-faire capitalism with the humanistic ends of political democracy. The central philosophical threads of political liberalism were reflected in the social policies advanced by Progressive Era social reformers and the New Deal legislation enacted during the first decade of the FDR administration but were not coalesced into a coherent moral theory until John Rawls's (1971) *Theory of Justice*. Although Rawls's theory of justice and the foundations it provides for a universal entitlement to health care will be expanded upon at a later point in this chapter, liberalism's central justification for health care as a social right of citizenship is predicated on the idea that democratic citizenship requires *fair equality of opportunity*, which in turn requires universal access to the means through which genuine fair equality of opportunity can be realized. Such means (which Rawls identifies as *primary goods*) include not only the liberty rights that are the central concern of libertarian political philosophy but certain social rights commensurate with the requirements of citizenship and fair equality of opportunity, including adequate provisions for education, material security, and health care (Rawls, 1971, p. 107; Rawls, 2001, pp. 58–59, 174–175).

The Capabilities Approach

The capabilities approach to social justice and human rights, formulated by economist Amartya Sen in response to what he viewed as the limitations of theories of justice originating from Western political philosophy (Sen, 2009), is based on two essential normative claims.[7] First, that the freedom to achieve well-being is of primary moral importance and, second, that the freedom to achieve well-being is "to be understood in terms of people's capabilities, that is their real opportunities to do and be what they have reason to value" (Robeyns, 2011, p. 1). In a further elaboration of Sen's capabilities approach framework, philosopher Martha Nussbaum included among her Ten Central Human Functional Capabilities that of "Bodily Health. Being able to have good health, including reproductive health; to be adequately nourished; to have adequate shelter" (Nussbaum, 2000, pp. 78–80). As argued by Venkatapuram (2011), the "Capability to be Healthy" (as a moral claim that defines the character of a just society) can only be realized through a combination of a range of civil, political, and social rights, including an extensive array of "health rights" that begin with universal rights to health care for the prevention and treatment of disease and disability (pp. 182–183).

T. H. MARSHALL AND JOHN RAWLS IN HISTORICAL, PERSONAL, AND INTELLECTUAL CONTEXTS

The arguments to be advanced in this book on a social right to health care originate in the remarkable convergences in the theories of T. H. Marshall (1893–1981) and John Rawls (1921–2002), two intellectual titans on the political foundations of the liberal welfare state. The writings of both illuminate the necessity of particular kinds of social rights as structural requisites to democratic citizenship. Despite their defining differences in disciplinary perspective, epistemologies, and points of departure, in some key respects, they arrived at a common destination through different intellectual pathways. That common ground can be thought of as a shared point of view, albeit based on very different theoretical justifications, on the nature of democratic societies and the necessity of certain kinds of social rights as essential to the status and powers of democratic citizenship and the viability of democratic institutions. In particular, it can be said that both Marshall and Rawls immersed themselves in the contradictions between various forms of inherited disadvantage and privilege, the egalitarian foundations of citizenship in a democratic society, and the integrity of democratic political institutions.

It is perhaps not at all coincidental that both Marshall and Rawls share some remarkable similarities in their personal biographies. Both Marshall and Rawls were gifted children of privileged backgrounds who, during their intellectually formative years, found themselves thrust into the paradoxes of social class and terrible world wars that were justified as essential to the defense of democracy. T. H. Marshall, by an accident of tourism during the outbreak of World War I, spent four years in Germany as an interned British national—sharing his plight with the large number of working-class Britons who were also caught in Germany at the war's outbreak. It is also likely that Marshall's considerable empathy with the struggles and aspirations of the British working class can also be traced to his early career beginnings at the London School of Economics in the 1920s as a tutor in social work—a position he held for several years before becoming a lecturer in economic history (Harris, 2010).

Like T. H. Marshall, John Rawls was born into privilege, educated at an elite university, but then transformed by his personal experiences of war. The child of an established and wealthy Baltimore family, Rawls completed an undergraduate degree at Princeton (class of 1943) and then, instead of pursuing either graduate studies in theology or the offer to join a Major League Baseball franchise as a pitcher, Rawls joined the U.S. Army as an ordinary enlisted man. According to his biographical memoir by Harvard colleague Hilary Putnam (2005), Rawls's wartime experiences of brutal combat in the Philippines (endured side-by-side with ordinary poor and working-class Americans) caused him to rethink his faith and his plans for a career as an Episcopal priest, so he instead returned to Princeton to complete his PhD in philosophy. It can also be said that, in common with Marshall, a large share of the substance of Rawls's development as a philosopher must be credited to his immersion into the deep waters of elite British academia. As a visiting scholar at Oxford in the early 1950s, Rawls associated with British luminaries such as Herbert Hart, Isaiah Berlin, and Stuart Hampshire. These associations, perhaps foregrounded by his harrowing wartime experiences as an ordinary soldier in service of his country, were the wellspring of the central ideas on democracy and social justice that later became fully crystalized in Rawls's (1971) A Theory of Justice (2005, pp. 115–116).[8]

Although the ideas of Marshall and Rawls on the nature of democratic citizenship and its structural requisites are in parts synonymous and on the whole complementary, each approaches the problem of reconciling political democracy with free-market capitalism with different epistemologically framed questions. Marshall, as the empirical sociologist, asks, "Does the evidence from history validate the hypothesis that basic equality, when enriched in substance and embodied in the formal rights of citizenship, is consistent with the inequalities of social class?" (Marshall & Bottomore, 1992, p. 7).

Whereas Rawls, the political philosopher, asks a hypothetical question rather than an empirical one: What principles and rules for governing the basic structure of a given society would arise from the deliberations undertaken by a group of rational actors, charged with the task of representing the interests of persons unknown to them, who are to be free and equal citizens of that society?[9] As will become apparent in the interrogation of Marshall and Rawls that follows, we have something akin to the convergence of two distinct epistemologies on (1) the nature of democratic citizenship in societies predicated upon the principles of political democracy and free-market capitalism and (2) the foundational requirements of democratic citizenship, that is, the social provisions that are crucial to what Rawls refers to as the "moral powers of citizens free and equal" and the permeable class structure that Marshall argues is essential to the stability of democratic societies.

T. H. MARSHALL ON THE FOUNDATIONAL REQUIREMENTS OF DEMOCRATIC CITIZENSHIP

Marshall's Theory of Democratic Citizenship in Historical Context

To gain a full appreciation of Marshall's theory of democratic citizenship and its implications for the essential social rights of citizenship that encompass universal health care, it is important to consider the historical context of the essay that defined his place in intellectual history, *Citizenship and Social Class*. When *Citizenship and Social Class* was first published in 1950, the military and geopolitical partnership between the United States, Great Britain, and the Soviet Union that had destroyed Nazi Germany and its allies had dissolved into two opposing blocs, with each seeking to dominate in the new world order and, if possible, destroy the other in a protracted struggle known as the Cold War. The so-called Western bloc of constitutional democracies with market economies, led by the

United States, Great Britain, and France, sought to advance democracy and free-market capitalism through military dominance and economic prosperity, while the so-called Eastern bloc, led by the Soviet Union, sought to advance communism through military might and postcolonial/Marxist political ideology.

Despite their opposing political ideologies and geopolitical aims, the strategic doctrines of the East and West blocs were fundamentally the same—in essence, military containment of the territorial expansion/incursion of the rival bloc until the inevitable collapse of the rival bloc due to the internal contradictions of its presumed to be fatally flawed political system. With respect to communist states, Cold War doctrine in the West pointed to the totalitarian character of communist regimes (as embodied in Stalinism) and the visible economic failures of state-owned production and centralized planning as evidence of communism's internal contradictions (as shown by the Soviet Union's dependence on Western wheat imports during the Cold War era). On the other hand, with respect to the flaws inherent in the political systems of Western democracies, communist doctrine pointed to the inherent contradictions between capitalism, popular democracy, and the social class oppression that is ordained by the nature of capitalism. As evidence, doctrinaire communists could point to the endemic poverty among the laboring classes, the vulnerability of workers and their dependents to the harsh incentives of laissez-faire capitalism, and the lack of material and social equality between the different social classes commiserate with democratic notions of equality in citizenship. It was Marshall's task to reconcile these contradictions, as aptly captured in the title of his 1950 monograph, *Citizenship and Social Class*.

A second aspect of historical context that is essential to the interpretation of Marshall's theory of democratic citizenship, if not his explicit purpose in formulating his theory, lies in the contrast between social welfare philosophies of the United States and Great Britain that were ascendant in the immediate post–World War II era. It should be remembered that in the immediate post–World War II decade, the United States and Great Britain, as the only Western bloc superpowers, were in close partnership in a global quest to advance free-market democracy against totalitarian socialism. Thus, their divergent approaches to welfare capitalism would be deeply influential in the shaping of the welfare states among the emergent democracies of the post–World War II/postcolonial world.

In Great Britain, where the Labour Party had triumphed in postwar national elections, the nation was moving toward full realization of the "cradle-to-grave" social security envisioned by the Beveridge Report to the British Parliament in 1942.[10] This was accomplished initially and primarily through the Family Allowance Bill (1945) and the founding of the National Health Service (1948), the first providing income subsidies for families with children and the second providing universal health care through compulsory social insurance.

In stark contrast to Great Britain, in the United States, the immediate postwar period had ushered in a newly elected Republican Party majority in Congress. Fueled and sanctioned by the "creeping communism" rhetoric of McCarthyism that was widely believed by the American public, the new Republican Congress was working to resist and, to the extent possible, reverse the New Deal policies that had been the domestic hallmark of the FDR administration and his Democratic Party successor, President Harry Truman. In addition to blocking Truman's attempt to expand the Social Security Act to encompass a social insurance fund for universal health care, the Republican-dominated Congress had overridden the veto of Truman to enact the Taft-Hartley Act (1947), which both severely restricted the collective bargaining, political, and organizing rights of labor and also forced labor unions to expel leaders who had been associated with socialist ideas that might be construed as communistic.

Thus, at the precise point in history when T. H. Marshall was formulating the lectures that became the text of *Citizenship and Social Class*, Great Britain's Labour government was laying the foundations of its "cradle-to-grave" public welfare state envisioned by the Beveridge Report, while in the United States, the conservative Republican Party (representing the interests of the capital class and laissez-faire economics) was seeking to make income and health security throughout the life course primarily a matter of employment-based insurance, meager means-based public assistance programs, and private charity (J. Klein, 2003). Even though both the United States and Great Britain ultimately stayed within the Esping-Andersen liberal welfare state typology as their social policies solidified over the post-World War II era, Great Britain remains (despite being encumbered by a deeply embedded class structure) much closer to a social democratic welfare regime than the United States in its universalistic antipoverty subsidies and health-care entitlements (Esping-Andersen, 1990). It is in defense of this British approach to welfare capitalism, which blends a high tolerance of social and income inequality with a strong public welfare state, that Marshall writes (and advocates of the American model of the residualist welfare state seek to repudiate).[11]

The Evolution of Democratic Citizenship in Great Britain

In many respects, Marshall was first and foremost a gifted and accomplished historian, as evidenced by excelling in his history exams at Cambridge and then, upon his return to Cambridge after the war, earning a fellowship for a thesis on the decline of the English guild system during the Enlightenment period (Harris, 2010, p. 8). Thus, he was well positioned to make coherent, in light of British political economic and social class history, the emergence of the post–World War II British welfare state as part and parcel of a larger evolution of democratic citizenship that was centuries in the making.

Marshall's *Citizenship and Social Class* is framed as a historically informed interrogation of what Marshall refers to as "a latent" sociological hypothesis embedded in a 1873 essay, *The Future of the Working Class*, by Victorian-era economist Alfred Marshall (Marshall & Bottomore, 1992, pp. 6–7).

According to T. H. Marshall, the latent sociological thesis embedded in Marshall's *Future of the Working Class* can be summarized as follows:

It postulates that there is a kind of basic human equality associated with the concept of full membership in a community—or, as I should say, of citizenship—which is not inconsistent with the inequalities which distinguish the various economic levels of the society. In other words, the inequality of the social class system may be acceptable provided the equality of citizenship is recognized. (p. 6)

This thesis, so says T. H. Marshall, invites four empirical questions (p. 7):

1. Is it evident that basic equality, when enriched in substance and embodied in the formal rights of citizenship, is consistent with the inequalities of social class?
2. Is it evident that basic equality, as a principle of democratic citizenship, is consistent with the principles of laissez faire that govern the market economy?
3. Is the shift from an emphasis on the *duties* of citizenship to the *rights* of citizenship, such as has been in evidence in recent history, inevitable and irreversible?

4. If it is true, as Alfred Marshall claims, that modern history is in part characterized by the gradual amelioration of class differences, are there limits to this modern drive toward social equality?

The easiest of these four questions to answer, again says T. H. Marshall, is the second question—he considers it simply obvious from the excesses of the nineteenth century that the principles of democratic citizenship are in conflict with unrestrained free-market capitalism. He responds to the other three empirical questions by proposing and then defending in light of recent British history his own thesis, i.e., that the modern drive toward social equality is but the latest phase of an evolution of citizenship that has been in continuous process since the Enlightenment (p. 7). In a wonderful turn of phrase that captures the essence of his historical empiricism, Marshall introduces the approach he takes to the defense of his thesis as "prepar[ing] the ground for an attack of the problems of today by digging into the subsoil of past history" (p. 7).

Marshall's Account of the Evolution of Democratic Citizenship

Although Marshall's simplified version of the evolution of democratic citizenship in Britain is not without its critiques and contrary evidence (Harris, 2010), he nonetheless makes a compelling case that democratic citizenship emerged in three stages over a period of roughly 250 years, with each stage representing a distinct and crucial dimension of democratic citizenship.[12] The first stage, corresponding primarily to the eighteenth century, saw the gradual realization of civil citizenship. Briefly stated, *civil* citizenship encompasses those rights that we would commonly refer to as liberty rights—freedoms of the person, religion, thought, and speech; property ownership; entrance into contracts; and rights to justice in accordance with due processes of law (p. 8). As evidence, Marshall refers to the right of habeas corpus, which (while it can be traced back to the twelfth century) emerged in its modern form in the Habeas Corpus Act of 1679, the Toleration Act of 1689 (which established religious freedom), the judicial recognition of the right to sell one's labor as a natural right in the mid-1700s, and the success of the freedom of the press movement in the early 1800s.

Political citizenship, which pertains to those rights essential to the exercise of one's political power (voting rights, the right to hold elective office), emerged during the 1800s as the bonds between economic status and voting rights were gradually broken through a series of reform acts, culminating in the Act of 1918, which enfranchised voting rights for men and women based on age rather than economic status, although until 1928, women's age of voting enfranchisement was thirty as opposed to twenty-one (pp. 12–13).

Finally, social citizenship, which encompasses those rights previously described as *social rights*, is viewed by Marshall as primarily a twentieth-century development. To expand on an earlier discussion at the beginning of this chapter, *social rights* are defined broadly to include the basic economic security provisions and human capital investments essential to what Marshall refers to as "the right to share to the full in the social heritage [of a given society] and to live the life of a civilized being according to the standards prevailing in the society" (p. 8). Social rights would thus include antipoverty provisions such as income and food assistance to the poor and human capital investments like public education and basic health care.

As Marshall describes it, however, social citizenship did not emerge in Britain until social rights became compatible with the civil and political rights of citizenship—as had not been with the case with social rights granted under the Poor Laws that had governed poor relief in England since the Elizabethan era. While the Poor Laws established a system whereby communities in England were required to make minimal provision for the destitute and in that sense granted the poor at least minimal social rights, the poor surrendered their civil and political rights in exchange—the penultimate example being relegated to the harsh conditions of the workhouse as an alternative to death by starvation. The demise of the Poor Laws occurred toward the end of the nineteenth century, when poverty was less and less seen as a defining trait of a particular social class but as an affront to the egalitarian notions of citizenship that gradually emerged in the wake of both civil and political citizenship and the amelioration of class differences in standards of living. To the latter, Marshall attributes the changes in modes of production and monetary income that decreased the income gaps between different classes of workers, the introduction of graduated direct taxation policies that reduced extremes of income inequality, and a shift of industrial production to a growing market of commoners with newly acquired tastes for products associated with popular notions of "the good life." Thus, in contrast to other narratives of the emergence of social rights and the welfare state, Marshall does not so much cite a chronological litany of articles of social legislation, as he describes in broad strokes Great Britain's profound social evolution. Social legislation is, in Marshall's narrative of the history of the British welfare state, a product of the societal evolution that created it and not per se its foundations. His thesis on the emergence of social rights as an *aspect*, not an *alternative* to full citizenship, is well captured in the following few sentences from his *Citizenship and Social Class*:

Social integration spread from the sphere of sentiment and patriotism into that of material enjoyment. The components of a civilized and cultured life, formally the monopoly of the few, were brought progressively within reach of the many, who were encouraged thereby to stretch out their hands to those that still eluded their grasp. The diminution of inequality strengthened the demand for its abolition, at least with regards to the essentials of social welfare. (p. 28)

It is this drive toward the realization of a right common to all citizens "to live the life of a civilized being according to the standards prevailing in the society" (p. 8) that provided the political foundations for the 1942 Beveridge Report and the social right provisions that later embodied its principles. As previously mentioned, prominent examples of these social right provisions included both the 1945 Family Allowance Bill and the 1948 National Health Service.

Social Citizenship Rights as Requisites to Democratic Citizenship and the Sustainability of Democratic Societies

While there is no doubt that T. H. Marshall's principal contribution to posterity is his theory that the rights and properties of democratic citizenship are manifested in three distinct dimensions (the civil, political, and the social), we would be doing him a disservice if we failed to acknowledge and illuminate his arguments concerning the ways in which certain social citizenship rights are crucial not only to the fulfillment of the civil and political rights of citizenship but also to the substantive meaning of democratic citizenship and to the long-term sustainability to democratic societies. These are the empirical arguments that, when joined with the philosophical arguments of John Rawls, satisfy the main purpose of this chapter.

The easiest connections made between social rights and other rights of democratic citizenship are those between the civil and political rights of democratic citizenship and the right to a public education—upon which Marshall imposes a very high threshold of adequacy. The right to a public education is not fulfilled merely by providing a child the right to go to school "but as the right of the adult citizen to have been educated" (Marshall & Bottomore, 1992, p. 16). In other words, such a right cannot be realized by providing access to a poorly equipped and substandard neighborhood school and a modest chance for a decent education for the most motivated and endowed but a school genuinely capable of producing educated citizens as its common standard of output. Marshall makes the point that civil rights are designed for use by reasonable and intelligent (meaning also educated) persons and that political democracy needs an educated electorate (p. 16). While he offers myriad arguments in support of the ways in which civil and political rights are predicated upon educational rights, Marshall's most concise is the observation that "the right to freedom of speech has little real substance if, from lack of education, you have nothing to say that is worth saying, and no means of making yourself heard if you say it" (p. 21). This same logic applies to the exercise of political rights as well, in that the substantive meaning of voting rights is grounded in the capacity to comprehend the political discourse and discern the electoral choices that reflect one's best interests and personal principles of just governance.

In making the connections between material social rights (such as income security, adequate housing, and health care) and democratic citizenship, Marshall places primary emphasis on the requisites of *full* citizenship status, as opposed to material requisites that are specific to the civil and political dimensions of citizenship. To appreciate the strength of the connections between material social rights and democratic citizenship, it is crucial to return to Marshall's original definition of citizenship, "as a status that is bestowed on those who are full members of a community" (p. 18). To be *full* members of a community, not only are citizens "equal with respect to the rights and duties with which the status is endowed" (p. 18), but they are equal with respect to their status as citizens, meaning that there is no hierarchy of citizenship status that parallels that of social class (p. 6).

While democratic citizenship is not wholly incompatible with a social class structure, Marshall points out that two requisites to this accommodation together provide the basis for material social rights: differences in social class status "can receive the stamp of legitimacy in terms of democratic citizenship provided they do not cut too deep, but occur in a population united in a single civilization; and provided they are not an expression of hereditary class privilege" (p. 44). As discussed previously, in Marshall's empirical analysis of post-seventeenth-century British history, the realization of equality of citizenship status emerged only as class differences in standards of living were ameliorated, initially through economic progress and redistributive taxation, and later through social rights that provided a modicum of material security throughout the life course. In contrast, the minimalist array of social rights that were intended to address only the extremes of poverty and destitution that prevailed until the end of the nineteenth century (referred to previously as the Poor Laws) not only reinforced the harsh prospects for the working class but also burdened the poor with a discounted identity as citizens that was commensurate with their status as dependents—a status that also entailed the surrender of their civil and political rights.

In sum, Marshall's empirical defense of social rights as a distinct feature of democratic citizenship is based on four essential justifications. The first justification, pertaining to the educational domain of social rights, argues that realization of the civil and political rights of citizenship is predicated on an educated citizenry. The second is that citizenship, defined as being afforded the status of full members of the community, is compatible with social inequalities if and only if such social inequalities do not result in extreme differences in the standards of living between the social classes, such that there is no basic standard of civilized living to which all citizens are entitled. The third justification pertains to social integration, the idea that all citizens, irrespective of social class status, share a common bond or, in Marshall's words, "a sense of community membership based on loyalty to a civilization which is a common possession" (p. 24). The fourth justification of social rights is based on the imperative of democratic citizenship that class structure must be reasonably permeable, meaning that citizenship confers equality of opportunity for social mobility and, furthermore, that a social class structure based on inherited privilege is incompatible with the concept of equal social worth. In this vein, Marshall makes the point that democratic governance, in the sense of equal political rights and representation irrespective of social class, was only realized in Britain as entrenched assumptions about intrinsic superiority of the upper-class elites waned in favor of notions of equal basic social worth (p. 22).

Marshall's Statement on the Particular Social Rights
of Democratic Citizenship

While Marshall's *Citizenship and Social Class* devotes some attention to the structural aspects of the educational and social services that comprise the substance of social rights, he does not offer a specific accounting of the particular social welfare entitlements that are essential to the requirements of democratic citizenship. Instead, Marshall speaks to the ends that social rights are to achieve:

What matters is that there is a general enrichment of the concrete substance of civilized life, a general reduction of risk and insecurity, an equalisation between the more and less fortunate at all levels—between the healthy and the sick, the employed and unemployed, the old and the active, the bachelor and the father of a large family. Equalisation is not so much between classes as between individuals within a population which is now treated for this purpose as though it were of one class. (p. 33)

The "one class" that Marshall refers to is persons bestowed with the status of citizen. Embedded in this concise statement are the justifications for such social rights as income subsidies for low-wage workers with dependent children, unemployment insurance, old age income commensurate with an adequate standard of living, and a *universal right to health care.*

JOHN RAWLS ON THE FOUNDATIONAL REQUIREMENTS
OF DEMOCRATIC CITIZENSHIP

Rawls's Theory of Justice in Historical Context

Preceding the 1971 publication of John Rawls's penultimate defense of political liberalism, *A Theory of Justice,* Americans had elected Richard Nixon as their president—in part due to widespread disenchantment with the Great Society programs that had been promulgated under the resurgence of political liberalism throughout the 1960s. While Nixon himself was more of a pragmatist in his domestic social policies than a right-wing ideologue, there is little question that his election represented a repudiation of the liberal notions of an activist federal government that could, through expansion of the public welfare state, eventually eradicate poverty and ameliorate the legacies of African American slavery. It was during the Nixon era that the term *liberal* became not a statement of one's political principles but a derogatory label that inferred naiveté, weakness of moral conviction, and fiscal irresponsibility. While liberalism as a political ideology thrived where it had endorsed programs that benefited the white middle class, liberalism's popularity waned in the late 1960s when social programs based on simplistic applications of liberal principles not only failed to reduce poverty but also became associated with unearned entitlements, nonmarital childbearing, and racially stereotyped welfare dependency (Gilens, 2000). In the early 1970s, as deindustrialization began to make itself felt in the declining wages of the American working class, the economic vitality of the nation's core industrial cities waned, and the cynicism about the effectiveness of the government as an agent of social progress deepened—in an instance of historical irony, political liberalism at last emerged with a coherent defense of its premises and principles in the brilliant treatise of a would-be professional baseball player turned Harvard professor of philosophy, John Rawls (Putnam, 2005).

Although Rawls's theory of justice was not fully developed until he was a middle-aged full professor of philosophy at Harvard, the essence of his philosophy of justice first appeared in the 1957 publication of his "Justice as Fairness" symposium paper in the *Journal of Philosophy*. It was in this seminal paper that the earliest forms of his two principles of justice first appeared—the first pertaining to equal basic liberties and the second to equality of opportunity. While in full development these two principles define the basic criteria for the just distribution of the rights and benefits of society, Rawls framed them within a conception of justice that is predicated on fair and mutually beneficial principles of reciprocity. At the time, this was a radical departure from the then-dominant utilitarian conception of justice in Western moral philosophy that presumes that justice is derived from some optimally efficient design of the social and political institutions charged with the task of distributing the benefits of society (Rawls, 1957). Rawls's conception of justice was later captured in his idea of a just society being, at its essence, "a fair system of cooperation" (Rawls, 2001)—a conception of society that is further illuminated in the next section, which provides the broad strokes of Rawls's theory of justice as it evolved in its final form, shortly before his death in 2002.

The Key Philosophical Premises of Rawls's Theory of Justice

What follows is not a full statement of Rawls's theory of justice but rather a synopsis of the fundamental ideas and premises that are crucial to the ways in which his principles of justice lead to the conclusion that the requirements of democratic citizenship extend to a positive right to health care. We begin with his vision of a just society being "a fair system of cooperation."

Society as a Fair System of Cooperation

While history is replete with examples of the different ways in which human societies form and evolve, Enlightenment political philosophy introduced the idea of voluntary human societies formed on the basis of mutual advantage, equality of status and rights, and reciprocity, which many might recognize as the essence of libertarian (as opposed to liberal) utopia.

Rawls introduced a crucial modification of this vision, the idea of a society formed as "a unified and fair system of cooperation for reciprocal advantage between free and equal persons" (Rawls, 2001, p. 22). What distinguishes Rawls's vision of a just society from the libertarian version is the inclusion of the term *fair*, by which Rawls means that the terms of cooperation are specified in accordance with agreed-upon principles of justice that do not advantage one person or group over others. This then leads us to consider the content of the principles of justice selected to determine the terms of cooperation and the process through which they are agreed upon.

The Original Position

At an earlier point in this chapter, when the epistemologies of Rawls and T. H. Marshall were being contrasted, the essence of Rawls's concept of the original position was described (without being defined as such) in terms of a fundamental question: What principles and rules for governing the basic structure of a given society would arise from the deliberations undertaken by a group of rational actors, charged with the task of representing the interests of persons unknown to them, who are to be free and equal citizens of that society? What is captured in this question is Rawls's illustration of the ideal circumstances of total objectivity and beneficence of intent that would, by logical deliberation among rational actors, lead to two principles of justice he ultimately advances. That is, the rational actors in this thought experiment would be forced to consider the possibility that the constituents they represent, with attributes and circumstances unknown to them, might occupy the least advantaged positions in their imagined society and therefore would be best served by principles of justice that would advance not only equal rights but also *fair* equality of opportunity.

It is this notion of *fair* equality of opportunity (a concept of equal opportunity that accounts for social and economic disadvantage) as opposed to a purely abstract de jure equality of opportunity that most sets Rawls's liberal vision of just governance apart from the more simplistic libertarian version of just governance that emerged from the Enlightenment era essays of John Locke, which later became embodied in the political philosophy of Thomas Jefferson.

The Moral Powers of Free and Equal Citizens

In the very essence of his theory of just democratic governance and citizenship, Rawls viewed such a society as a "fair system of cooperation" just described, predicated on a social contract, whereby citizens as persons free and equal possess two "moral powers." The first moral power concerns what Marshall regarded as the *political* dimension of democratic citizenship, that is, possessing the capacities essential to the pursuit of whatever might be individual conceptualizations of political and social justice. The second moral power entails what Marshall would include in the *civil* dimension of citizenship—the capacity "to have, to revise, and rationally to pursue a conception of the good"—that is, the capacities essential to the imagining and pursuit of whatever might be individual preferences of the good in life or whatever an individual might regard as "a fully worthwhile life" (Rawls, 2001, p. 19).

Primary Goods

Rawls (2001) defines *primary goods* as those "things needed and required by persons seen in the light of the political conception of persons who are fully cooperating members of society, and not merely human beings" (p. 58). That is, primary goods are not merely rights and resources that might be desirable or rational to want, but they are the rights and resources essential to the status and realization of citizenship. Primary goods include not only civil and political rights but also social rights such as the right to an education commiserate with the requirements of political citizenship and the right to health care sufficient to "underwrite fair equality of opportunity" (p. 174). One category of primary goods that is particularly relevant to the convergence of Rawls and Marshall on the social rights of citizenship is the category of primary goods that Rawls refers to as "the social bases of self-respect," by which he means those aspects of basic social institutions essential to persons possessing "a lively sense of their worth as persons and able to advance their ends with self-confidence" (p. 59). In sum, a general way to think about primary goods is that they comprise the rights and resources of society that are the central concern of Rawls's principles of justice.

Rawls's Two Principles of Justice

In Rawls's vision of democratic society as a fair system of cooperation, the basic institutional arrangements of such a society would be guided by two principles of justice, which, to recap, would be those principles of justice that would arise naturally from deliberations undertaken by a group of rational actors, charged with the task of representing the interests of persons unknown to them, who are to be free and equal citizens of that society. In Rawls's final (2001) version of his theory of justice, these two principles are stated as follows (p. 43):

1. Each person has the same indefeasible claim to a fully adequate scheme of equal basic liberties, which scheme is compatible with the same scheme of liberties for all; and
2. Social and economic inequalities are to satisfy two conditions: first, they are to be attached to offices and positions open to all under conditions of fair equality of opportunity; and second, they are to be of the greatest benefit to the least-advantaged members of society.

In illuminating our interpretation of these principles of justice, Rawls emphasizes that the first principle (the so-called equal basic liberties principle) is prior to the second in order of importance and that within his second principle of justice, "fair equality of opportunity" is superior in order of priority to the so-called difference principle—the concern that social and economic inequalities "be of the greatest benefit to the least advantaged."

Although the case can be made that the equal realization of some kinds of liberty rights is to some extent predicated on specific social rights,[13] it is

Rawls's second principle of justice that provides the primary justifications in support of social rights—including the right to health care.

The Bases of Social Citizenship Rights in Rawls's Theory of Justice

In contrast to Marshall, Rawls prefers to address social rights through logical inference, as opposed to delving deeply into the specific social rights that derive from his theory. This makes sense if it is considered that the specific content of social rights must be continually adapted to the requirements of justice as society evolves. Thus, Rawls sees the specific content of social rights as a product of a just society's political and social institutions, negotiated and then renegotiated by citizens in response to the substantive interpretation of the agreed-upon principles of justice under conditions of constant social change (Rawls, 2001, pp. 50–51). That said, Rawls's theory of justice provides a solid foundation for an array of general social rights through three pillars of justification: as they are essential to citizenship status, as they are essential to the capacities to exercise the moral powers of citizenship, and as they are essential to fair equality of opportunity.

Social Rights as Requisite to the Status of Citizen
To begin, all social rights fall within Rawls's definition of primary goods—those things needed and required by persons seen in the light of their status as citizens and "not merely human beings" (Rawls, 2001, p. 58). Thus, such social rights as education, health care, and a modicum of material security commensurate with the requirements of a decent standard of living are not provided on purely humanitarian grounds but because they are essential to the very nature of a citizen being a "fully cooperating member of society" who is not only free but also equal in citizenship status (p. 58). That is, one who is afforded recognition, dignity, and the capacity to participate as a member of society. By this understanding of citizenship (one accorded status as a fully cooperating member of society), a homeless disabled veteran who is denied shelter and medical care because his condition has not been classified as "service connected" has been relegated to a status that is subordinate to that of full citizen—this inconsistency providing the basis for social rights pertaining to a modicum of income security, affordable decent housing, and adequate health care. Not because he is a veteran, but because he is a citizen.

Social Rights as Requisite to the Capacities Essential to the Exercise of the Moral Powers of Citizenship

To recap, Rawls identified two moral powers of citizenship: the first deals with possessing the capacities essential to the pursuit of whatever might be individual conceptualizations of political and social justice, and the second involves the capacities essential to the imagining and pursuit of whatever might be individual preferences of the good in life (Rawls, 2001, pp. 18–19). Also as mentioned previously, the first capacity corresponds to what Marshall refers to as political citizenship, while the second pertains more to the civil dimension of citizenship. Both capacities entail investments in human capital not only through education but also in other requisites of human development such as adequate shelter, nutrition, safety of social environment, and health care. These vital human capital investments fall within what Rawls refers to as "the requisite institutions of background justice"—the structural arrangements that are indispensable to the development of the basic capabilities essential to the exercise of the moral powers of citizenship (Rawls, 2001, pp. 170–171). While a skeptic might quibble and suggest that social rights predicated on the development of basic capabilities are relevant only to special rights to children, the impoverished circumstances of children cannot be separated from that of their parents— unless we are prepared to resurrect orphanages. Similarly, the developmental needs and well-being of children are inextricably bound within the social circumstances of their neighbors and the social conditions prevalent within their neighborhoods. Finally, Rawls also makes it clear that the entitlements (social rights) that are crucial to what he refers to as "basic capabilities" (the capabilities that are essential to the moral powers of citizenship) are relevant over the complete life irrespective of fortune and social position (p. 171).

Social Rights as Requisites to Fair Equality of Opportunity

The most salient case for social rights is their relevance to *fair* equality of opportunity contained in Rawls's second principle of justice, which (to recap) is a conceptualization of equality of opportunity that recognizes and accounts for the burdens and impediments of social and economic disadvantage (Rawls, 2001, p. 43). This requirement of justice, because it makes it incumbent upon governments to ameliorate both the structural disadvantages to equality of opportunity (such as social class) and those that arise from personal misfortune (such as disablement or ill health), provides the foundation for an array of social rights. In educational terms, it suggests that not only should a child from a poor family be provided a basic education commensurate with that required for the exercise of political citizenship but that the child's poverty be of no more relevance to his or her prospects for an eventual education in law or medicine than another child's wealth. In terms of material circumstances, the "fair equality of opportunity" requisite means that differences in the real incomes between families should not be so large as to preclude the ability of any family so motivated to pursue a better life with some genuine prospect for success. Finally, there is the linkage between fair equality of opportunity and access to health care—a connection that provides perhaps the strongest justification for a universal right to health care.

CONVERGENT THEMES IN MARSHALL AND RAWLS ON THE JUSTIFICATION OF CERTAIN SOCIAL RIGHTS, INCLUDING A UNIVERSAL RIGHT TO HEALTH CARE

Despite the omission of any reference to T. H. Marshall's 1950 classic *Citizenship and Social Class* in either John Rawls's *Theory of Justice* (1971) or the final version of his theory of justice published just after his death (*Justice as Fairness: A Restatement*), their ideas on the nature of democratic citizenship and its structural requisites are in many respects overlapping and complementary in important ways. Despite also their two very different epistemologies and historical contexts, the discussion that follows will illuminate the ways in which the theories of these two giants of progressive political thought converge on the justifications for particular social rights— including the universal right to health care. We begin with a synopsis of the convergent themes in the theories of Marshall and Rawls as they pertain to the nature of democratic citizenship and its requisites.

Convergent Themes in the Nature of Democratic Citizenship and Its Requisites

Although there are many areas of agreement on the nature of citizenship in a democratic society and its structural requisites, Marshall and Rawls's theories neither totally converge nor really fall within the same class of social theories. We are reminded that Marshall, the sociologist, was seek-

TABLE 3.1
Convergent Themes in Marshall and Rawls Relevant to the Justification of Social Rights

Convergent theme	T. H. Marshall	John Rawls
Nature of democratic society	Sustainable compromise	Fair system of cooperation
Nature of democratic citizenship	Political citizenship	First moral power of citizens
Nature of democratic citizenship	Civil citizenship	Second moral power of citizens
Requisites to citizenship status	Decent standard of living	Social bases of self-respect
Requisites to exercise of civil citizenship	Capacity for civil citizenship	Capacity for conception of the good
Requisites to exercise of political citizenship	Capacity for political citizenship	Capacity for sense of justice
Requisites to permeable class structure	Social mobility	Fair equality of opportunity
Requisites to collective sense of social equality	Amelioration of social class	The difference principle

Source: Author's compilation.

ing to explain the emergence of the liberal welfare state in Great Britain and justify its necessity as a way to reconcile the contradictions between an entrenched class structure and democratic governance, whereas Rawls, the political philosopher, was seeking to formulate a theoretical justification of the political liberalism that had emerged in the United States in the wake of the 1930s Great Depression. While Rawls characterized the ideal of democratic society as a "fair system of cooperation between persons free and equal," Marshall wrote of a de facto democratic society seeking to sustain political stability and social progress in the face of endemic economic inequality and class conflict. Although a comprehensive synthesis of Marshall's *Citizenship and Social Class* and Rawls's *A Theory of Justice* that would consider all the implications for democratic political philosophy and its derivatives in social rights might encompass volumes, the purpose here is limited to an abbreviated accounting of the main domains of convergence that are particularly relevant to the justification of social rights, as shown in table 3.1. As this discussion proceeds, each of these convergent themes will be briefly illuminated, along with the justifications for social rights that follow.

The Nature of Democratic Society

Both Marshall and Rawls envision democratic society as an egalitarian liberal democracy—that is, a form of democratic governance that fuses together the principles of constitutional democracy, free-market economics, and egalitarian social philosophy. Marshall, the sociologist and historical empiricist, viewed the egalitarian liberal democracy and its attendant social rights as representing an evolvement of civil society that by the twentieth century had stumbled upon a workable and stable compromise between the principles of laissez-faire capitalism and egalitarian notions of social class. Notably, Marshall does not credit the brilliance of Western political philosophers for discovery of this stable compromise but views the emergence of the egalitarian democratic state as a reflection of evolutionary collective social behavior that is not dictated by logic but by simple functional necessity and adaptive compromise (Marshall & Bottomore, 1992, pp. 48–49). Rawls's vision of democratic society as a "fair system of cooperation" also represents a compromise between free-market capitalism and egalitarian social philosophy—but one justified instead on the basis of formal moral theory (Rawls, 1957, 1971, 2001). Despite their differing epistemologies and rules of evidence for their arguments, both Marshall and Rawls converge on a view of democratic society as one that includes social rights as the means crucial to reconciling the contradictions between capitalism, genuine equality of opportunity, and extremes of social inequality that would endanger political democracy.

The Nature of Democratic Citizenship
The essence of both of Marshall's first two dimensions of citizenship, civil citizenship and political citizenship, is encompassed within Rawls's two moral powers of citizens, although Rawls places the political dimension of citizenship in advance of the civil one. Recall that Marshall describes the political dimension of citizenship as involving "the right to participate in the exercise of political power" (Marshall & Bottomore, 1992, p. 10), whereas Rawls defines the first moral power of citizens as "the capacity to understand, to apply, and act from (and not merely in accordance with) the principles of political justice that specify the fair terms of social cooperation" (Rawls, 2001, pp. 18–19). Importantly, Rawls's use of the term *capacity* is applied to both comprehension and action, the latter of which clearly entails the right to participate in the exercise of political power, which in democratic society entails voting rights and the right to hold elected offices. The civil dimension of citizenship, which Marshall defines as encompassing both liberty rights (freedom of speech, to own property, to work at one's chosen occupation) and the right to seek justice, resides within Rawls's second moral power of citizens.

Rawls defines this second moral power as the "the capacity to have, revise, and rationally pursue a conception of the good" or "what is regarded as a fully worthwhile life" (p. 19). While the right to seek justice is not explicitly identified in Rawls's second moral power, it is implied in the meaning of possessing the capacity to have and pursue one's conception of the good.

Social Rights as Requisites to Citizenship Status

Both Marshall and Rawls employ a conceptualization of citizenship status that goes well beyond simply qualifying for certain rights and protections, and incurring certain obligations. To both Marshall and Rawls, to be bestowed with the status of citizen means that one has claim to a certain modicum of individual dignity and respect that goes with being regarded a "full member" of the community or society that confers that status (Marshall & Bottomore, 1992, p. 18). Deep poverty, or being enmired in a state of existence that is inconsistent with the prevailing norms of adequate material circumstances, is inconsistent with the qualities of dignity, equal social worth, and full membership of community with which the status of citizen is imbued—or, as Marshall, puts it "the stuff of which the status is made" (p. 18). Thus, it is that Marshall arrives at his central thesis, that social inequalities and the status differences they represent are only legitimate with respect to democratic citizenship status to the extent they "do not cut too deep, but occur within a population united in a single civilization" (p. 44). By any reasonable interpretation, this suggests that citizenship status is predicated upon a decent standard of living within the prevailing norms of a given democratic society.

Rawls brings us to this same conclusion but through a different path—in essence, by including among his categories of primary goods (those rights and resources essential to the status and realization of citizenship) "*the social bases of self-respect*, understood as those aspects of basic institutions normally essential if citizens are to have a lively sense of their worth as persons and to be able to advance their ends with self-confidence" (Rawls, 2001, p. 59). By basic institutions, Rawls is referring to the social institutions through which human development and well-being are advanced, which includes not only the education system but also other kinds of social institutions designed to advance human development and well-being, including those that function to ensure a minimum standard of material existence commensurate with the status and requirements of citizenship (p. 57).

Social Rights as Requisites to the Exercise of Civil and Political Citizenship

Both Marshall and Rawls make a clear distinction between the de jure conceptualization of the rights and liberties of citizenship and the more demanding de facto conceptualization of the rights and liberties of citizenship—the latter requiring possession of the *capacities* essential to the realization of rights and liberties. Marshall, for his part, succinctly illustrates this distinction when he points out (in an excerpt also cited previously) "[that] the right to freedom of speech has little substance if, from lack of education, you have nothing to say that is worth saying, and no means of making yourself heard if you say it" (Marshall & Bottomore, 1992, p. 21). Although Marshall makes this point in reference to a civil right, the phrase "making yourself heard" implies also the political dimension of citizenship. Despite Amartya Sen's critique that Rawls's theory is primarily concerned with the *means* necessary to act as persons "free and equal" in the pursuit of their individual conceptualizations of the good, rather than development of the *capacities* (or human capabilities) to do so (Sen, 2009), it is crucial to point out that when Rawls speaks specifically to the ability to exercise the two moral powers of citizenship, he speaks also to the social rights that are crucial to the development of *capacities* (Rawls, 2001, pp. 170–176).

Specific Social Rights

It must be acknowledged that, outside of education, neither Marshall nor Rawls devotes great attention to illuminating what by logical inference are the myriad connections between *specific social rights* and the *specific capacities* that are essential to the civil and political dimensions of citizenship. In Rawls's case, he makes it clear enough that such critical connections exist in his discussions of the basic structure of a just society and social institutions that provide the means essential to the development and realization of the moral powers of citizens (Rawls, 1971, p. 304; Rawls, 2001, pp. 56–57). As to Marshall, while he prefers to make his primary case for social rights outside of education on the basis of citizenship status as opposed to specific capacities (Marshall & Bottomore, 1992, p. 33), he does extend this reasoning to capacities that are essential to the realization of political rights, citing the particular example of the capacity among the working class to question the political privilege of elites (p. 22).

Social Rights as Requisite to a Permeable Class Structure

Social mobility, broadly defined as the movement of individuals or groups from one socioeconomic position to another (Giddens, 2009), is intrinsic to assumptions of individual and political equality, going back to Enlightenment philosopher John Locke. In contrast, societies with a rigid class structure are predicated on the conviction that social class differences reflect real differences in the natural endowments and predilections of individuals occupying their different positions in the social hierarchy. While societies with a rigid class structure can imitate popular democracy through such provisions of universal voting rights, to the extent that class structure is impermeable, the real mechanisms of political power reside with the elites who are presumed to be "born to rule." As noted by Marshall, such was the case in nineteenth-century Great Britain prior to the amelioration of class differences in standards of living and literacy, which over time eroded the obstacles of social class to the more full realization of citizenship status and political power (Marshall & Bottomore, 1992). Thus, the achievement and sustainment of political democracy require the social rights essential to a permeable class structure or, as Marshall puts it, those social right requisites to social mobility and "the elimination of inherited privilege" as the primary basis of social inequalities (p. 39).

Marshall establishes the case for the relationship between social citizenship rights and social mobility entirely on the right to an education commensurate with ability as opposed to class privilege. This is valid, of course, but low-hanging fruit. While it is unfortunate that Marshall's essay did not go further to illuminate the relationship between other kinds of social rights and social mobility (such as material security in childhood and health care), Rawls corrects this oversight by making not only education but also health care requisite to *fair equality of opportunity*, which in the end is sine qua non to social mobility (Rawls, 2001, p. 174).

Social Rights as Requisite to a Collective Sense of Social Equality

The final convergent theme relevant to the justification of social rights to be considered is that of social equality, or citizens possessing a shared sense of equal social worth despite whatever differences may exist in material wealth or social position. Distinct from equality in citizenship status, which as discussed previously requires a social minimum commensurate with the prevailing norm for a "decent standard of living," sustaining a collective sense of equal social worth requires that social class distinctions be minimized, both in their substantive differences and in their bases of legitimacy. Marshall refers to this imperative as the amelioration of social class differences, which in the case of twentieth-century Great Britain was accomplished by redistributive taxation and certain essential social rights that advanced a sense of "the fundamental equality of all citizens and not the inequalities of earnings or occupational grade" (Marshall & Bottomore, 1992, pp. 7, 48). For Rawls, the justifications of redistributive taxation and social rights that are tied to the minimization of social class reside primarily in his second principle of justice, the so-called difference principle, which limits the circumstances under which social and economic inequalities are accepted as just. To recap, Rawls's "difference principle" reads as follows (Rawls, 2001, p. 42): "Social and economic inequalities are to satisfy two conditions: first, they are to be attached to offices and positions under conditions of fair equality of opportunity; and second, they are to be to the greatest benefit to the least-advantaged members of society (the difference principle)."

In sum, despite their different epistemological justifications, both Marshall and Rawls converge on their conviction that the collective sense of social equality that is essential to the nature of a democratic society can only be reconciled with social and economic inequalities to the extent that they are both modest and malleable. In institutional terms, this means that the inequalities in material circumstances and basic security that are produced as an inevitable feature of the market economy must be continuously offset by transfers from the more to the less advantaged. Empirically, while the precise structure of these transfers varies considerably from one democracy to another, for the most egalitarian democracies, they always entail an extensive array of social rights (Esping-Andersen, 1990; Garfinkel et al., 2010).

TOWARD A SYNTHESIS OF MARSHALL AND RAWLS ON UNIVERSAL HEALTH CARE AS REQUISITE TO DEMOCRATIC CITIZENSHIP

At this point, this chapter has now accomplished its primary task, which is to show why, from the standpoint of progressive democratic political philosophy, some kinds of social rights (defined broadly as economic security provisions and human capital investments that are granted to all citizens) are essential both to the moral powers of democratic citizenship and to a permeable class structure—the latter necessary to the reconciliation of democracy with capitalism. We now turn to the special case of health care as a universal right of citizenship, which attends to the central purpose of this book as a whole.

As discussed previously, there are many rationales for universal health care that range from faith-based and secular humanism to global economic competitiveness. However convincing each of these justifications may be, they do little to directly rebut the libertarian contention that health care as a social right of citizenship is inconsistent with the democratic citizenship envisioned by the authors of the Constitution, which is predicated on the idea of full self-ownership and limited government (Boaz, 1997).[14] This rebuttal is left to the more nuanced understanding of the requisites of democratic citizenship and democratic society provided by the preceding synthesis of T. H. Marshall and John Rawls on the nature and requisites of democratic citizenship and democratic society. Within this fusion of Marshall and Rawls, at least four areas of convergence provide a clear justification for health care as a universal right of citizenship.

The first of these is *citizenship status*, which incorporates Marshall's argument that being accorded equal citizenship status has a substantive component in basic material well-being and protection from risk (both subsumed under the notion of a "decent standard of living" commensurate with the requisites of a unified civilization) and Rawls's argument that free and equal citizenship means one is accorded the means necessary to "the social basis of self-respect." To the extent that any citizen is denied essential health care on the basis of any number of extraneous factors (e.g., age, income, employment opportunities, state or county of residence), that person's status as a citizen free and equal is impugned.

The second area of convergence relevant specifically to health care as a social right is where access to essential health care becomes requisite to the *moral powers of citizenship*, particularly *political citizenship*. Both Marshall and Rawls illuminate the distinction between the de jure and de facto possession of political citizenship, the latter of which requires not just status but intellectual capacities essential to reason and action. According to both Marshall and Rawls, the development of such intellectual capacities provides, for one, the justification for basic education as a social right of citizenship. Based on this same foundation, the case that is made for basic education as a social right of political citizenship can also be extended to health care. To cite just one illustrative example, it should be amply evident that recovery of the cognitive capacities essential to the exercise of political citizenship following a cerebrovascular accident (or stroke) is greatly influenced by both the availability and quality of rehabilitative health care. Yet, within the United States, where health care is not yet a social right of citizenship, the availability and quality of rehabilitative health care following a stroke (and ergo equal protection of political citizenship capacities) are greatly determined by such factors as race, ethnicity, age, gender, and income (Freburger et al., 2011).

The third area of convergence relevant to health care as a social right is the role of health care as an important requisite to sustaining a permeable class structure, which in turn is essential to the reconciliation of political democracy and capitalism (Marshall & Bottomore, 1992). As noted previously, while Marshall does not refer specifically to health care as a social right essential to social mobility, he complements Rawls by providing the empirical case for social rights in general as requisite to a permeable class structure. Rawls, for his part, makes the specific case for health care as requisite to a permeable class structure through reference to the fair equality of opportunity clause in his second principle of justice. Fair equality of opportunity is of course sine qua non to social mobility as an imperative feature of democratic societies. To cite Rawls specifically on this crucial point: "Medical care, as with primary goods generally, is to meet the needs and requirements of citizens as free and equal. Such care falls under the means necessary to underwrite fair equality of opportunity and our capacity to take advantage of our basic rights and liberties, and thus be normal and fully cooperating members of society over a complete life" (Rawls, 2001, p. 174).

The fourth and final area of convergence relevant to the justification of health care as a social right concerns health care's contribution to a collective sense of social equality. To recap, both Marshall and Rawls converge on the finding, through their different epistemologies, that democracy is compatible with social and economic inequalities only to the extent that such inequalities are modest and malleable. Fixed and more extreme social and economic inequalities erode the shared conviction among all strata of society that the least and most advantaged of society share, as Marshall puts it, "a kind of basic human equality, associated with full community membership" (Marshall & Bottomore, 1992, p. 45). In this sense, then, health care as a privilege afforded to the fortunate and advantaged undermines a collective sense of basic social equality, whereas health care as a social right of citizenship underscores the shared conviction that at some very basic level, all members of society possess equal value. While this argument converges on humanistic justifications for health care as a social right, it should be emphasized that its roots reside in the theories of democracy and democratic citizenship advanced by Marshall and Rawls.

CONCLUDING REMARKS: FOUR PRINCIPLES ON THE SUBSTANTIVE FOUNDATIONS OF A SOCIAL RIGHT TO HEALTH CARE

By one definition of a social right to health care, wherein it refers to a general entitlement to health care for acute illnesses and injuries, this policy milestone was actually reached nearly three decades ago during the presidency of Ronald Reagan with the passage of the 1986 Emergency Medical Treatment and Labor Act (EMTALA). EMTALA requires that hospitals with emergency departments provide a medical screening examination and any necessary urgent care to any and all individuals upon request, regardless of ability to pay. While few would agree that the EMTALA mandate constitutes what is commonly meant by a social right to health care, it represents one end of a continuum that ranges from a very minimalist right to health care to the realization of a utopian social right to health care that is fully comprehensive with respect to any and all health-care needs and also wholly devoid of disparities in either accessibility or quality. This book is not about the requisites of a health-care utopia but the substantive foundations of a social right to health care as defined by the core requirements of democratic citizenship and the sustainability of political democracy.

As per the preceding synthesis of Marshall and Rawls, these core requirements pertain to citizenship status, the exercise of political citizenship, the realization of fair equality of opportunity (also conceptualized as a permeable class structure), and the achievement and preservation of a collective sense of social equality. Also, as per the earlier discussion on the conceptualization of a social right to health care (under the Defining Health and Health Care section), the substantive foundations to the social right to health care include the disease- and disability-specific responses and claims to health affecting goods and services that are essential to the realization and preservation of normal human functioning in the context of a modern political democracy. I now bring these ideas together in four principles that guide this book's analysis of not only the ACA but also future stages and the ends to be realized in the nation's progression toward a social right to health care commensurate with the requirements of democracy.

• *Principle I: The substantive requirements of a social right to health care as justified by the nature of citizenship status.* Citizenship status has two substantive components, one pertaining to material security and the other to status equality. With respect to material security, an adequately realized health-care right must provide economic protections from the financial burdens of illness and health-care needs that are crucial for the optimal realization of the normal range of human functioning (Daniels, 2008). With respect to equality of status, to the extent that citizens encounter substantial disparities in either health-care quality or access on the basis of any number of extraneous factors (such as age, income, employment opportunities, state or county of residence), their status as free and equal citizens is compromised.

• *Principle II: The substantive requirements of a social right to health care as justified by the capacities essential to the exercise of political citizenship.* Political citizenship entails both particular rights (such as the right to vote or hold political office) and particular capacities (such as the capacity to discern what is in one's best interest, the ability to communicate a point of view). The substantive foundations of a social right to health care, as pertaining to the exercise of political citizenship, are concerned with the disease- and disability-specific responses and claims to health affecting goods and services that are necessary to the development and preservation of capacities that are essential to the exercise of political citizenship. These essential capacities encompass the normal range of human functioning in cognition (thought, comprehension, learning, and memory), interpretive and expressive communication, and, to some extent, the physical ability to both access public spaces and endure the rigors of engaging in political activism and holding public office.

• *Principle III: The substantive requirements of a social right to health care as justified by the realization of fair equality of opportunity and the sustainment of a permeable class structure.* To the extent that persons or particular groups are encumbered by a disproportionate share of disease, injury, and disability, their share of the normal opportunity range for the resources and benefits of society (fair equality of opportunity) is similarly encumbered (Daniels, 2008). The substantive foundations of a social right to health care, as pertaining to the realization of fair equality of opportunity, require that distribution of the disease- and disability-specific responses and claims to health affecting goods and services are commensurate with equal shares of the normal opportunity range. By extension, this same principle applies to the substantive foundations of a social right to health care essential to the realization of social mobility for individuals and groups, which requires fair equality of opportunity.

• *Principle IV: The substantive requirements of a social right to health care as justified by the realization of a collective sense of social equality.* To the extent that either health-care access or quality is experienced or viewed as a privilege afforded to the fortunate and advantaged, the collective sense of basic social equality is undermined. Conversely, to the extent that equity health-care access and quality are promoted as a social right of citizenship, so is the shared conviction that at some very basic level, all members of society possess equal value. Disparities in the distribution of the disease- and disability-specific responses and claims to health affecting goods, other than those that are intended to offset disadvantages in the burden of disease, injury, and disability borne by individuals and groups, are inconsistent with the substantive foundations of a social right to health care.

Chapter Four

A PRINCIPLED CRITIQUE OF THE ACA AND THE ACA IN AN EVOLUTIONARY PERSPECTIVE

In his landmark *Just Health: Meeting Health Needs Fairly* (2008), health-care policy ethicist Norman Daniels suggests that the health needs commensurate with adequate protection of fair equality of opportunity might be met under a range of institutional structures, with no theoretically implied preferences for either private or public approaches to health systems financing and administration (p. 144). Instead, consistent with the conceptualization of particular health-care reforms as social experiments, he proposes a framework for the evidence-based appraisal of health system reforms based on what he identifies as "Benchmarks of Fairness" that reflect the central concerns of justice as fairness: equity, efficiency, and accountability (pp. 245–254). In reduced form, this is the approach to the principled analysis of the ACA undertaken in this chapter, modified to address the concerns of four principles on the substantive foundation to a social right to health care set forth at the conclusion of chapter 3. In doing so, I also make use of several of Daniels's ideas as developed in *Just Health*, specifically the relationship between normal human (species) functioning and the normal opportunity range, as well as health needs (as opposed to demands or preferences).

However, there are four important ways in which the ideas advanced in this book contrast with Daniels's foundational work in *Just Health*. First, the ideas advanced in this book are concerned with a social right to health *care* as opposed to health, which, while overlapping in important respects, leads to a far more limited analysis. Second, this book provides a particular focus on the ACA as an evolutionary stage in policy progression toward a substantively robust social right to health care, whereas Daniels was concerned with the development of an ethical framework that might be applied to a range of social policies and institutional arrangements relevant to the just distribution of resources essential to health. Third, the analytic framework applied to the ACA is based on the contrast between specific provisions of the ACA and the policy aims that are consistent with the substantive foundations of a social right to health care, as opposed to the set of generally applicable benchmarks advanced by Daniels. Fourth, Daniels's analysis was based on an extension of Rawls's theory of justice as fairness, whereas the theoretical basis of this book's analysis is a synthesis of Rawls's theory of justice and Marshall's theory of the substantive requisites of democratic citizenship.

These differences aside, this book is in general agreement with Daniels on the essentials of a social right to health care, such as would be derived from Rawls's theory of justice as fairness and complemented by T. H. Marshall's theory of the requisites of democratic citizenship and political democracy. This book's synthesis of the theories of Rawls, Daniels, and Marshall on a social right to health care is stated as follows: *A social right to health care is defined as universal comprehensive health insurance coverage, with adequate and equal risk protection, for those health-care needs that are essential to the optimal realization and preservation of the normal range of functioning, and fair equality of opportunity.*

A PRINCIPLED ANALYSIS OF THE ACA

The analytical framework shown in table 4.1 represents the progression from the justifications to a social right to health care advanced at the conclusion of chapter 3 to four core health-care policy aims relevant to fulfilling the substantive requirements intrinsic to each justification.

Before delving into each justification to a social right to health care shown in table 4.1, along with their substantive requirements and the core health-care policy aims that are implied, some key concepts embedded in the table's content require some illumination. These key concepts include the idea of a fair distribution, equity, health needs, functional requisites, and compensatory entitlements.

TABLE 4.1
A Framework for the Principled Analysis of the ACA

Justifications to a social right to health care	Substantive requirement	Core health-care policy aims
As essential to citizenship status	Economic protections from the financial burdens of illness and health-care needs	1. Universal comprehensive health insurance with adequate and equal risk protection
	Equity in health-care access and quality	2. Amelioration of disparities in health-care access and quality
As essential to the exercise of political citizenship	Fair distribution of disease- and disability-specific health-care services, technologies, and public health investments necessary for the promotion and protection of the functional requisites essential to the exercise of political citizenship	3. Equitable distribution of: (a) preventative, curative, rehabilitative, and adaptive health-care services/technologies specific to health needs (b) public health investments and interventions 4. Compensatory entitlements and investments in health-care services and public health infrastructure/ interventions for individuals, groups, and populations adversely affected by health disparities
As essential to fair equality of opportunity	Fair distribution of disease- and disability-specific health-care services, technologies, and public health investments necessary for the promotion and protection of the functional requisites essential to the exercise of political citizenship	3. Equitable distribution of: (a) preventative, curative, rehabilitative, and adaptive health-care services/technologies specific to health needs (b) public health investments and interventions 4. Compensatory entitlements and investments in health-care services and public health infrastructure/ interventions for individuals, groups, and populations adversely affected by health disparities
As essential to a collective sense of social equality	Equity in health-care access and quality	2. Amelioration of disparities in health-care access and quality

Source: Author's compilation.

The Fair Distribution of Health-Care Resources, Equity, and Compensatory Entitlements

As applied here, the idea of fairness entails two requirements. The first pertains to equity, meaning that persons, groups, and populations that are equal with respect to health needs possess an equal entitlement to the health-care resources that are specific to those needs. The second pertains to *compensatory entitlements*, which acknowledge that some individuals, groups, and populations carry a disproportionate burden of disease and disability as a reflection and "embodiment" of their disadvantaged position in society (Krieger, 2002; Link & Phelan, 1996).[1] While the origins of such health disparities may lie outside of the health-care system (as in poverty, racial segregation, historical trauma), to the extent that they can be mitigated by targeted compensatory health-care entitlements (such as intensive diabetes prevention and treatment programs on tribal reservations with a disproportionate prevalence of diabetes), such compensatory entitlements are justified by functional requisites of (1) the exercise of political citizenship and (2) fair equality of opportunity.

Functional Requisites and Health-Care Needs

As argued by Rawls (2001, pp. 174–175) and elaborated upon in Daniels (2008, pp. 29–31), the moral importance of a social right to health care (as part and parcel of the resources essential to meeting health needs) is based on health's place as a crucial determinant of the capacities essential to fair equality of opportunity. That is, fair equality of opportunity (as equally unencumbered access to a democratic society's normal opportunity range) has functional requisites, such as the normal range of abilities in cognition and in interpretive and expressive communication. Rather than delineating an exhaustive list of the specific functional requisites to either fair equality of opportunity or (by logical extension) the exercise of political citizenship, it is accepted that Daniels (2008, p. 30) is correct in his argument that the normal range of opportunity is predicated on the resources essential to the protection of the "normal range of human functioning." This argument is also extended to the conceptualization of "health needs," which Daniels (2008) defines as "those things we need in order to maintain, restore, or provide the functional equivalents (where possible) to normal species functioning" (p. 42). Health-care needs are (by extension) those services, technologies, and public health investments and measures that we (in the individual and collective sense) need to maintain, restore, or provide for the functional requisites essential to both fair equality of opportunity and the exercise of political citizenship. It is also worth noting that there is a clear and crucial distinction between health care that falls under the rubric of health needs and health care that is delivered or demanded based on other considerations. Health services and public health provisions that fall within the special class of health needs are those evaluated as essential to the functional requisites to fair equality of opportunity and political citizenship and thus have a particular "urgency" or moral importance that justifies their inclusion in a social right to health care (Daniels, 2008, p. 42; Rawls, 2001, pp. 174–175), whereas health care that is based on other considerations (such as socially constructed versions of optimal health, happiness, or physical attractiveness) is treated as a commodity that falls outside of the substantive requisites of a social right to health care.

With these key concepts in mind, we now consider each justification to a social right to health care shown in table 4.1, along with their substantive requirements and related core health-care policy aims.

The Core Health-Care Policy Aims Derived from Citizenship Status

As stated in principle I (and elaborated on in chapter 3), citizenship status has two substantive components, one pertaining to material security and the other to status equality. Specific to core health-care policy aim 1, to the extent that individuals possessing citizenship status are placed at risk for financially catastrophic health-care expenditures, the aspect of citizenship status pertaining to a basic modicum of material security is jeopardized. Second, to the extent that there are significant disparities in the economic protections against the financial burdens of illness and health-care needs, equity in citizenship status is undermined. Considered together, these two risks to the full realization of citizenship status create the necessity of adequate and comprehensive health insurance coverage as a social right of citizenship. As used here, the term *adequate* refers to a level of risk protection essential to financial security, meaning that the costs associated with health care are not a threat or impediment to the realization of a decent standard of living commensurate within the prevailing social norms.

The term *comprehensive* pertains to the necessity of a broad scope of coverage that is inclusive of all health conditions, health-care needs, and related health-care services and technologies.

Specific to core health-care policy aim 2 (as elaborated upon in chapter 3), in democratic societies, equality of citizenship status is intrinsic to the meaning of citizenship status. It therefore follows that to the extent citizens possessing a common social right to health care encounter substantial disparities in either health-care quality or access on the basis of any number of attributes and circumstances (e.g., age, race, income, employment opportunities, state or county of residence), their de facto status as free and equal citizens is compromised. While the origins of disparities in health-care access and quality often arise from structural disadvantages that lie outside of the organization of the health-care system, health-care financing and delivery systems can be organized in ways that mitigate, replicate, or exacerbate the effects of a wide range of structural disadvantages to health-care access and quality. Thus, the amelioration of disparities in health-care access and quality must be a core health-care policy aim.

The Core Health Policy Aims Derived from the Exercise of Political Citizenship

As discussed in chapter 3, political citizenship pertains to those rights essential to the exercise of one's political power (voting rights, the right to hold elective offices) and, as stated by Rawls, "the capacity to understand, to apply and to act from (not merely in accordance with) the principles of political justice that specify the fair terms of social cooperation" (Rawls, 2001, pp. 18–19). Specific to core health-care policy aim 3, the substantive foundations of a social right to health care, as pertaining to the exercise of political citizenship, are concerned with the *fair distribution* of disease- and disability-specific responses and health affecting services, technologies, and public health investments that are necessary to the development and preservation of capacities that are essential to the exercise of political citizenship. These essential capacities encompass the "normal range of human functioning" in cognition (thought, comprehension, learning, and memory), interpretive and expressive communication, and, to some extent, the physical ability to both access public spaces and endure the rigors of engaging in political activism and holding public office (Daniels, 2008). By *fair distribution*, two things are being said. The first is that disease and disability responses and the broad range of public health investments and measures are a finite resource and therefore subject to principles of distributive justice. The second is that the particular principles of distributive justice are those advanced by John Rawls in accordance with his theory of justice as fairness. That is, since health-care needs are defined as essential to the functional requisites of political citizenship, all citizens have equal standing with respect to claims to the resources encompassed within health-care needs. Put another way, like needs for medical care between citizens who are regarded as free and equal are provided under principles of equity—equal shares of finite medical care resources for equal needs (Rawls, 2001, pp. 175–176). Thus, core health-care policy aim 3 speaks to "the equitable distribution of a) the preventative, curative, rehabilitative, and adaptive health care services/technologies specific to health needs and b) public health investments and measures."[2]

Consistent with Rawls's conceptualization of justice as fairness, core health-care policy aim 4 holds that departures from a simple principle of equity are justified when it is necessary to counter the effects of extreme structural disadvantages on health. To cite one example among many, the profound health effects of decades of racial segregation and concentrated poverty cannot wholly be countered or quickly reversed by the sudden realization of equity in comprehensive health insurance coverage and the quality of health services. To the extent that extremes in the burdens of disease carried by a group or community reflect extremes in structural disadvantage, the compensatory health-care entitlements and public health investments that contribute to the normal functioning capacities essential to political citizenship are not only justified but also imperative. In this respect, core health-care policy aim 4 is akin to the explicit goal of the (now permanently reauthorized) Indian Health Care Improvement Act to elevate the health status of American Indians and Alaska Natives to parity with the U.S. population as a whole, with special entitlements and investments inclusive of cancer care, diabetes prevention and treatment, and higher subsidies for the purchase of health insurance (Perry & Foster, 2010). The distinction is that while the special entitlements and public health investments of the Indian Health Improvement Act are based on the fulfillment of treaty rights to health care for indigenous peoples, under core health-care policy aim 4, they would also be justified under the more general and inclusive functional requisites of political citizenship.

The Core Health-Care Policy Aims Derived from
Fair Equality of Opportunity

As shown in table 4.1 (middle column), the functional requisites to fair
equality of opportunity are assumed to be identical to those essential to the
exercise of political citizenship; hence, policy aims 3 and 4 apply to fair
equality of opportunity just as they do for political citizenship. It is considered self-evident, for example, that the intellectual and communicative capacities essential to political activism and the holding of political office
would also be essential to the realization of fair equality of opportunity in
the labor market. While it is conceivable that functional requisites to fair
equality of opportunity might be distinct from those essential to political
citizenship, it seems that both would be impeded by any significant departure from the normal range of capacities.

The Core Health-Care Policy Aims Derived from a
Collective Sense of Social Equality

Another compelling justification of core health-care policy aim 2 (the amelioration of disparities in health-care access and quality) is based on the
crucial importance of a collective and inclusive conviction of genuine
social equality as an aspect of full democratic citizenship, defined in chapter 3 as citizens possessing a shared sense of equal social worth despite
whatever differences may exist in material wealth or social position. As
argued by Marshall, the essence of democratic citizenship is predicated
upon "a kind of basic human equality, associated with full community
membership" (Marshall & Bottomore, 1992, p. 45). The relevance of core
health-care policy aim 2 to a shared sense of equal worth is that an inclusive sense of equal worth is undermined to the extent that American society
is rife with significant disparities in health-care access and health-care
quality.

As an analogy, the social norms that govern social behavior in the typical emergency department waiting room are based on the expectation that
patients will tolerate long waits for care as long as (1) they are being
accorded the consideration they have a right to expect as patients in need
of care and (2) they will be attended to in accordance with the seriousness
and immediacy of their medical problem. For the most part, this social
convention of equity of patient status but differential response by medical

urgency works—even seriously ill patients can be incredibly tolerant of delayed care as long as they believe they are being accorded due respect and fair consideration commensurate with their "patient in need of care status" and the relative urgency of their medical problem. In the social order of the typical hospital emergency department, there is a kind of collective acceptance of prolonged personal suffering and inconvenience predicated on communitarian notions of basic equality and the common good that enables emergency medical care to function, which in remarkable respects mirrors the foundations of democratic society.

ANALYSIS OF THE ACA AND THE FOUR CORE HEALTH POLICY AIMS

Core Health-Care Policy Aim 1: Universal Comprehensive Health Insurance with Adequate and Equal Risk Protection

Analysis of this core health-care policy aim first requires that the requisites of citizenship status be formally defined. Rather than adopt the very narrow standard of legal citizenship status by either birth or naturalization, a theoretical definition of citizenship will be used in accordance with a synthesis of Marshall's and Rawls's ideas on the basic meaning of the construct. Marshall (in Marshall & Bottomore, 1992, p. 18) defines citizenship as "a status bestowed on those who are full members of a community," with the added caveat that "all who possess the status are equal with respect to the rights and duties with which the status is endowed." Rawls's conceptualization of citizenship is essentially the equivalent, in that he speaks of citizens as being "free and equal persons," as "fully cooperating members of society," and (in his first principle of justice) as having the "same indefeasible claim to a fully adequate scheme of equal basic liberties" (Rawls, 2001, pp. 8, 42).[3] This theoretical construction of citizenship would encompass those in the United States accorded legal citizenship by right of birth or naturalization as well as those accorded status as permanent U.S. residents. However, the citizenship criteria of "free and equal" and "equal with respect to rights and duties" would exclude undocumented workers and their dependents, despite their myriad and indispensable contributions to the national economy and the fiscal sustainability of such entitlement programs as Social Security and Medicare. This injustice, embedded as it is in the definitional paradox of citizenship and the particular health-care policy considerations that should apply to undocumented workers and their dependents, will be taken up in the book's final chapter.

With this broad definition of citizenship in mind, we begin by comparing the nation's population of uninsured with a presumptive right to health care, as it is has been estimated to be in 2019 in the absence of the ACA, with the population of uninsured under the assumption that the ACA is fully implemented as originally passed by Congress and signed into law by President Obama. These estimates are based on an analysis of the ACA's health insurance coverage effects prepared by the CMS in early 2010 and the Census Bureau's 2012 Population Projections for the years 2015 through 2060. In absence of the ACA, CMS estimates suggest that the uninsured population with a presumptive social right to health care would rise to 52 million by 2019 (calculated as 57 million uninsured less 5 million undocumented uninsured), or about or 17.5 percent of the national population of citizens and legal residents (CMS, 2010; U.S. Census Bureau, 2013). Under the assumption that the ACA is fully implemented as intended by Congress, CMS estimates suggest that by 2019, the uninsured population with a presumptive social right to health care would fall to 18 million or 5.5 percent of the national population of citizens and legal residents (CMS, 2010; U.S. Census Bureau, 2013). Put another way, were the ACA to be fully implemented as legislated, by 2019, about 95 percent of the nation's population of citizens and legal residents would be covered by either public or private health insurance (including publicly subsidized private health insurance). While this would be a very encouraging development, the United States would still remain among the bottom four of thirty-four modern democracies in the proportion of the population covered by either public or private health insurance (OECD, 2013b).

However, it is very clear that the ACA will fall well short of its policy aims at full implementation due in large part to two factors. The first is the U.S. Supreme Court ruling in 2012 that held that the ACA's provisions that would coerce states into expanding Medicaid coverage to previously ineligible uninsured persons were unconstitutional, thus leaving the individual states to decide whether to accept the ACA's fully subsidized expansions of Medicaid enrollment.[4] The second factor, related to the first, is deep-seated ideological and partisan resistance against the ACA's expansion of the American welfare state. Thus, by 2014, only half of the nation's fifty states had chosen to expand Medicaid coverage to millions of the uninsured who would otherwise have been eligible, despite the ACA's provisions that the costs of Medicaid expansion would be fully subsidized by federal funds. As estimated by the Henry J. Kaiser Family Foundation, this leaves 7.6 million uninsured adults who would have been eligible for Medicaid coverage under the ACA without insurance, largely because the most politically conservative and oppositional states have a disproportionate share of the nation's poor and low-income populations (KFF, 2014).

Other aspects of either the ACA or the social and political context of its legislation also call into question the ACA's capacity to fulfill its health insurance coverage goals by 2019. First among them is the ACA's health insurance market assumption that both the state-level health insurance exchanges and the federal health insurance exchange (aka the health insurance marketplace) would both be implemented and basically work as planned—in time to foster enough public trust to ensure the voluntary health insurance enrollment needed to enable the ACA to achieve its insurance coverage targets. A second worrisome aspect of the ACA's health insurance market assumptions (related to the first) is the ACA's premise that a large share of the uninsured who can afford at least subsidized health insurance, particularly young adults, will elect to purchase health insurance as an alternative to paying the tax penalty for electing not to obtain health insurance coverage. Aside from its direct effects on expanding health insurance coverage to a larger share of the national population, the success of the "individual mandate" provision of the ACA in promoting health insurance enrollment is also particularly crucial to the balance between healthy young persons and less healthy older persons that is essential to the affordability of health insurance premiums.[5] Finally, but not least, is the ACA's reliance on goodwill and cooperation of state-level bureaucrats and political appointees who are ultimately charged with implementing many of the specifics of the ACA's provisions, particularly the provisions related to both Medicaid enrollment and the health insurance market reforms intended to promote health insurance enrollment. While this analysis of the ACA's policy aims does not take into account the possibility of repeal by Congress, it does consider the ACA's vulnerability to "death from 1,000 cuts" at the state level (Skocpol, 2010).

This part of the analysis of the ACA pertains not only to universal coverage but also to comprehensive universal coverage—the term *comprehensive* pertaining to the necessity of a broad scope of coverage that is inclusive of all health conditions, health-care needs, and related health-care services and technologies. In this respect, the ACA is a considerable advancement over the status quo, which can be characterized by large discretion among the individual states in the extent to which the health insurance plans (other than those large employer insurance plans that fell under federal regulation through the Employment Retirement and Income Security Act or ERISA) were reviewed and regulated with respect to the adequacy of their health insurance benefits relative to health-care needs. As a result, even individuals *with* health insurance have long faced significant risks for catastrophic medical debts and barriers to access related to inadequate insurance coverage, either in terms of benefits for specific health-care needs or maximum overall risk protection (Seifert & Rukavina, 2006). To counter this problem, the ACA requires, effective 2014, that the "essential health benefits" of individual and employment-based insurance plans provide a large array of minimum health insurance benefits under ten general categories inclusive of ambulatory care, emergency services, hospitalization, laboratory services, maternity and newborn care, mental health and addiction services, prescription drugs, prevention and wellness services, and chronic disease care. Although these requirements do not extend to insurance plans that existed before the passage of the ACA in March 2010 or self-insurance plans regulated under ERISA, it is assumed that over time, the "essential health benefits" under the ACA will encompass all health insurance plans.

Adequate and Equal Risk Protection

As discussed previously, the meaning of *adequate* risk protection is that the costs associated with health care are not a threat or impediment to the realization of a decent standard of living commensurate within the prevailing social norms. *Equal* risk protection means that this same level of risk protection applies to all citizens. Under the traditional employment-based insurance system, labor force stratification in occupational status, income, and benefits has been replicated in the level of risk protection provided by the health insurance benefits available to lower-status, lower-wage employees, and employees who were not covered under collective bargaining agreements. In addition, individuals with preexisting health conditions were largely precluded from acquiring affordable health insurance. Under the ACA, aside from eliminating the preexisting condition exclusions from insurance coverage, there are four levels of risk protection from which individuals and employers may choose, ranging from the minimum of 60 percent of total expenditure coverage for the essential health benefit expenditures to 90 percent coverage of total expenditures. Thus, while the ACA represents a significant advancement over the pre-ACA status quo in the provision of *adequate* protection (through the elimination of preexisting exclusions of health insurance coverage and also the minimum levels or financial risk protection required of individual and employment-based insurance plans), it falls well short of anything akin to *equal* protection. Presumably, lower-income individuals and lower-wage employers will be far more likely to purchase the minimum protection plans that leave as much as 40 percent of health-care expenditures uncovered, while more advantaged workers and their dependents will be more likely to be represented among those with all but 10 percent of expenditures covered.

Summary of the ACA's Achievement of Core Health-Care Policy Aim 1

While the ACA is likely to reduce the number of Americans who are presumed to have a presumptive right to comprehensive health care that provides adequate and equal risk protection, in light of the ACA's inability to mandate its expanded Medicaid coverage provisions, it seems that by 2019, as many as 25 million may be uninsured (as opposed to the ACA's assumed reduction to 18 million), thus suggesting that a decade after the passage of the ACA, only 92 percent of the nation's citizens and legal residents would have either public or private health insurance coverage. This would leave the United States among the bottom four of thirty-four modern democracies in the proportion of the population with health insurance coverage (OECD, 2013b) and is well short of the achievement of the core health policy aim pertaining to universal coverage, even when excluding consideration of undocumented workers and their dependents. On the other hand, the comprehensive coverage component of core health-care policy aim 1 is largely if not wholly achieved by the ACA's "essential health benefits" requirement that will ultimately apply to all health insurance plans.

Finally, the adequate and equal risk protection component of core health-care policy aim 1 is (like the universal coverage component) only partially realized—that is, the ACA only partially mitigates the linkage between social stratification in the labor market and social stratification in adequate risk protection from the financial burdens of health care.

Core Health-Care Policy Aim 2: Amelioration of Disparities in
Health-Care Access and Quality

Amelioration of Disparities in Health-Care Access

Assuming that the earlier CMS projections are essentially correct and
then adjusting for states that have refused to expand Medicaid coverage, the
ACA should reduce the number of uninsured by some 25 million by 2019.
Insomuch as the lack of health insurance coverage is a principal barrier to
health-care access in the United States, the ACA represents a significant advancement of this core policy aim. That acknowledged, it must also be said
that the ACA's reliance on increased Medicaid enrollment as a means of
health insurance coverage extends impediments to health-care access that
are tied to stigma associated with Medicaid coverage and the reluctance of
a large share of health-care providers to accept either Medicaid coverage
or Medicaid patients (Raykar et al., 2014; Stuber & Kronebusch, 2004). In
contrast to Medicare and private insurance, which have high levels of participation, physicians generally find Medicaid to pay very low fees and to
be administratively burdensome. While there are promising indications
that the provisions of the ACA that bring Medicaid payments closer to
Medicare rates of reimbursement may increase the willingness of at least
primary care providers to accept new Medicaid patients (Decker, 2013),
in contrast to Medicare reimbursement rates, reimbursement rates for
Medicaid remain highly vulnerable to politically motivated entitlement
reductions.

It also should be acknowledged that among the states that have refused
to take advantage of the ACA's Medicaid expansion provisions, there is the
distinct possibility that the ACA may have the effect of reducing access to
health care for the most disadvantaged poor relying on safety net hospitals,
due to the ACA's reduction of "disproportionate share hospital payment"
(DSH) funding as a mechanism for financing the presumed expansion of
Medicaid. In a nutshell, safety net hospitals that provide a disproportionate share of uncompensated care to the poor rely on Medicaid DSH payments to sustain their financial solvency. Under the ACA, these DSH
funds (which totaled $17.4 billion in 2011) are to be reduced by $17.1 billion
by 2020. In states that have expanded Medicaid, new Medicaid revenue for
treating poor and low-income individuals who are newly eligible for Medicaid is expected to offset the DSH reduction. However, in states that have

refused to expand Medicaid, the safety net hospitals may be in real danger of insolvency due to DSH funding reductions that were supposed to be offset by expanded Medicaid enrollment (Kaiser Commission on Medicaid and the Uninsured, 2013a). Averting this threat to the health-care safety net requires either action from Congress to amend the DSH funding reductions in states that have not expanded Medicaid or a major shift among the recalcitrant states toward the embracement of the ACA's provisions to expand Medicaid eligibility. The political prospects for either are dubious at best.

Amelioration of Disparities in Health-Care Quality
To the extent that the ACA is implemented as originally signed into law, there are a number of ways in which the ACA should dramatically reduce disparities in health-care quality that are associated with race, ethnicity, and socioeconomic status. First and foremost is the reduction in disparities in the quality of care that are likely to take place as the ACA connects newly insured patients to a regular source of primary health care as an alternative to reliance on the emergency medicine system and urgent care clinics.

Research has shown that when low-income adults have medical insurance and are able to access a "medical home," they are more likely to be up to date with preventative care health screenings and also report greater satisfaction with the quality of their care (Berenson et al., 2012).[6]

Second, aside from channeling formally uninsured populations toward primary care providers through insurance coverage, the ACA makes significant investments in the development of innovative primary care models that target disadvantaged populations and communities, such as Section 2703, which offers states the option to receive an enhanced federal match rate for expanding or implementing medical home programs for Medicaid beneficiaries with chronic conditions (Berenson et al., 2012). The ACA provision that increases the Medicaid reimbursement rate to providers is also likely to increase the quality of care provided to poor and low-income patients.

Third, the ACA's health insurance market reforms that establish a national standard for comprehensive health insurance benefits (described previously as the ACA's "essential health benefits") will reduce disparities in the scope of coverage for needed health-care services that have long existed between the employment-based insurance plans of low-income and high-income workers, which has a direct and obvious relationship to the amelioration of disparities in health-care quality.

Finally, embedded in the ACA are a number of policy strategies that are intended to elevate the reduction of a wide range of persistent health-care disparities (e.g., race, ethnicity, gender, age, income, geography). These include (but are not limited to) enhanced patient characteristic data collection in federally funded health centers and programs, elevating the National Center for Minority Health and Health Disparities (NCMHD) to full institute status within the National Institutes of Health (NIH) and increasing NCMHD funding, expanding grant programs designed to attract and retain diverse health professionals and also funding to health professionals who agree to work in underserved areas (such as American Indian reservations and rural communities), and providing an oral health campaign intended to reduce racial and ethnic disparities in oral health (Robert Wood Johnson Foundation, 2011). Of particular significance to the reduction of health and health-care disparities among Native Americans and Alaska Natives, the ACA makes permanent the reauthorization of the Indian Health Care Improvement Act, which empowers Congress to fund health-care services for American Indians and Alaska Natives through the Indian Health Service and has as its explicit policy aim the complete elimination of health disparities between indigenous peoples and the U.S. population as a whole (American Indian Health and Family Services, 2010).

Despite these promising inroads to the amelioration of health-care disparities in quality of care, there may be limits to the reduction of disparities in the quality of care that are imposed by the ACA's reliance on a different form of insurance coverage for the poor and low-income populations. Medicaid, as a means-based entitlement program that has had a long history of stigma and underpayment to providers, is particularly problematic (Stuber & Kronebusch, 2004). Historically, Medicaid coverage has not provided the same level of consumer choice in primary care providers as has either the typical health insurance plan or Medicare, and Medicaid patients are more likely to encounter disparities in access to specialty care than are privately insured patients (Government Accountability Office [GAO], 2011; Raykar et al., 2014). While some studies show that adult Medicaid patients are less likely to receive appropriate care than privately insured patients, the evidence is more mixed where there are controls for the sociodemographic characteristics of patients (Calvin et al., 2006; Kaiser Commission on Medicaid and the Uninsured, 2013b).

Another area where the ACA's impacts on disparities in the quality of health care are limited has to do with the amelioration of disparities in health-care system infrastructure that affect not only access to care but also quality of care. Since the 1970s, investments in hospital facilities and clinics have tended to favor communities with a high proportion of insured patients as opposed to low-income communities with higher levels of health-care need, thus leaving low-income and poor communities with more antiquated facilities and technologies (Almgren & Ferguson, 1999; Carrier et al., 2012). In addition, the closure of safety net hospitals or acquisition of failing safety net hospitals by for-profit hospital corporations over recent decades has adversely affected both health-care access and quality of care for racial minorities and poor communities (Almgren & Ferguson, 1999; Bazzoli et al., 2012). There is also evidence to suggest that the expansions in Medicaid coverage in low-income communities are unlikely to create incentives for hospital investments in disadvantaged communities, even though the health-care needs are greater (Freedman et al., 2014). Related to this is the concern that a large share of the hospitals that comprise the nation's safety net health-care system, because they operate at the margins of solvency in aging facilities, is quite literally crumbling (Berggren, 2005; Taylor, 2001). While the health insurance coverage expansions under the ACA may help some distressed hospitals to become more solvent, the ACA does not provide the targeted investments in the hospital infrastructure of poor communities that would be needed to offset decades of disparities in hospital preservation and modernization.

Summary of the ACA's Prospects for the Achievement of Core Health-Care Policy Aim 2

Depending on the pace and the extent of its implementation, the ACA has enormous potential to greatly ameliorate the disparities in health-care access and quality that have been endemic throughout the American health-care system. As pointed out previously, as of the midpoint of the ACA's decade-long plan of implementation it appears that the ACA will reduce the number of uninsured by about 25 million by 2019, with obvious implications for the reduction of disparities in both health-care access and health-care quality. In addition, the ACA has multiple provisions that specifically target the origins and structural mechanisms of disparities in health-care quality that have adversely affected racial and ethnic minorities, women, and indigenous peoples.

Paradoxically, the ACA has the potential of increasing geographic disparities in health care due to its inability to mandate that states expand their Medicaid programs, thus leaving the low-income adults in those states that oppose the ACA without a viable path to affordable health care. In addition, the safety net hospitals in those oppositional states are placed in more jeopardy because they lack the increased Medicaid revenue to offset reductions in federal subsidies for uncompensated care (National Association of Urban Hospitals, 2012).[7]

With respect to the amelioration of the disparities in health-care infrastructure that are crucial determinants of health-care quality and access, the ACA's likely impact is at best mixed. On one hand, the ACA includes multiple provisions for health-care workforce investments that target disadvantaged populations and communities, such as scholarship, loan forgiveness, and grant programs to support capacity building in underserved areas, and $11 billion in additional funding for community health centers. On the other hand, the ACA does not provide funds to modernize and replace the aging hospital buildings and clinic facilities that comprise a large and crucial share of the nation's crumbling health-care safety net (Institute of Medicine, 2000)—a problem that will be made worse by the $17 billion reduction in DSH payments to struggling safety net hospitals that will be phased in over the balance of the ACA's first decade absent corrective actions by Congress.

Despite these limitations, it can be said that taken as a whole, the ACA holds great promise as social legislation that will significantly (if not even greatly) reduce the disparities in health-care access and quality that have characterized the American health-care system throughout the modern era of medicine. In this sense, the ACA is evaluated as highly responsive to core health-care policy aim 2.

Core Health-Care Policy Aim 3: Equitable Distribution of
Preventative, Curative, Rehabilitative, and Adaptive Health-Care
Services/Technologies Specific to Health Needs and
Public Health Investments and Interventions

The Equitable Distribution of Health-Care Services and Technologies
To recap, the equitable distribution of health-care services and technologies specific to health-care needs requires that all citizens with equivalent health-care needs are entitled to equal shares of the nation's limited health-care

resources. Hypothetically and ideally, this standard of equity would be achieved if (1) all citizens possessed the same health insurance card that would entitle them to the same insurance plan benefits irrespective of education, place of employment and occupation, race, gender, or any other characteristic other than their medical condition and specific health-care needs, (2) there were no significant disparities in the geographic distribution of health-care resources, and (3) the processes of diagnosis and treatment planning were devoid of all forms of discrimination (both interpersonal and institutional). No nation has achieved this standard of equity, although Sweden's health-care system is ranked as the most equitable based on measures that are based on the "equal care for equal needs" principle (Davis et al., 2014).[8] Because the ACA preserves and in many respects extends the employment-based health insurance system that is supplemented by both means-tested and social insurance public health-care entitlements, it also continues into the foreseeable future the disequities in health-care access and quality that are based on the disparities in health-care benefits available from different employment-based insurance plans, Medicare, and Medicaid. With respect to employment-based insurance, the analysis of the ACA's potential to achieve the equitable distribution of health-care services and technologies is largely the same as that applied to the chapter's early analysis of the ACA's adequacy with respect to equal risk protection, which points to the enduring relationship between social stratification in the labor market and social stratification in health care. While the ACA mitigates this relationship to a significant extent through its provisions that establish a national standard for minimum health insurance benefits that will benefit lower-wage workers, it retains a tiered health insurance benefit structure (identified as the platinum, gold, silver, bronze, and catastrophic plan categories) that in effect will retain the relationship between socioeconomic status and the level of entitlement to health care. With respect to Medicaid (also as pointed out at an earlier point in this chapter), it is unlikely that the ACA will wholly eliminate the sources of barriers to care encountered by Medicaid patients relative to privately insured patients or patients insured by Medicare. Finally, with respect to Medicare, it is at best a partial social insurance program that only pays for 60 percent of the health-care expenditures of older adults (even excluding long-term care expenditures), leaving the largest share of the remainder to out-of-pocket resources and private supplemental insurance (Fronstin et al., 2012).

As a result, even among Medicare recipients, socioeconomic status affects health-care access and quality (Rogowski et al., 2008).

The Equitable Distribution of Public Health Interventions and Measures

The appraisal of the ACA's potential to advance the equitable distribution of public health interventions and measures might best be contextualized in light of Paul Starr's *The Social Transformation of American Medicine* (1982), his definitive history of the path to American exceptionalism in health care. In this seminal work, Starr devotes considerable space to a rather bleak narrative of the marginalization of the public health component of the nation's health-care system over the twentieth century in favor of the advancement of medical free enterprise and the commodification of health care. According to Starr, whereas at the end of the nineteenth century, public health's centrality on American health care seemed assured and its future limitless, within a few decades, it became clear that "public health in America was to be relegated to a secondary status: less prestigious than clinical medicine, less amply financed, and blocked from assuming the higher-level functions of coordination and direction that might have been developed had it not been banished from medical care" (p. 197). In the brief summary of the ACA's public health provisions that follows, it becomes apparent that the ACA goes a very long way toward reversing the past century of public health's marginalization and in many respects places public health at the forefront of the policy strategies and societal investments to realize advancements in both population health and clinical health care.

There are over forty major public health provisions in the ACA that include tens of billions in funding for community transformation grants targeting the prevention and amelioration of chronic diseases, major investments in federally funded community health centers and school-based health clinics, childhood obesity prevention programs, employment-based wellness programs, and perhaps most critically funds to support the development of a "National Prevention Strategy" under the auspices of Health and Human Services (National Association of City and County Health Officials [NACCHO], 2012). Prominent among the ACA's public health investments are $9.75 billion for community-based prevention programs under the Prevention and Public Health Fund title that strengthens the role and capacity of local health departments in promoting population health,[9] invests funds in public health training fellowships and preventative health-care practice, and improves the nation's public health laboratory infra-structure for the detection, prevention, and control of infectious diseases (Centers for Disease Control and Prevention [CDC], 2013b; NACCHO, 2012). Also prominent is the ACA's investment of $11 billion in additional funds for operational and capital investments in new and renovated com-munity health-care facilities (Health Resources and Services Administra-tion [HRSA], 2013).

From the standpoint of *equity in public health investments and interven-tions*, the funding allocation procedures and requirements for ACA's pub-lic health programs are designed to strike a balance between investments in the nation's public health programs and infrastructure that will benefit the national population as a whole (both wealthy and poor communities benefit from public health advancements in the prevention, detection, and control of infectious diseases and investments in preventative medicine practice) and targeted public health investments to disadvantaged popula-tions and communities, such as funds for capacity building for Federally Qualified Community Health Centers and training fellowships to prepare and incentivize clinicians to practice in poor communities and safety net health-care settings.

Summary of the ACA's Prospects for the Achievement of Core Health-Care Policy Aim 3

Because the ACA essentially preserves the disequities in health-care ser-vices and technologies that are embedded in the employment-based health insurance system, a means-based public health-care coverage for the poor, and a social insurance program for older adults that covers only some 60 percent of actual health-care costs, its prospects for the achievement of core health-care policy aim 3 are inherently limited—notwithstanding the ACA representing a major improvement over the status quo. With respect to public health investments and measures, the equity evaluation of the ACA is far more favorable. While a detailed critique of the individual pub-lic health provisions of the ACA can uncover a variety of weaknesses with respect to the equity principle (such as the adequacy of specific investments relative to the public health needs of particular groups and communities), it is evident that the ACA represents a historically unprecedented advance-ment in the equitable distribution of public health investments and measures, a judgment that also reflects the position of the American Public Health Association (APHA, 2012).

Core Health-Care Policy Aim 4: Compensatory Entitlements and Investments in Health-Care Services and Public Health Infrastructure/Interventions

When the ACA was signed into law in 2010, the age-adjusted death rate for African Americans was 27 percent in excess of that for whites (Miniño, 2011). Among the members of the Lakota tribe of Pine Ridge Reservation in South Dakota, the age-adjusted death rate was 67 percent in excess of that the whites (South Dakota Department of Public Health [SDDPH], 2012). These dramatic disparities in health help contextualize and frame the analysis that follows of the ACA's adequacy with respect to compensatory investments in health services and public health infrastructure for groups and populations adversely affected by health disparities.

Compensatory Investments in Health Services

Among the disadvantaged populations and communities that rely on the hospitals, clinics, and programs that are a part of the public health component of the health-care system, there is large overlap between compensatory investments in health services and compensatory investments in public health infrastructure. In general, compensatory health service investments pertain to "downstream" funds that are allocated to the facility, workforce, and technological components of the diagnosis and treatment of individuals affected by health disparities (such as a member of a tribal community manifesting the symptoms of diabetes, which is disproportionately prevalent among Native Americans), whereas compensatory public health infrastructure investments entail resources targeted toward "upstream" population health strategies that are intended to reduce disparities in disease risk and prevalence (such as improving the diabetes surveillance infrastructure in tribal communities and addressing the nutritional disparities that are antecedent to the onset of diabetes).[10]

With this distinction in mind, the ACA has a number of provisions that entail compensatory investments in the facility, workforce, and technological components of health care that are intended to ameliorate the individual-level manifestations of health disparities. With respect to capital components of compensatory health service investments (facilities and technology), the most significant direct investment is the ACA's $11 billion allocation to the Community Health Center Fund referred to briefly in the preceding section. The largest share of the Community Health Care Center Fund ($9.5 billion) is directed to support ongoing health center operations, create new health center sites in medically underserved areas, and expand preventive and primary health-care services at already existing health center sites. The remaining $1.5 billion is allocated to investments in new construction and renovation that will enhance the quality of care and increase the service capacity of the nation's community health centers (HRSA, 2013). One particularly crucial compensatory investment embedded in the Community Health Center Fund component of the ACA is the capacity building of school-based health centers in underserved communities, which is estimated to provide health care to an additional 875,000 children at high risk for health disparities (HRSA, 2013).

A second major compensatory investment in health services is the ACA's workforce development initiatives, which encompass an entire subtitle of the ACA (Health Care Workforce, Subtitle E, Title VI, Sections 5001–5701). Notably, the language in the Health Care Workforce subtitle places particular emphasis on the health-care workforce investments that are critical to particularly low-income, underserved, uninsured, minority, health disparity, and rural populations (Reid & Wong, 2011). Within this section of the ACA, there are two basic health-care workforce development strategies for enhanced services to disadvantaged populations and communities: (1) education and training programs for providers with a particular commitment to underserved populations and communities (such as funding for interdisciplinary, community-based linkages for community-based training programs to increase the number of primary care providers serving in underserved areas) and (2) specialized training investments for providers to better enable them to effectively serve populations and communities adversely affected by health and health-care disparities, such as funding to colleges to provide mental and behavioral health education and training that addresses the needs of individuals and groups from different racial, ethnic, cultural, geographic, religious, linguistic, and class backgrounds.

A third major compensatory investment in health services that pertains to indigenous Americans is the (previously referenced) permanent reauthorization of the Indian Health Care Improvement Act, which in and of itself represents a major compensatory commitment to the health and well-being of indigenous Americans. Aside from this landmark provision of the ACA, within this permanent reauthorization, there are several amendments aimed at enhancing health services to tribal reservations and for Native Americans and Alaska Natives living in urban areas. These include empowering tribal organizations and urban Indian organizations to apply for grant and contract programs (for which these entities were previously not eligible), expanded mental health services to create comprehensive behavioral health and treatment programs and youth suicide prevention programs, and funding for modular facility demonstration projects that are intended to enhance service delivery to underserved indigenous communities (Congressional Research Service [CRS], 2010).

Finally, there are also myriad minor but important provisions of the ACA that should be counted among compensatory investments. For example, the ACA's quality improvement provisions (Section 3013) include a particular emphasis on the development of measures that evaluate the equity of services across populations and geographic areas affected by health disparities and investments in enhanced maternal, infant, and child health services to low-income and at-risk families (Center for Healthcare Research and Transformation [CHRT], 2012).

Compensatory Investments in Public Health Infrastructure

Most of the ACA's compensatory investments in public health infrastructure are embedded in the Prevention and Public Health Fund (Section 4002 of the ACA), which was allocated $5 billion for the years 2010–2014 and then $2 billion thereafter as permanent annual appropriation (CRS, 2013). Included in the ACA's Prevention and Public Health Fund is the "Community Transformation Grant" program, which directs the CDC to issue competitive community grants to states, local governments, tribal organizations, and other community-based organizations to implement and evaluate community prevention programs, including strategies to reduce health disparities (Reid & Wong, 2011). Another crucial compensatory public health infrastructure investment pertains to enhanced data collection (ACA, Section 4302) that would encompass the demographic and functional correlates of health disparities, which, as pointed out by Reid and Wong (2011), "is a necessary precondition to developing workable prevention and treatment strategies" (p. 3). This data collection provision of the

ACA, because it extends to any federally conducted or supported health-care activity, program, or survey, in this respect is a transformative compensatory investment. A third public health infrastructure investment worthy of highlighting is the ACA's National Diabetes Prevention Program (ACA, Section 10501g), because it targets the populations and communities with a disproportionate prevalence of type II diabetes—among them African Americans, Hispanics, and American Indians (Reid & Wong, 2011). This provision of the ACA promotes the development of collaborative diabetes prevention strategies and activities among federal agencies, community-based organizations, health-care providers, health insurance companies, and other key entities with the overall aim of reducing the prevalence of diabetes and disparities in risk and incidence.

Summary of the ACA's Prospects for the Achievement of Core Health-Care Policy Aim 4

Consistent with the coverage and access provisions for the amelioration of health disparities discussed in connection with core health-care policy aim 2, the ACA places significant emphasis on health services and public health investments that target populations and communities carrying a disproportionate burden of disease and premature mortality. These include investments in facilities, workforce, and technology that are essential to health-care capacity building in poor communities, as well as public health-care infrastructure investments in epidemiological and health services data, community-based prevention programs, and macro-level disease prevention strategies.

This acknowledged, there is a fundamental vulnerability to the ACA's ambitious long-term program of compensatory investments in health services and public health infrastructure that has to do with the distinction between mandatory and discretionary funding that is built into the ACA. That is, although many of the ACA's prevention programs have mandatory funding through the ACA's Prevention and Public Health Fund, a large share of the ACA's compensatory investments in health services and public health measures is actually discretionary as opposed to mandatory (Reid & Wong, 2011). In contrast to mandatory provisions of the ACA, which refer to programs and entitlements that are both authorized and statutorily funded, discretionary provisions are authorized but not appropriated, thus leaving Congress the option of either supporting or undercutting the ACA's many discretionary provisions that represent compensatory investments in the health and health care of disadvantaged populations. Such discretionary provisions of the ACA include funding for school-based health centers, nurse-managed health clinics that provide comprehensive primary health care and wellness services to vulnerable or underserved populations, a substantial share of the workforce development grants, the entire section of the ACA (4302, Part a) pertaining to health disparities data collection and analysis, and the entirety of the National Diabetes Prevention Program (CRS, 2011). It therefore must be said that in the final analysis, the ACA's adequacy with respect to core health-care policy aim 4 is at best tenuous—conditioned as it is on the will of a divided and recalcitrant Congress to fund many of the ACA's provisions representing a genuinely substantive commitment to a social right to health care.

CONCLUDING REMARKS:
THE ACA IN EVOLUTIONARY PERSPECTIVE

In chapter 1, it was established that American exceptionalism in health care is attributable to the convergence of policy compromises that have been crafted to reconcile the liberal–libertarian streams in American political consciousness, the capacity of the AMA to frame the national discourse on health care at a critical juncture in national history, and the phenomenon of path dependence in social policy.

Subsequent chapters provide both the historical context for the emergence of the ACA and a framework through which the ACA can be evaluated against the requisites of political democracy, leading ultimately to the conclusion in this chapter that, from this penultimate perspective, the ACA falls well short of assuring the necessary social right to health care, despite its appraisal by both its friends and foes as a triumph of liberalism. Were the nation's journey toward a more encompassing social right to health care to end with the ACA, even at full implementation, scholars a generation from now will still be debating the antecedents to the enduring American exceptionalism in health care. As discussed in the concluding section of chapter 1, the premise of this book (and in particular the chapters that follow this one) is that this is not the dismal future that awaits us. To recapitulate the primary reasons why this is so, it is because:

1. the gains of the ACA with respect to expanded health-care coverage and access are here to stay;

2.   the idea of universal health insurance coverage as a social right of citizenship, as affirmed by the ACA being signed into law as an act of Congress, is here to stay;

3.   the above notwithstanding, the ACA is inadequate to the task of providing all Americans with a social right to health care; and

4.   the status quo, even with the ACA in place, is unsustainable; in particular, the impending collapse of the Medicare Hospital Insurance Trust Fund[11] will push the nation toward fundamental reforms in health-care delivery and financing that will inevitably encompass all payers and age groups in the next new era of health-care reform, in contrast to previous eras, and will be framed within the idea of health care as a social right of citizenship—and this is perhaps the ACA's most enduring legacy.

So it is that the ACA should be viewed as a very large step in an evolutionary progression toward the substantive realization of a social right to health care, rather than that the health-care policy structure is capable of delivering on that right. This leaves us to ponder just what national health-care policy must look like to fulfill that elusive substantive realization to a social right to health care, which is the task of the next chapter.

Chapter Five

A PRINCIPLED APPROACH TO RADICAL
HEALTH-CARE FINANCE REFORM

Chapter 4 concluded with the conviction that, even should the ACA be fully implemented as signed into law, the nation's "three-legged stool" approach to health-care financing that combines employment-based insurance, social insurance for the aged, and means-tested coverage for low-income populations is unsustainable.

This reality is made manifest in the predicted collapse of the Medicare Hospital Insurance Trust Fund even with the cost containment provisions of the ACA fully implemented (as discussed in chapter 1) and also made inevitable by the contradiction between the continued health-care policy hegemony of health-care industry stakeholder groups and the dubious long-term fiscal sustainability of the ACA's mixed public and private system of health-care financing. So what might replace the system of health-care finance that has prevailed for the past half century, and equally critically, what should? Delving into this two-part question and then answering it in a way that balances the principles of health-care reform advanced in previous chapters with the pragmatics of the possible can be aided by some comparative analysis of the ways in which other modern democracies have financed a social right to health care in the context of a market economy.

HEALTH SYSTEM TYPOLOGIES AND ALTERNATIVE APPROACHES
TO THE FINANCING OF A SOCIAL RIGHT TO HEALTH CARE

Critics of the U.S. health-care system are fond of noting that the United States is the only modern democracy that fails to provide its citizens with universal coverage. This is mostly accurate; among the member states of the Organization for Cooperation and Development (OECD), only the United States and Mexico have failed to provide universal health insurance coverage for core health services (OECD, 2013a). While it can be said that most modern democracies provide universal health care through public health insurance coverage, this obscures an important distinction between universal public health insurance coverage for core health services and universal public coverage for all health expenditures. If the latter definition of universal coverage is used, a far more complex pattern emerges wherein it becomes apparent that almost all modern democracies rely on a mixture of public and private health-care coverage for health-care services, with a wide range of philosophies with respect to the relative roles of private versus public health insurance.

One way this variation becomes readily apparent is through the examination of data on the share of total health expenditures among the "universal coverage" nations that actually paid either directly out of pocket or through the purchase of private health insurance. For example, Wendt's (2009) analysis of health-care financing approaches among a sample of thirteen Western European countries that are listed by the OECD as providing "universal health insurance coverage" (that is, at least 99 percent of the total population covered by health insurance for core health services) reveals that the average share of the total health expenditures that are paid for out of pocket (either directly or through the purchase of private health insurance) is nearly 19 percent (OECD, 2013a; Wendt, 2009). Among these OECD member states with universal health care, France provides the most public health insurance protection, with only 6.5 percent of total health expenditures uncovered by public health insurance, while in Greece, 42 percent of health expenditures are uncovered by public health insurance (Wendt, 2009). Even among the Scandinavian countries in this sample (Sweden and Denmark), the share of total health expenditures that are uncovered by public health insurance exceeds 15 percent (Wendt, 2009). Clearly, if all health expenditures are considered as opposed to just those that are considered core health services (primary and specialty physician consultations, diagnostic services, hospital care and surgical/medical treatments), private insurance coverage is a crucial component of health care financing, even among the most generous of welfare states.

As it happens, private health can assume any one of four health-care financing roles: as the *primary* source of health insurance coverage (as it does in the United States), as *complementary* to public health insurance that pays for the cost-sharing component of the basic health services covered under the public plan, as *duplicate* health insurance for faster access/more provider choice for basic health services, or as *supplemental* insurance for the coverage of health services that are not covered by public health insurance plans. In nations with a strong egalitarian ethos like France and Denmark, private health insurance plays a significant role in the health-care system but only as a means of defraying out-of-pocket costs of the basic services all are entitled to as opposed to a means of providing the more affluent with a higher level of convenience/choice or access to more health services. In fact, in France, complementary private insurance covers 96 percent of the national population (OECD, 2013a). In other countries with either a more deeply embedded social class tradition and/or inadequately financed public health-care services, both duplicative and supplemental forms of private health insurance coverage are quite common.

For example, in Australia, just over 50 percent of the nation's population is covered by private insurance that provides either more convenience/choice or access to more services (OECD, 2013a). The comparative analysis of health systems that provide universal coverage becomes even more complex when other important aspects aside from the relative roles of public versus private health insurance are considered, such as the basis of entitlement to health care (need, citizenship, payment into social insurance) and the range of choice between health-care providers and easy access to specialists. In Wendt's (2009) comparative analysis of Western European health systems that addressed these and other essential considerations,[1] a three-system typology emerged that is very instructive with respect to the kinds of policy choices that provide the substantive trade-offs that are inevitable to the realization of a social right to health care.

Briefly stated, Type I, which Wendt (2009) identifies as the *health service provision-oriented type* (inclusive of Austria, Belgium, France, Germany, and Luxembourg), refers to a health system that places particular emphasis on a high number of health-care providers, relatively unfettered access to a range of providers, and modest out-of-pocket expenditures (either for direct payment or supplementary private health insurance). Type II, identified as the *universal coverage-controlled access type* (inclusive of Denmark, Great Britain, Sweden, Italy, and Ireland), is characterized by its emphasis on an inclusive egalitarian health-care system that provides a common standard of publicly financed health care at a cost of convenience of access and choice of providers. In this type of system, there is a low prevalence of private insurance coverage and also low out-of-pocket expenditures. The Type III system, which Wendt (2009) labels as the *low-budget restricted access type* (inclusive of Portugal, Spain, and Finland), refers to a health system where national per-capita health expenditures are low, as are the number of providers, and out-of-pocket health expenditures are high, thus restricting access to care for the low income and poor. However, this type also has a high degree of regulation, both in the patients' choice of primary care doctors and also via regulation of primary care physician salaries.

With the respect to the core health care policy aims advanced in chapter 4 (in particular core health-care policy aim 1: the achievement of universal comprehensive health insurance coverage with adequate and equal risk protection), it should be evident that anything approximating the Type III approach is unacceptable, even if it were feasible from the standpoint of the political economy of the American health-care system, which it clearly is not. It is really about whether the next stage of national health-care reform beyond the ACA should or even could move toward a Type I health service provision-oriented system or toward a more egalitarian Type II universal coverage-controlled access system.

Delving deeply into this pivotal policy crossroads requires some contextual appraisal as to which particular direction is more viable and sustainable within the social and political parameters of the American welfare state and therefore more likely to achieve the four core health-care reform aims advanced in the preceding chapter.

APPRAISING THE BOUNDARIES OF A SOCIAL RIGHT TO HEALTH CARE IN THE AMERICAN VERSION OF THE LIBERAL WELFARE STATE

In an interview with the editorial staff of the journal *Managed Care* three years after the ACA was signed into law, Princeton health-care economist Uwe Reinhart was asked if he saw an evolution toward a single-payer system in the United States. His response was an emphatic "no," in keeping with his viewpoint published elsewhere (E. Klein, 2014) that the U.S. Congress was too corrupted by money from vested interests in the health-care industry to create and oversee a compulsory social insurance fund for health care. Rather, Reinhart suggested that the evolution toward a three-tiered system is far more plausible, which he described as a public health-care tier that provided a minimal standard of health services to the poor, a preferred provider network tier for the middle class, and a "boutique" medicine tier for the elites—one where the wealthy and privileged would not be forced to mix with the rest of humanity ("A Conversation," 2013).

While Reinhart's portrait of the nation's health-care system of the future is a bleak one by the standards of the more egalitarian traditions of American progressivism, it is in many respects consistent with decades of public opinion and also the basic characteristics of the American version of the welfare state. With respect to public opinion on what might be called at least a minimalist right to health care (which holds that most Americans believe that it is the responsibility of the government to make sure all Americans have access to needed health care), most find a separate system of subsidized health care for the poor more acceptable than a single-payer system or, in essence, a social insurance plan that would provide an equal level of health insurance coverage for all (Blendon, Martilla, et al., 1994; Blendon et al., 2006). As to the American version of the welfare state (that falls within the authoritative Esping-Andersen typology of the liberal welfare state), there is strong preference for private-sector and labor market provisions for material and health security, means-tested programs of assistance for the poor, and a minimalist role of government (Esping-Andersen, 1990). This is in contrast to Esping-Andersen's social democratic typology of the welfare state that places strong emphasis on a high standard of minimal material and health security that is universal and egalitarian, such as would be typified by the Scandinavian countries (Esping-Andersen, 1990). However, even among other liberal welfare state regimes such as the United Kingdom, Canada, and Australia, the United States is a more extreme case of the general type, which has prompted scholars for decades to interrogate the social and political origins of American exceptionalism in social welfare (Garfinkel et al., 2010; Massey, 2009; Skocpol, 1992). The origins of American exceptionalism in social welfare have powerful implications for the most feasible path to the achievement of the core policy aims for health-care reform.

The Reluctant Welfare State

Although there are a variety of ways that American exceptionalism in social welfare has been defined and characterized in the comparative social policy literature, perhaps the version that best captures the essence of American exceptionalism is Bruce Jansson's notion of the "reluctant welfare state" (Jansson, 1988), by which he means a welfare state that develops belatedly relative to its Western European counterparts, has meager social expenditures as a proportion of its economic productivity, has a fragmented institutional structure, has unstable social programs and benefits, emphasizes minimal means-tested benefits in its antipoverty programs, and maintains a system of taxation that promotes rather than ameliorates income inequality. Specific indices of the nation's reluctant welfare state include the level of public social spending as a percentage of the gross domestic product (just 71 percent of the OECD average),[2] the nation's historical tolerance for high levels of child poverty (50 percent in excess of the OECD average),[3] the nation's level of income inequality (23 percent in excess of the OECD average, a level exceeded only by Turkey, Chile, and Mexico), and of course the fact that the United States stands alone among the OECD member states that does not provide universal health-care coverage as a social right of citizenship (Harvard School of Public Health, 2012; OECD, 2014c, 2014d). Among the four main social provision pillars that comprise the welfare state (income security, health security, social service support, and education), there is only one where the American version of the welfare state has been historically generous relative to its European counterparts rather than reluctant—public education (Garfinkel et al., 2010). However, as will be seen in the discussion that follows, there is a coherence to this seeming inconsistency that has to do with a particular ideological cornerstone of the nation's reluctant welfare state—an ideological cornerstone that is a crucial limiting factor to a more egalitarian approach to the financing of a social right to health care.

The Boundaries of Egalitarianism in Social Welfare

In contrast to the reasons for American exceptionalism in health care highlighted in chapter 1 (which emphasize the historical influence of the medical profession, path dependence in social policy, and libertarian notions of predatory governance), American exceptionalism in social welfare is more deeply rooted not only in the libertarianism but also in structural aspects of the nation's political system, in its ethnic and racial heterogeneity, and in the pathological derivatives of racial and ethnic diversity in racism and "otherness." In particular, the politics of race have weakened both the power of labor and the capacity of the federal government to provide for a national minimum standard of material and health security (Massey, 2009). In addition, there is also both the national history and prevailing notion of a fairly permeable social class structure, which is rooted both in the nation's Jeffersonian vision of a land of equal opportunity and its development as a society shaped by waves of upwardly mobile immigrants (Hirschman, 2005; Shklar, 1991). Collectively and in many ways synergistically, all of these origins of American exceptionalism in social welfare undermine the prospects for an approach to the financing of a social health care that embraces egalitarianism in either health-care access or quality. We will begin with interrogating the role of racism and "otherness" in determining the substance and boundaries of social rights generally.

As noted by prominent scholars of race and social policy (such as Massey, 2009) as well as others (Lieberman, 2001; Nakano-Glenn, 2002), the nation's history of racial and ethnic subordination is pivotal to the understanding of American exceptionalism in social welfare policy, beginning with the foundations of the American welfare state in the New Deal legislation that, at the behest of Southern members of Congress, (1) disenfranchised African Americans and other minorities (such as agricultural wage workers, sharecroppers, and domestic servants) from old age social insurance and (2) ceded to the individual states the authority to determine the eligibility criteria and benefit levels of the nation's primary antipoverty program—formally Aid to Dependent Children and now known as Temporary Assistance to Needy Families. Even fifty years after the passage of the Civil Rights Act of 1964 and eighty years after the Social Security Act of 1935, impoverished African American families are disproportionately disenrolled from public assistance due to the discretion given to states and the complicity of low-level bureaucrats given the authority to determine which families are excluded from the nation's most basic social safety net (Schram et al., 2009; Soss et al., 2001).

Another explanation for the nation's reluctant welfare state is the lack of a radical labor tradition and strong unions that in other nations have been fundamental to development of a robust social safety net (Jansson,

1988; Skocpol, 1992), which is also in large part attributable to the nation's history of racial subordination. As argued by Massey (2009), the labor movement was weakened by the race-based exclusion of African Americans and other minorities from unions and by racially differentiated collective-bargaining agreements. Also, the preservation of the Jim Crow status quo motivated populist Southern Democrats to join with pro-business Republicans in the passage (over President Truman's veto) of the infamous 1947 Taft-Hartley Act—legislation that eviscerated the power of unions to both organize and bargain for higher wages and thus be a political force for a more adequate public social safety net (J. Klein, 2003; Massey, 2009).[4]

With respect specifically to the historical influence of race in the shaping of the American welfare state's exclusionary health-care system, there is a relationship between racial stratification in the labor market, racial stratification in the availability and adequacy of employment benefits for health care, and the legacy of racially segregated health care that still endures (J. Klein, 2003; Serwer, 2009). While some have argued that there is progression toward a so-called postracial society that is more or less synonymous with a progression toward more egalitarian social institutions, there is a counternarrative that racism, and its correlates in a lack of an inclusive citizenship and genuine social equality, is far more consistent with the evidence—such as the historically unprecedented rate of black male incarceration, ironically at the point that the nation elected its first African American president (Bonilla-Silva & Dietrich, 2011). It is that correlate of racism and "otherness," the lack of an inclusive sense of shared citizenship and genuine social equality, that precludes the realization of equity in social rights, whether in education, basic material security, and health care.

The second major origin of American exceptionalism in social welfare, derived from the nation's ability to sustain a permeable social class structure for most immigrant groups over much of its history, is characterized by the popular belief that in America, birth is not destiny—that upward mobility is a matter of individual endowments and efforts to "get ahead in life" (Hirschman, 2005). Thus, Americans tend to be less concerned about the nation's high-level income inequality relative to other democracies with much lower levels of income inequality and tend to see poverty either in individual or racial terms (Bullock, 2006; Gilens, 2000; Pew Research Center, 2013). Americans are also unaware of the fact that relative to other prosperous democracies (including the Scandinavian countries, Canada, Australia, New Zealand, Germany, Japan, and France), the United States actually has lower social mobility[5] (Corak, 2013). A corollary to the myth of a readily permeable class structure is the tolerance, if not outright embracement, of a range of material and social inequalities as a matter of merit rather than unearned privilege or fortune of birth. This myth, as well as the general tolerance of inequalities it fosters, is perhaps best captured in the libertarian mantra that "our society should guarantee equality of opportunity, but not equality of result" (Strauss, 1992, p. 171).[6]

The Boundaries of Egalitarianism and Public Consensus in the Substance of a Social Right to Health Care

It would seem that the broad acceptance of the material and social inequalities that originate in the nation's history of racism and "otherness," when combined with the justifications of inequalities based on the myths of equality of opportunity and genuine meritocracy, all but preclude a social right to health care that is egalitarian—that is, a right to health care completely equitable with respect to access, quality, and shared cost. While Americans at least ideologically reject the legitimacy of disparities in health care that are clearly attributable to race, in terms of national health-care policy, they clearly tolerate de facto racially segregated health care, just as they tolerate de facto racially segregated public schools. Disparities in health care that arise from social class are far more acceptable, both de jure and de facto. Two quotes from leading health economist Uwe Reinhart are illustrative in this regard. First, there is this one, from a PBS interview in 2000:

If you look who are the uninsured, my answer often is they are the people that make America great. They're the people who get up in the morning, they work very hard, they make our life comfortable for the upper classes. They drive us. They fill our gas tanks. They're very proud people. And they usually don't beg. I mean they're really tough customers, but when they're sick, they don't really want to stand in the Medicaid line.

They want what every other working stiff has, which is private insurance. My own sense is that while these people take care of us, serve us food, drive us when they're healthy and make our life comfortable, we owe it to them morally to look after them when they get sick. We ought to pay taxes to help these people.

Then there is this second quote, from a 2013 interview with the editorial staff of *Managed Care* ("A Conversation," 2013, p. 1):

I mean, why should a corporate CEO, when he gets sick, be in a ward when they never mix with humanity as you and I know it? They have their limos, their jets. They have mansions and presidential suites in the Ritz when they go to Washington. It would be almost cruel to say, "When you get sick, we stick you in a ward." I don't mind that they have a little suite—every hospital in America has that.

While it may seem that Reinhart (a staunch proponent of universal health insurance coverage) is being incredibly inconsistent, both quotes arise from a coherent appraisal of the limits of egalitarianism in health care in a society predicated upon the inherent justice of class privilege. Reinhart in fact believes that a system of universal health insurance in the United States is not only a moral imperative but also well within reach politically—albeit under the assumption of a tiered health-care system that is consistent with the realities of social class in America (Reinhart, 2013). That is also the viewpoint of this book, despite a more egalitarian perspective on what ought to be in the interests of genuine political democracy.

However, social class is not the only limiting factor to a wholly egalitarian and undifferentiated substantive social right to health care. Cultural heterogeneity and the complementary functions of health-care consumerism are also a limiting consideration to a social right to health care that realizes complete uniformity in health-care financing and benefits.

The Problem of Public Consensus in a Social Right to Health Care

The substantive features of a social right to health care involve two primary considerations: the level of health insurance protection against the financial burden of health-care costs and the array of benefits encompassed in health insurance coverage. The first consideration, the level of protection against the financial burden of health-care costs, in essence comprises the degree of financial risk for the full costs of catastrophic health-care expenditures one is willing to assume (as in the so-called out-of-pocket maximum) and the relative amount of the required copays for a range of health-care services and products (doctor visits, lab tests, pharmacy prescriptions, etc.). Obviously, the health insurance plans that provide the highest level of insurance coverage of health-care costs are also those that have the highest insurance premiums—all other factors such as the age and smoking history of the insured being equal.

Among the American public, widely divergent preferences for the level of health insurance coverage reflect not only what health insurance consumers consider affordable but also the degree to which they are willing to risk the financial burden of unplanned health-care expenditures, as in "Why do I need gold standard health insurance plan, I hate going to the doctor?" (Blumberg et al., 2013). This is the rationale behind the ACA's tiered approach to standardized health insurance plans, otherwise known as the bronze, silver, gold, and platinum plans.

The second consideration, the array of benefits encompassed in health insurance coverage, refers to the health-care services and products that a given insurance plan will pay all or a part of as "allowable" expenditures. During the early decades of the growth of the private and dominantly not-for-profit health insurance industry (from the 1940s through the 1960s), the array of health insurance benefit coverage was restrictive with respect to the kinds of providers, services, and products covered (for example, only medical doctors for physician services as opposed to naturopaths) but wide open with respect to the specific providers chosen. However, since the mid-1960s, the kinds of providers, services, and products covered by health insurance have expanded almost exponentially, driven by a combination of technological innovation, health-care provider marketing, tax-subsidized health insurance benefits, and escalating consumer demands for health-care services and products. In essence, the widespread availability of health insurance (fostered by government tax and labor market policies as well as collective bargaining for health benefits) fueled the public demand for more health care and a broader array of health-care services, which in turn fueled the demand for both a broader array of health insurance benefits and more kinds of health insurance plans with different benefit packages, all catering to diverse preferences for health care (Weisbrod, 1991). In short, while in the 1950s and 1960s, it might have been possible to achieve a public and political consensus on a uniform set of comprehensive health-care benefits that would be essential for adequate financial protection, the evolvement of a consumer-oriented health-care economy in subsequent decades unleashed the full power of the nation's cultural, religious, and political heterogeneity as an obstacle to a national insurance plan with a standardized level of insurance protection and covered benefits.

The Boundaries of a Social Right to Health Care Imposed
by the Private Health Insurance Industry

A notable feature of the American version of the liberal welfare state is that its
two major social insurance funds, the Old-Age and Survivors Insurance
(OASI) benefit and the Medicare Hospital Insurance Trust Fund, were shaped
by the nation's insurance industry to be inadequate to the financial security
needs of the nation's older adults (J. Klein, 2003). With respect to the OASI
fund, the 1939 amendments to the Social Security Act established a cap on
survivors' benefits that would not exceed 80 percent of the wage laborer's average earnings and exempted from the definition of taxable wages employer
contributions to retirement, unemployment, or disability benefits, thus ensuring an underfunded OASI fund and the necessity of private-sector pension
funds that were a major source of the insurance industry's business revenue
(J. Klein, 2003). Essential to passage of the 1965 Medicare entitlement legislation were provisions that delegated Medicare program claims administration
to the private health insurance industry (a very lucrative arrangement) and
gaps in Medicare program coverage that would ensure the viability of a vibrant private supplementary insurance market (Berkowitz, 2008; Starr, 1982).
More recently, at the behest of the health insurance industry's influence in
Congress, the final version of the ACA was stripped of its public health insurance option as a condition of its passage (Noah, 2009).[7] In the sense that the
legislative past of health-care reform is indeed a prologue to the future (as
suggested by Berkowitz, 2008), it is difficult to imagine a more formidable
obstacle to a social right to health care *in the absence of a major role for private health insurance* than the $900 billion health insurance industry—an
industry that in 2013 spent $24 million in lobbying expenditures alone (Cen-
ter for Responsive Politics, 2014; CMS, 2014c).[8]

THE EMERGENT AMERICAN APPROACH TO THE FINANCING
OF A SOCIAL RIGHT TO HEALTH CARE: EMBEDDED SOCIAL
STRATIFICATION, HETEROGENEITY, AND PATH DEPENDENCE

The take-home points of the preceding discussion of the boundaries of
a realizable social right to health care, in light of the nation's social, economic, and political context, can be summarized as follows:

  1. The United States is not Sweden. Although egalitarian in its Jeffersonian ideals of civil and political citizenship, it is a nation that has a high

tolerance of social and economic inequalities that is justified by latent racism and enduring libertarian notions of unfettered equal opportunity, the myth of robust social mobility, and the prevalence of beliefs about individual origins of poverty and wealth. It is also a nation comprising a highly heterogeneous population with respect to race, ethnicity, religion, and deeply embedded cultural orientations toward health and health care. These contextual factors are formidable if not insurmountable obstacles to a single-tiered health-care system with the uniform array of health-care benefits that characterizes the Scandinavian model of health care.

2. By the late 1960s, the nation's employment-based insurance system and its new health-care entitlement programs (principally Medicare), in combination with technological innovations in health-care services and products, sophisticated health-care marketing, and the political clout of the health-care industry, had let the genie of rampant health-care consumerism and tax-subsidized health-care entrepreneurialism out of the bottle, thus precluding the possibility of a public consensus on an affordable and uniform set of comprehensive health-care benefits that could have served as the foundation of a general entitlement to health care.

3. Beginning with the New Deal legislation of the 1930s and ever more since, the private component of the American welfare state, represented by the insurance industry, has effectively used its deep pockets and ideological arsenal to set the limits of the public welfare state. Nowhere has this been more evident than in health-care entitlement legislation. While President Truman in 1945 could have realistically advanced a proposal for a social insurance fund for health care that was sufficiently comprehensive to preclude more than a secondary role for private health insurance, that moment passed with the nation's embracement of the employment-based health insurance during the 1950s. Simply put, the $900 billion private health insurance industry that rose to dominance after the Truman era is here to stay.

Although there are other formidable considerations, these are the principal contextual limits that shape the boundaries of what is feasible in health-care financing that will yield some version of a social right to health care for all Americans. The worst-case scenario for the form of this social right to health care, aside from the status quo of a piecemeal implementation of the ACA, is eminent health economist Uwe Reinhart's predicted vision of a three-tiered health-care system comprising a poorly funded public health-care tier that would provide a minimal standard of health services to the poor, a preferred provider network tier for the middle class, and "boutique" medicine tier for the elites (see "A Conversation," 2013). The best-case scenario for a far more equitable vision of health-care financing, which this book advances as both optimal and feasible in light of the four core health-care policy aims developed in chapter 4, is what amounts to a "soft" two-tiered health-care system—that is, a health-care system financed by (1) a universal social insurance fund that provides a basic scheme of health insurance benefits commensurate with adequate financial risk protection and the functional requisites of democratic citizenship and (2) a vibrant voluntary complementary insurance market that caters to individual and social class demands for more convenience and a broader array of health insurance benefits. While this vision of a hybrid social insurance/private complementary insurance approach might appear to be no more than an extension of the current system of financing health care for the nation's older adults, a kind of universal Medicare, there are three important differences:

1.   In contrast to Medicare as we know it, which is dominated by a traditional fee-for-service payment model for approved services, technologies, and treatments that fuels unnecessary health-care utilization and fragmented health care, the health-care financing mechanisms of the proposed universal social insurance fund would be integrated with an outcomes-based health-care delivery system, such as has already been advanced as essential to the future solvency of the current Medicare program and, to a limited extent, already implemented under the ACA (The Brookings Institution, 2014).

2.   Also in contrast to Medicare as we know it, there would be an individual and family household cap on out-of-pocket expenditures that is means tested—also akin to current proposals for Medicare reform that include a so-called catastrophic cap (The Brookings Institution, 2014).

3.   As a final contrast to the current version of Medicare, the "catastrophic cap" would be set at a level of income and assets that would preclude the necessity of purchasing private market supplemental insurance as a hedge against unaffordable health-care expenditures and medical bankruptcy. That is, the role of private supplemental insurance would be complementary (in the sense of providing a mechanism for the financing of a broader array of nonessential health-care services and a high standard of personal convenience for those who demand and are willing to pay

for it) rather than as the supplementary private component that is essential to realize an adequate level of health insurance risk protection and access to comprehensive health care.

In sum, what has been proposed is the broad outline of an approach to the financing of health care that is a credible alternative to the unrealizable egalitarian ideal of a wholly uniform comprehensive social insurance fund and the repugnant three-tiered approach that relegates the poor to minimalist and stigmatized health care. It is a rational approach to health-care financing that balances the desirability of a basic and adequate social right to health care with the twin realities of a nonegalitarian and heterogeneous society and an entrenched health insurance industry that thrives on both cultural diversity and social stratification. The next task of this chapter is to address whether the proposed approach is ideologically acceptable.

RECONCILING THE CORE HEALTH-CARE POLICY AIMS WITH A "SOFT" TWO-TIERED HEALTH-CARE SYSTEM

As defined here, a "soft" two-tiered health care system is one where the qualitative differences between the two levels of health care are not so extreme as to compromise either (1) equal and adequate financial risk protection in the event of catastrophic health-care expenditures or (2) the availability and quality of health care for health needs that are crucial to the normal range of human functioning (as defined by Daniels, 2008, and elaborated upon in chapter 4). A "soft" two-tiered system is also one that is not strictly reflective of differences in social class or other aspects of social stratification but to a large extent reflects nonhierarchical differences in individual preferences for investments in personal health care, health insurance risk protection, the scope of health-care services available, and the emphasis on personal convenience relative to cost. A "soft" two-tiered system reflects the phenomenon that many of us (irrespective of race, income, education, or any other attribute associated with advantage) as a matter of personal preference would gladly trade the occasional inconvenience of a crowded doctor's waiting room or a limited selection of health-care providers for lower health insurance costs and the chance to spend our money on other things. It also accommodates a significant role for private health insurance as means of siphoning off consumption demands for an ever broader array of health services and more convenience under the guise of "a reasonable standard of basic health care" that would in the end make public health insurance an unaffordable entitlement (Gruber, 2009). Finally, because the lower tier of a "soft" two-tiered system is neither exclusively nor dominantly composed of the poor and marginalized of society, the social stigma attached to two-tiered health care is greatly minimized. This is very different from the more pejorative conceptualization of a two-tiered health-care system where the low income and poor possess a far more limited entitlement to health care than the middle and upper classes, as represented by the distinction between private insurance coverage and Medicaid ("A New Prescription," 2011).

With this definition in mind, it is evident that "soft" two-tiered systems are quite prevalent among modern democracies with universal health insurance coverage. For example, included among the many OECD member nations with a significant role of private health insurance as a supplement to public health insurance coverage (defined as paying for services that are not covered by the public health insurance plan, such as dental care and pharmaceutical products) are the Netherlands (covering 89 percent of the population), Israel (80 percent), Canada (68 percent), Australia (34 percent), and Finland (14 percent) (OECD, 2013a). Less prevalent among OECD member states is a strong preference among the public for the use of private insurance as a means of gaining faster and more convenient private-sector access to medical services where there are waiting times in public systems. In fact, some countries (like Canada) have regulations that prohibit the use of private insurance for publicly insured medical and hospital services to preclude the eventual development of a two-tiered system with inferior services for the low income and poor (Hurley & Guindon, 2008).[9] While it is unlikely that such a restricted use for private health insurance would be either legislatively or constitutionally feasible in the United States, such government policies do speak to the importance of sustaining a high standard of access and care quality in the publicly funded health-care services, which is only possible to the extent (1) that the public health insurance plan is adequately funded so as to preclude the necessity of private health insurance as a means of accessing essential health care and (2) private health insurance is treated as a commodity rather than as an extension of a public entitlement to a higher standard of health care.

Framed by these considerations, in the next section of the chapter, I present the essential features of a two-tiered health-care financing scheme that funds a basic scheme of comprehensive health-care services as a social right of citizenship, while preserving a place for private health insurance for the health-care services and products that are classified as desirable rather than essential.

Tier I: Limited Entitlement Social Insurance Trust Fund for Basic Health Care

Expenditures for preventative, curative, rehabilitative, and adaptive health services, technologies, and products that are deemed essential to the realization and preservation of the normal range of functioning will be covered under a compulsory social insurance fund under amendments to the Social Security Act that will (1) remove the age and income criteria from existing health-care entitlements and (2) merge the separate parts of Medicare into a single social insurance fund for health care. Copayments for covered health-care expenditures are permissible but subject to an individual and family household cap commensurate with the elimination of income-based disparities in health-care access and quality. Both covered services and the specific rules for copayments and caps will be established through evidence-based public deliberation and congressional action, as guided by three policy imperatives: (1) adequate and equal risk protection, (2) optimal amelioration of disparities in health-care access and quality, and (3) fiscal sustainability.

Tier II: The Unsubsidized Voluntary Private Health Insurance Market

Expenditures for health-care services, technologies, and products that are not deemed essential to the realization and preservation of the normal range of functioning will be the province of individual out-of-pocket payments and the voluntary private health insurance market, as will be the individual and family household copayments for health-care services deemed allowable under the public basic health-care plan. The only restrictions placed on the private health insurance market (other than those necessary for consumer protection, the fostering and protection of competitive markets, and health information security) are (1) those that will be necessary to ensure fee and reimbursement parity between the public health-care plan and private insurance plans with respect to equivalent health-care services, technologies, and products and (2) the disallowance of either direct or indirect tax subsidies for the costs of individual or

group private health insurance coverage, except where it is deemed beneficial to the accessibility, quality, and solvency of publicly funded health-
care entitlements.

Explanations and Caveats

This two-tiered approach to the financing of health care is based on two
primary considerations. The first is the practical impossibility of achieving
a high standard of uniformity of health insurance coverage, health-care access, and health-care quality in a heterogeneous and complexly stratified
society inhabiting a vast continent. The second is the entrenched health
insurance industry and the related culture of health-care consumerism
that is also deeply embedded in American society. As argued in this
chapter and also previously by Harvard University health-care economist
Jonathan Gruber (2009, p. 12), the best plausible alternative is an explicit
two-tiered health-care system, whereby society sets minimum standards
in the scope of public health-care coverage, access, and quality but then
allows individuals to purchase higher levels of coverage, access, or quality
using their own resources (either directly or through a vibrant private insurance market). Where this specific proposal for a two-tiered system goes
beyond Gruber's explicit two-tiered approach is its insistence on a high
threshold regarding what is defined as minimum in each of these areas—
in essence, a scope of health-care coverage commensurate with (1) the realization and preservation of the normal range of functioning and (2) a level
of insurance protection sufficient to eliminate income-based disparities
in health-care access and quality.

Under the proposed scheme, copayments have three crucial functions.
The first is to inhibit the use of unnecessary health care, consistent with
findings from decades of research on health consumption behavior (Shi &
Singh, 2001). The second is to promote equity of financial burden for those
health-care services that are deemed essential. One aspect of this is
obvious—that is, copayments in general can be adjusted to income level,
thus to a limited extent placing a higher burden of payment for essential
health care on the more affluent. Another way that copayments might be
used to promote equity is less obvious, such as having income-adjusted
copayments for long-term care services at the older age ranges, thus incentivizing adults to invest in personal resources for long-term care needs during their working years and easing some of the burden for long-term care

expenditures on the younger generations. The third function of copayments is to promote the fiscal sustainability of the social insurance fund for health care by placing a threshold on the tax-subsidized component of health-care expenditures.

With respect to the private insurance market, or what might be termed the upper-tier component of the health-care financing proposal, it should be noted that unlike Canada, there is no specific restriction against private health insurance for health-care services that are covered under the public plan, thus allowing for some level of more rapid or convenient access to health services for those willing to purchase private insurance with those benefits. This is viewed as a pragmatic concession to the convergence of an entrenched health insurance industry and the nation's weak commitment to egalitarian health care. However, the mandated fee and payment parity for equivalent services between public and private insurance is likely to have broader political appeal among the general public, and it goes a long way toward constraining the extent to which there is disparity between publicly insured and privately insured essential health services. Although the broad-scale elimination of tax subsidies for private health insurance coverage will be difficult to accomplish politically due to the power of the health insurance industry, the public is unlikely to be particularly averse to this provision to the extent that the public health insurance benefits are affordable and comprehensive. Finally, putting in place a caveat for the use of tax subsidies for specific kinds of private health insurance that lend viability to the sustainability of public health-care entitlements (like long-term care insurance) adds some essential flexibility to the overall two-tiered approach.

PROSPECTS FOR THE EVOLVEMENT OF THE TWO-TIERED APPROACH

In early 2013, conservative health policy pundit John Goodman published an online essay in *Forbes.com* that predicted the evolution of a two-tiered health-care system, aided and abetted by the ACA, that would be akin to an "even worse" version of the Canadian health-care system, by which he meant a system that employs long lines and wait times to ration care for average Americans and concierge care for those able and willing to pay for it. The basis of his dire prediction was the crisis-level imbalance between supply and demand that will result from adding 32 million Americans covered by health insurance against a dwindling supply of physicians—as evidenced by the growing share of physicians electing to practice as salaried employ-ees of hospital systems and the number of disenchanted physicians choos-ing early retirement. Goodman cites as his reference case the experience of the pre-ACA health-care reform experiment of the Massachusetts Com-monwealth Care plan, which he describes in disastrous terms. Goodman's narrative of the future of health-care reform in America is crisp, convinc-ing, and chilling. The problem with his analysis is that he uses the suppos-edly failed experiment with universal health insurance coverage in Massa-chusetts as his example.

In fact, during the first five years of health-care reform in Massachu-setts, the numbers of uninsured in the state declined between 60 and 70 percent while actual wait times for family and internal medicine medi-cal appointments remained basically unchanged—this according to data from the Massachusetts Medical Society (Gruber, 2011). Also, public opin-ion surveys conducted jointly by the *Boston Globe* and Harvard School of Public Health five years after the implementation of the Massachusetts health reform showed that (1) 68 percent of state residents saw the health reform law as successful and (2) only 14 percent viewed the health reform law as detrimental to their health care (Blendon et al., 2014). In sum, the pursuit of publicly subsidized universal health insurance is not synony-mous with an inevitable progression toward a two-tiered system of health care characterized by a low standard of health care for either the general public or the poor. The question is whether a social insurance approach for an adequate first-tier basic comprehensive health-care entitlement is (1) fiscally feasible and (2) in the long run politically viable.

The Fiscal Feasibility of a Social Insurance Fund for a Basic Comprehensive Health-Care Entitlement

The term *social insurance for health care* can refer to a health-care financ-ing approach that has multiple social insurance funds for health care that together cover a national population or to a single national insur-ance fund. As used here, the term *social insurance for health care* refers to a system of mandatory contributions to a single national insurance risk pool that funds a core set of health-care coverage benefits inclusive of physician services, diagnostic technology, pharmaceuticals, and hos-pital care—more commonly known as the single-payer system (White, 2009).

While advocates of the single-payer system for the United States generally point to the savings that can be realized by the elimination of the costly administrative bureaucracies of the multipayer health insurance industry, the ability to negotiate fair and consistent provider fees, and the opportunities to coordinate and streamline care under a single-payment umbrella, the findings from comparative health systems research suggest that the savings from single-payer versus multipayer approaches to health-care financing are both modest and highly variable (Glied, 2009). Also, the proposed preservation of a private insurance market will to some extent limit the ability to reduce administrative costs associated with insurance claims management. These cautionary notes aside, it is still likely that in the context of the United States where both the administrative costs associated with the insurance industry and the perverse incentives that lead to higher health-care prices abound, substantial savings can be realized with the consolidation of the largest share of health-care needs and expenditures into a single insurance fund (Anderson & Hussey, 2004).

As to the specific mechanisms of financing, University of Massachusetts economist Gerald Friedman's analysis of the single-payer health-care plan introduced annually to Congress by Rep. John Conyers (D-MI) serves as a plausible example. Known as the Expanded and Improved Medicare for All Act (HR 676), this legislation proposes to replace the "three-legged stool" of employment-based private insurance for workers and their dependents, Medicaid for the poor, and Medicare for older adults with a social insurance fund that provides comprehensive health care for all Americans. Friedman makes a credible case for the financial feasibility of the Medicare for All Act's funding scheme, a strategy that would in its essence combine progressive taxation with the elimination of employment-based insurance tax subsidies as the primary revenue sources and thereby eliminate the regressive sources of health insurance financing, particularly employer and employee contributions to health insurance premiums. At the individual and household level, Friedman's analysis predicts that this health-care financing approach would yield a substantial net reduction in the combination of out-of-pocket and health insurance premium expenditures for households with incomes under $220,00/year in 2014 dollars, with only 5 percent of American households paying more (Friedman, 2013). While Friedman's analysis of the single-payer approach advocated in Conyers's Medicare for All Act does not consider the impact of the retention of a vibrant private health insurance market for supplemental benefits, analysis of the two-tiered single-payer/private supplemental insurance market that is prevalent among OECD countries does not suggest the two are incompatible (Hussey & Anderson, 2003).

Public Attitudes Toward Single-Payer Financing

Contrary to political rhetoric that conflates skepticism of government with the idea of a national health insurance, as the employment-based health insurance system has devolved, there seems to have been a shift among the American public toward majority support for abandonment of the employment-based insurance system for some version of a single-payer system—with the margin of majority support depending on the framing of the question. In this regard, the question wording and results from a nationally representative survey of American adults sponsored by the Associated Press during the months preceding the 2008 presidential election

QUESTION 1

(LISTED AS ITEM ISS114 ON THE SURVEY INSTRUMENT): WHICH COMES CLOSEST TO YOUR VIEW?

The United States should continue the current health insurance system in which most people get their health insurance from private employers, but some people have no insurance [34%]

The United States should adopt a universal health insurance program in which everyone is covered under a program like Medicare that is run by the government and financed by taxpayers [65%]

QUESTION 2

(LISTED AS ISS115 ON THE SURVEY INSTRUMENT):

Do you consider yourself a supporter of a single-payer health care system, that is a national health plan financed by taxpayers in which all Americans would get their insurance from a single government plan, or not? [Yes 54%] [No 44%]

are illuminating (the questions posed are cited verbatim, with the response percentages in bold).[10]

First and foremost, it is evident that between 54 percent and 65 percent of the public support the idea of a single-payer system as an alternative to the pre-ACA status quo. This is in dramatic contrast to the weak support of single-payer system among the American public at the beginning of the decade (from surveys conducted between 1998 and 2002), which varied between 36 and 42 percent in favor of a single-payer plan (Blendon et al., 2006).[11] Second, the margin of majority support is significantly larger when the term *like Medicare* is used to describe the single-payer system, which speaks to the Medicare program's political popularity and its power as a concrete example of a national social insurance entitlement to health care funded by progressive taxation.[12] That said, the level of public support for a single-payer plan to the exclusion of the option of obtaining health insurance coverage through private insurance appears to be much softer. In this respect, a Kaiser Family Foundation poll conducted in 2009 that contrasted "Having a national health plan—or single-payer plan—in which all Americans would get their insurance from a single government plan" with "Creating a government-administered public health insurance option *similar to Medicare* to compete with private insurance plans" is particularly instructive. The single-payer alone alternative, when contrasted with a single-payer plan that would need to compete with private insurance options, received only 40 percent favorable support, whereas the competitive market alternative garnered 58 percent approval (Kaiser Health Tracking Poll, 2009). This finding is also consistent with the observation that the majority share of Americans favoring a single-payer approach appears composed of those who are just "somewhat in favor" as well as those who are "strongly in favor" (Kaiser Health Tracking Poll, 2009). These are points that will be revisited as the most plausible paths to a single-payer system are considered.

Of equal importance to the prospects for a national single-payer plan is the definitive and historically unprecedented shift toward majority support of the idea of national health insurance as an alternative to the status quo of a mixed public/private approach *among physicians* that occurred over the most recent decade. In 2002, researchers from the Indiana School of Medicine conducted a random sample study of physicians listed in the American Medical Association Masterfile and found that 49 percent favored national health insurance, a development of seismic significance in and of itself. When the survey was replicated in 2007 and then published in the prestigious *Annals of Internal Medicine*, the share of physicians in favor of national health insurance had moved to 59 percent (Carroll & Ackerman, 2008). Significantly, the wording used in the survey question was "national health insurance," which, unlike "universal health care," clearly connotes federalized single-payer financing. It seems likely that this shift toward acceptance of national health insurance among physicians, historically its most powerful and vociferous opponents, represents a combination of several factors: disillusionment with a health-care system dominated by a bureaucratic cacophony of third-party payers, growth in the size of the uninsured population, and the different sentiments of younger generations of physicians socialized to the idea of universal health insurance as a common public good if not a social right. The shifting gender balance in the medical profession is also a likely factor, with women tending to be more supportive of mandated universal health (University of Delaware, 2012). With respect to the likelihood of the growing groundswell of support of a national single-payer plan among physicians being sustained, the advocacy of a single-payer approach to health-care financing reform by the American Medical Student Association (AMSA) suggests that it will be (AMSA, 2008).

In sum, the era of health-care reform that witnessed the emergence of the ACA had within it a remarkable and historically unprecedented convergence of support for a national single-payer health insurance plan from both a majority share of the public and the medical profession. To the extent that a single-payer plan is identified as an expanded version of Medicare or as a voluntary option to private health insurance, it appears more likely to garner a critical mass of public support. That said, it is also very clear that despite the growing appeal of a single-payer approach among both the public and the medical profession, there remains a strong level of preference for the choice and flexibility associated with the option of choosing private insurance.

Alternative Paths to Single-Payer Health Insurance

When asked during a 2013 PBS-sponsored media luncheon whether the ACA was in effect a step toward the eventual goal of a single-payer system, then Senate Majority Leader Harry Reid (D-NV) said, "Yes, yes. Absolutely, yes" (Roy, 2013). Reid's stunningly frank reply took his audience by surprise, because among the frequent attacks on the ACA is the accusation that it is intended as the first step toward a single-payer government-run insurance plan. Reid's abandonment of utterly any pretense to the contrary, particularly at the point where his political party's control of the Senate hung on the balance, is tantamount to his party's open declaration of war on the future of the health insurance industry's grip on the nation's health-care system—something that Reid must certainly have known.

Considering the political stakes, why was Reid willing to be so blunt in his embracement of a single-payer insurance plan as the ultimate future for the country? First, of course, would be his genuine belief in the inevitability of the nation's progression toward some version of a single-payer system. Second is his insider's knowledge that the partisan battles over every step of the ACA's implementation are in reality a proxy war over the idea of health insurance coverage as an entitlement of American citizenship—a war that Reid could reasonably conclude had already been won with the passage of the ACA in 2010. This is evidenced by the fact that by March 2014, four years after the ACA was signed into law, those Americans in favor of repealing the ACA were outnumbered by those in favor of retaining it by a margin of 2:1 (Kaiser Family Foundation Health Tracking Poll, 2014).[13] It is also the case that over the past three decades, the mainstream public opinion polls have shown that the majority of the public have continued to believe that it is the responsibility of the government to make sure that all Americans have health insurance coverage (Blendon & Benson, 2001; Gallup Poll, 2014). In sum, Reid had ample reason to be confident that he could blurt out what he saw as the truth about the ACA—that is, the ACA being but a very large interim step toward a single-payer system as opposed to the final version of an adequate social right to health care.

Assuming Reid is correct about not only the plausibility but also the inevitability of a national single-payer health insurance plan, how might it become realized? It is suggested here that there are three possible paths. The first is in some respects the most simple path but also the most politically unlikely, which is a sweeping legislation that would expand the Medicare program's health insurance coverage to all ages—some version of the so-called Medicare for All approach as represented in the congressional legislation (HR 626) introduced by Rep. Conyers annually and also killed in committee annually. Although the notion of Medicare for all is the most appealing and intuitive to the general public, it is also a radical expansion of the welfare state that, as of 2013, garnered only limited support even among congressional Democrats (when introduced in 2013, Rep. Conyers's

HR 626 had only sixty cosponsors among the 199 Democrats elected to the House of Representatives). As dismal as this might seem in the near future, at the point that Congress is forced to grapple with fundamental Medicare reform necessitated by the collapse of the Medicare Hospital Insurance Trust Fund (which the 2014 Medicare Board of Trustees Report predicts will occur by 2030),[14] the financial solvency of Medicare might well involve its becoming a fund that pools the insurance risks of the entire population and not just older adults (Friedman, 2013).

A second path, more incremental, is the introduction and gradual expansion of a single-payer public option—the provision of the original ACA legislation that was removed at the behest of the health insurance industry lobby.[15] As Congress turns from the futile and theatrical partisan battles over the repeal of the ACA to the public's preference for improvements, it reopens the door to reintroducing the public option provision that is popular among liberals in exchange for other kinds of concessions more to the liking of the health-care policy priorities of conservatives (such as tort reform). Such negotiations are not only quite possible but also very likely at the point when repeal of the ACA loses its traction as a credible political ploy. Despite claims to the contrary by the political right, the public option component of the ACA was actually quite popular—garnering an average of 57 percent favorable support across twenty-eight public opinion polls conducted at the time the public option provision of the ACA was being debated (Politifact.com, 2012). The health insurance industry and the AMA,[16] both vigorous opponents of the original ACA's inclusion of a public health insurance option, contended that the ability of the federal government to use its market clout to lower health-care prices would eventually lead to its ability to dominate the health insurance market through its lower costs and thus usher in a single-payer plan system (Mankiw, 2009). They were correct in their arguments that a Medicare-like public option could become a kind of Trojan horse for a progression to a single-payer system, and to the extent that Congress can be swayed by public opinion as it reopens negotiations over revisions to the ACA, it remains so.

The third plausible path to a single-payer system is a populist state-by-state single-payer movement that both demonstrates the advantages of a single-payer plan in access and cost control and energizes a national dialogue on the case for a "Medicare for All" social insurance fund for health care. Although several states have had either popular initiatives on the ballot or legislation introduced that would create a state-based single-payer plan (including Hawaii, New York, Oregon, Washington, California, Pennsylvania, and Ohio), the most recent near miss of a state actually enacting a state-based single-payer plan occurred in Vermont between 2011 and 2014. Its lessons, though, are sobering.

Based on the findings from a financial feasibility study by a Harvard University health economist that the Vermont legislature had authorized in 2010 that predicted substantially reduced health expenditures under a single-payer public plan (Hsiao, 2011), in 2011 the Vermont legislature passed legislation that established a path to universal enrollment in Green Mountain Care for all Vermont residents by the year 2017—in essence, a plan based on a quasi-competitive public and private partnership that allowed residents to choose Green Mountain Care as either their primary health insurance or the option to enroll in employment-based insurance with Green Mountain Care as secondary insurance (State of Vermont, 2014). Interestingly, this hybrid approach to a single-payer plan fit with data from national polling that indicated a preference for a single-payer option that is competitive with and accommodates the choice of private health insurance coverage (Kaiser Health Tracking Poll, 2009). However, in late 2014, Vermont Governor Peter Shumlin announced that the Green Mountain Care initiative had to be abandoned. In doing so, Shumlin cited findings from his staff that contradicted the optimistic projections of cost savings of 25 percent with estimated costs savings estimates of less than 2 percent, along with a projected tax increase of as much as 11.5 percent to employers and 9.5 percent for individuals (McDonough, 2015). A more critical look at the reasons for Shumlin's abandonment of the Vermont single-payer plan suggests that Vermont's overall health-care spending would have declined under the plan, as would have health-care expenditures for families with annual incomes under $150,000. In addition, the tax increases for employers and individuals that caused Shumlin to abandon his support for the plan would have been offset by reductions in health insurance premium costs, but these reductions would have been largely invisible to most workers and too heavy a lift politically (McDonough, 2015). Clearly, the lesson learned in Vermont is that while political vision and financial feasibility are necessary to the enactment of a single-payer plan, these are insufficient in the absence of a sophisticated public information strategy that informs everyday health consumers and voters about the ways in which they pay more for their health care under employment-based insurance than through public financing.

CONCLUDING REMARKS

While this chapter makes the general case for the social and political feasibility of a two-tiered health-care system, one that provides robust first-tier comprehensive health-care coverage as a basic social right, its falls short of predicting any particular path to its evolvement or a timeline to its realization. The best that can be said is that crisis promotes change, as it did with the emergence of the ACA in the wake of a deep recession and the failures of employment-based insurance, and that the next foreseeable crisis in health care will be upon us as the massive Medicare program can no longer pays its bills—now projected to happen by 2030 (Board of Trustees Medicare Hospital Insurance Trust Fund, 2014). This may seem like a distant point in the future, but it really is not—not when considering the kinds of changes that will need to take place in the nation's orientation toward sustainable health-care financing to avert this crisis.

The sense of urgency for the next stage of health-care reform, although it should come from Congress and the next occupant of the White House, may come instead from the state governments struggling to sustain even their pre-ACA commitments to health-care entitlements in the face of rising health-care costs. This could tip the balance toward the adoption of single-payer reforms in progressive leaning states like California and Vermont that have a history of near misses with single-payer reform legislation.[17] On the other hand, as suggested by Harvard School of Public Health policy scholar John McDonough, it may be that as the costs of Medicare, Medicaid, and the ACA health insurance purchase subsidies balloon under the nation's mixed public and private financing system, the nation's political leaders may at last grasp the "inanity of running multiple complex systems to insure different classes of Americans" (McDonough, 2015, p. 1585). Whatever the ultimate path to some version of a single-payer system, I believe that Harry Reid was correct in his conviction that the ACA, far from being an alternative to a single-payer system, is but a crucial step toward its evolvement.

Chapter Six

A PRINCIPLED APPROACH TO ESSENTIAL
HEALTH-CARE DELIVERY SYSTEM REFORMS

The task of this chapter is to establish the general features of health-care delivery reforms that will both fulfill the core criteria of equitability, sustainability, and feasibility and be adaptable to the two-tiered health-care financing structure described in chapter 5. To recap, as defined in chapter 5, a two-tiered health-care financing structure refers to an approach to national health-care financing that provides a universal first-tier public health insurance plan that is funded through a social insurance trust fund for basic health care and then a second tier of unsubsidized voluntary health insurance coverage for health care that is considered more than basic—that is, health care that might be desirable but not deemed essential to the realization and preservation of the normal range of functioning. It was emphasized that the two-tiered system of health-care financing would be characterized as a "soft" two-tiered system, meaning that the system is one where the qualitative differences between the two levels of health care are not so extreme as to compromise either (1) equal and adequate financial risk protection in the event of catastrophic health-care expenditures or (2) the availability and quality of health care for health needs that are crucial to the normal range of human functioning (as defined by Daniels, 2008, and elaborated upon in chapter 4). A "soft" two-tiered system is also one in which differences between the first and second tiers are not defined primarily by social class so much as by nonhierarchical differences in individual preferences for investments in personal health care, health insurance risk protection, the scope of nonessential health-care services available, and the emphasis on personal convenience relative to cost.[1]

This chapter is based on three core assumptions. First, the provider component of the nation's health-care system will continue its trend toward consolidation into large health-care systems that are horizontally and vertically integrated, presenting both dangers and opportunities for the future of health-care delivery reforms. Second, there is no clear dividing line between health-care financing reform and health-care delivery reform; health-care delivery reforms will necessarily involve payment systems that will better align financial incentives with cost control, quality of care, and health outcomes. Third, in health-care delivery, resource constraints are not necessarily a barrier to innovation but paradoxically can serve as the very foundation of innovation.

SOME ESSENTIAL CONTEXTUAL CONSIDERATIONS IN HEALTH-CARE SYSTEM DELIVERY REFORM

The Geography of Health-Care Disparities

Although preceding chapters of this book have focused on disparities in health-care access and quality by race and class, in many respects, disparities in health care by geography are more pronounced (Goodman et al., 2010). Because access to primary care and hospital services are widely accepted as crucial health system determinants of health outcomes, it is these two geographic disparities that are highlighted.

Geographic Disparities in Primary Care Physicians

A cornerstone of the ACA's health-care delivery reform strategy is to increase the number of primary care physicians (PCPs) available to provide care for both the newly insured patients and the insured population. Toward this end, decades of evidence suggests that in both developed and developing countries, enhanced access to primary care is associated with better population health outcomes, decreased rates of hospital and emergency department usage, and the mitigation of socioeconomic disadvantages on health (Shi, 2012). However, as with other core health-care resources, the supply of PCPs is grossly maldistributed relative to resource equity and need. With respect to resource equity between states, the number of PCPs per 100,000 persons ranges from a high of 135 in Massachusetts to a low of 63 in Oklahoma. The states with the highest numbers of PCPs relative to population size are concentrated almost entirely in the Mid-Atlantic and Northeast states, while states with the lowest levels of PCP supply tend to be in the South and in the Mountain West regions, which in significant part reflects the tendency of PCPs to be located in urban counties (Cunningham, 2011). Other factors that are associated with a higher number of PCPs relative to the population size include (predictably enough) lower numbers of uninsured patients and lower poverty rates (Cunningham, 2011). Insomuch as higher levels of poverty and higher numbers of the uninsured are associated with poorer population health, these determinants of PCP resourcing run completely contrary to population health needs. While there is no generally agreed-upon minimum PCP to population ratio, the Health Resources and Services Administration (HRSA), as the federal agency charged with the task of determining critical areas for targeted health-care infrastructure investments, defines a primary care Health Professional Shortage Area (HPSA) as a local area having fewer than twenty-nine PCPs per 100,000 persons. Using this figure as the threshold for a severe shortage of PCPs, as of 2014, there were 6,100 designated primary care HPSAs in the nation (HRSA, 2015). Clearly, any substantively meaningful reforms of the nation's health-care delivery system must significantly reduce this key indicator of geographic disparities in PCP resources.

Geographic Disparities in Hospital Resources

One of the hallmarks of the American health-care system is the remarkable degree of variation in hospital resources, typically measured as the number of acute care hospital beds per 1,000 persons. At the state level, that number varies from a high of 4.9 beds per 1,000 in South Dakota to a low of 1.7 beds per 1,000 in the state of Oregon (Kaiser Family Foundation State Health Facts, 2013). That noted, it is not the differences in the raw number of hospital beds per 1,000 that matter with respect to access to critical health-care resources so much as factors such as the distribution of beds in high-quality hospitals and also the distribution of hospital beds by forms of hospital ownership. For example, in states like Oregon with both high-quality hospitals and shorter length of hospital stays, fewer hospital beds per 1,000 are needed to achieve more optimal population health outcomes. Oregon's hospitals are also dominantly public or not-for-profit, which generally translates to better access to care for low-income and uninsured populations (Thorpe et al., 2000). However, if the ownership status of hospital beds is considered, then a very different picture emerges with respect to the national distribution of hospital beds. For example, in states like Nevada, Tennessee, Oklahoma, Texas, and Florida, with a high concentration of for-profit hospitals, the numbers of public and nonprofit hospital beds per 1,000 are well below the national average. In Nevada, there are .8 public or nonprofit hospital beds per 1,000, against the national average of 2.1 per 1,000 (Kaiser Family Foundation State Health Facts, 2013).

Significantly, there is also a clear relationship between the geographic distribution of public and nonprofit hospital beds and the level of income inequality. That is, there is a positive correlation between the state levels of income inequality and the share of hospital beds that are owned by for-profit entities. When there is a high level of income inequality in a given state, that state is more likely to have a larger share of its hospital resources under for-profit ownership and control.[2] There is also a relationship between the political embracement of for-profit hospital care and a high level of tolerance for lack of access to health care for the low income and poor. For example, of the five states with the highest share of their hospitals under for-profit ownership (Nevada, Tennessee, Oklahoma, Texas, and Florida), as of year 5 of the ACA's implementation, all but Nevada had declined to expand Medicaid coverage to the low-income uninsured, despite the ACA's provision of federal funds that would have enabled them to do so (Kaiser Family Foundation, 2015).

There is also a troubling relationship between racial segregation, the geography of poor-quality hospitals, and racial disparities in health outcomes. For example, in a national study of coronary artery bypass graft (CABG) surgery outcomes among 173,925 Medicare patients, it was found that nonwhite patients had 33 percent higher risk-adjusted mortality rates after CABG surgery than white patients and that differences in hospital quality explained 35 percent of the observed disparity in mortality rates (Rangrass et al., 2013). It has also been shown that African Americans living in the most segregated areas of the nation's urban landscape are between 41 and 96 percent more likely than white patients to undergo surgery at low-quality hospitals, even when there is spatial proximity to high-quality hospitals (Dimick et al., 2013).

Disparities in the Usual Sources of Care, the Quality of Care,
and Unmet Health Needs by Race and Class

For racial minorities and those at the margin economically, there is a kind
of devil's triangle of interrelated health-care disparities that is promulgated
by the structure of the nation's health-care delivery system, represented by
three indicators: disparities in the usual source of care, in the quality of
provider communication, and in unmet health-care needs.

Disparities in the usual source of care. It is well established that individuals and groups with a usual source of health care experience better health
outcomes than those who do not and also have superior preventative health
care (AHRQ, 2014a; Corbie-Smith et al., 2002), as opposed to health care
that is provided on an episodic basis by a haphazardly selected urgent care
clinic or an overcrowded hospital emergency department. Although improved health insurance coverage substantially increases the likelihood of
having a usual source of health care, even four years after the implementation of the ACA, African Americans, Native Americans/Alaska Natives,
and Hispanics are substantially less likely to report having a usual source
of ongoing care than are whites (AHRQ, 2014a).

The same is true of low-income individuals and groups, with the poor
and low income being substantially less likely to have a usual source of
health care (with 78 percent of the poor having a usual source of care compared to 92 percent of persons with high income) (AHRQ, 2014a, p. 241).

Provider communication. While there are many measures of quality of
care, there is none more significant or in many respects more challenging
than patient and provider communication, which is pivotal to a shared
understanding of patients' health problems and health-care needs, the range
of optimal treatment options and related risks and benefits, and patients'
sense of empowerment and confidence in their provider that facilitates
engagement in care and treatment adherence. A critical quality deficit of the
current fragmented health-care delivery system is the extent to which race
and income both continue to play a large role in the extent to which patients
are likely to experience negative communications with their health-care
providers. Although the overall share of patients reporting poor communication with their health-care providers declined significantly between
2000 and 2010, as of 2010, both African Americans and Hispanics were
about 44 percent more likely to report poor communication with their

health-care providers, with low-income patients across racial groups also reporting a substantially higher likelihood of poor communication with their providers (AHRQ, 2014a).

Unmet health-care needs. It has been well established that race and class both play a role in unmet health needs, defined typically as either the delay or failure to gain access to needed health care (Institute of Medicine, 2002). For example, in one comprehensive study of 32,374 adults that considered several core indicators of unmet health needs, investigators found that low-income persons (relative to high-income persons and controlling for race) were 58 percent more likely not to access needed medical care, two times more likely not to have a prescription filled, 77 percent more likely to delay needed mental health care, and 65 percent more likely to delay needed dental care (Shi & Stevens, 2005). It was also found, consistent with the disadvantages associated with Medicaid coverage discussed in chapter 3, that persons with public health insurance coverage were also substantially less likely to access needed health, mental health, and dental care relative to persons with private health insurance. The relationship between race and unmet health needs was shown to be a complex one that was mediated by the prevalence of impediments to health-care access or access risk factors (low income, not having health insurance, and lacking a regular source of care), with all three nonwhite groups included in the study (Asians, Hispanics, and African Americans) having high levels of all three health-care access risk factors (Shi & Stevens, 2005).

Geographic Variations in Health-Care Expenditures

Another hallmark of the American health-care system that speaks to its incredibly diverse and seemingly haphazard delivery system is the extent to which there is wide geographic variation in health-care expenditures that are unrelated to either population characteristics or health outcomes. Indeed, one of the central rationales for the preference of a privatized approach to health-care delivery is the idea that in health care, as in other sectors of the economy, competition will consistently produce superior products (better health-care outcomes) at lower cost. While decades of research on the American health-care system, including cross-national health system studies, have debunked the myth that privatized health-care delivery promotes cost and quality-based competition in a way that yields collective population health benefits, the illusion of doing more to privatize health care as the panacea to rising health-care costs persists.

The most comprehensive data on the geographic variations in health-care expenditures that are unrelated to either population characteristics or more optimal health outcomes come from the Dartmouth Atlas of Health Care, a two-decade-old project carried out by the Dartmouth Institute for Health Policy and Clinical Practice. For example, in 2012, the variation in total annual Medicare program expenditures per beneficiary (and controlling for price, age, race, and sex) ranged from a high of $14,165 in Miami, Florida, to a low of $7,028 in Grand Junction, Colorado—a difference of $7,137 or more than the total spent per beneficiary in a lower-cost location. The number of expected years of healthy life expectancy after age sixty-five in Florida and Colorado is virtually identical at 15.4 versus 15.3 years; thus, it cannot be concluded that somehow doubling the Medicare expenditures per beneficiary yields any net benefits in health outcomes (CDC, 2013a; Dartmouth Institute for Health Policy and Clinical Practice, 2012).

Moreover, in their comprehensive review of the evidence on the quality of health-care differences between low Medicare spending and high Medicare spending regions of the country, the Dartmouth Atlas researchers concluded that (1) differences in spending between regions were explained almost entirely by differences in the volume of services provided, (2) Medicare beneficiaries in high-spending regions do not receive either more "effective care" or more "preference-sensitive" care, and (3) higher spending does not result in better health-care outcomes, such as survival following a heart attack or optimal recovery from a hip fracture (Fisher et al., 2009).

Finally, if increased emphasis on private-sector solutions to rising health-care costs were an effective policy strategy, we should expect to see lower health-care expenditures per beneficiary in states with the largest share of their hospital systems under for-profit ownership. Quite the opposite is true; annual Medicare expenditures per beneficiary are actually substantially higher than the national average in nine of the ten states with the largest shares of hospital beds under for-profit ownership (Dartmouth Institute for Health Policy and Clinical Practice, 2012; Kaiser Family Foundation State Health Facts, 2013). This observation is consistent with prior research that shows that for-profit hospital ownership is associated with higher and not lower Medicare costs (Silverman et al., 1999), which may be attributable to their emphasis on service profitability over clinical need or added value to health outcomes (Horwitz, 2005). That the concentration and growth of for-profit hospitals is strongest in those regions in the country with higher levels of income inequality suggests that there is geography of disparities in needs-based health care that is worsening under the current political economy of health care.

The Consolidation of Hospital Systems Into Vertically Integrated Health-Care Networks

Among the institutional legacies of the political economy of health care in America over the recent decades is the emergence of multihospital systems as a replacement for what had been a national landscape dotted with thousands of independently owned and operated community hospitals. This trend can be traced to the restructuring of the private health insurance industry in the early 1980s from a community-based risk pooling system to one that became employer based, which incentivized formally independent hospitals to merge and consolidate their inpatient and outpatient services into integrated networks that could then competitively bid for health insurance provider contracts as preferred provider organizations (PPOs). In addition, both innovations in acute health-care medicine and technology and related changes in covered services led to a shrinking demand for hospital services in favor of outpatient services, as seen in the 33 percent decline in the number of hospital days (per million) between 1981 and 2011 and the closure of roughly 15 percent of the nation's hospitals over this same period (Cutler & Morton, 2013).

While today some 60 percent of the nation's hospitals are now part of an integrated health-care network under either joint ownership or control, the pace of hospital network consolidation is accelerating toward complete extinction of the independent community hospital and, of equal significance, the independent community clinic. During the five years between 2007 and 2012, there were thirty-two hospital merger and acquisition deals announced that involved 17 percent (or 835) of the nation's nearly 5,000 hospitals (Cutler & Morton, 2013). A core assumption of the discussion that follows on principled health-care delivery system reform is that these integrated health care networks are here to stay, and integrated care networks will therefore comprise the essential provider building block of the health-care delivery system of the future. With this core assumption in mind, it is worthwhile to illuminate the essential features of these integrated health-care networks, particularly their strengths and weaknesses with respect to what must be some of the essential objectives of health-care delivery system reform—cost containment and equity in both health-care access and quality.

As summarized by Cutler and Morton (2013), many of the integrated care networks that have become the dominant provider structure over recent decades are akin to the hub of a wagon wheel, with a large academic medical center at the center with surrounding "spokes" that extend out to other community hospitals that act as feeder sources to the more specialized and cutting-edge care of the academic medical center. Formally independent community hospitals thereby derive competitive advantages through their affiliation with the status and name recognition of the highly prestigious academic medical center "hub" (p. 1964).[3] While these affiliations or outright ownership and control relationships between health-care network hospitals are defined as "horizontal" integration, the "vertical integration" aspect of integrated care networks is represented in the ownership interests or contractual affiliations with community clinics and physicians providing primary and specialized health care, allied health professionals providing such services as physical therapy and mental health care, rehabilitation facilities, long-term and end-of-life care facilities, and home health agencies (Cutler & Morton, 2013; Hernandez, 2000).

Integrated Health-Care Networks: Implications for Health-Care Cost Containment and Improved Equity in Health-Care Access and Quality

With respect to both health-care cost containment and equity of access to high-quality health care, the optimistic scenario would see local health-care markets gradually consolidate from a fragmented patchwork of independent community providers seeking to promote the utilization of their services to well-insured patients, largely irrespective of holistic health outcomes, to a small number of vertically integrated health-care networks that would compete for private and governmental health insurance plans on the basis of health-care cost and objective metrics of health-care quality (both in terms of processes and outcomes). This, in fact, is the vision of the ACA's promotion of accountable care organizations as a key component of its health-care cost containment and quality reforms for the Medicare program[4] (Rittenhouse et al., 2009).

Two policy achievements are key to the realization of this more optimistic scenario. First, that the ACA ultimately will be successful in its health insurance enrollment targets that will see 93 percent of Americans covered by either public or private health insurance by 2020, thus promoting access for the poor and low income into the integrated health-care networks serving the middle class. Second, that the ACA's health-care delivery reforms pioneered with Medicare beneficiaries and providers will (1) prove to be successful and (2) transform health-care delivery for the working age population and their dependents.

The pessimistic scenario would instead see many of the nation's roughly 300 local health-care markets[5] be characterized by consolidation into three or so integrated health-care networks that would, with each in control of key local hospitals, make it very difficult for employers and health insurance underwriters to exclude any one network from price and quality competitive contracts—in effect, imposing the kinds of restraint on competition that could both lead to higher prices at lower quality and also invite federal antitrust litigation. In fact, there is evidence that in some local health-care markets, this has occurred (Cutler & Morton, 2013). Also, the inability to exclude high-price/high-prestige hospitals from local integrated networks may also impose a limit to price-based competition if not quality-based competition. Another element of this more pessimistic scenario is the inability of local safety net hospitals to find an integrated care network with which to merge, due to their antiquated facilities and disproportionate shares of uninsured patients. Finally, there is the potential of separate and unequal quality of care if there is a hierarchy of integrated care networks that emerges that mirrors social stratification in the labor market, with low-cost/limited-benefit health insurance plans and primary medicine clinics with a high proportion of Medicaid patients acting as the selection mechanism into low-cost and low-quality health-care networks.

Summary Comments on the Contextual Considerations in Health-Care System Delivery Reform

There are four take-home points from the preceding discussion of the contextual considerations in health-care system delivery reform. The first is that the realization of a higher level of equity of access to high-quality health care will require major national investments in health-care system capacity building in underresourced communities and underserved populations. The second is that amelioration of disparities in having access to high-quality primary care, particularly those that pertain to class and race, must be central to the evolutionary priorities of health-care system delivery reform. The third take-home point is that the enormous geographic variation in health-care expenditures in the absence of clear evidence of improved outcomes actually holds great promise for the realization of a fiscally sustainable high-quality health-care system. The fourth take-home point is that local integrated health-care networks have already evolved to become the health-care provider structures of the foreseeable future. Over the past three decades, this local provider structure has become as deeply embedded in the nation's health-care system as had the private health insurance industry in the 1950s and thus must serve as the basic building block of the health-care delivery system of the future in ways that promote the ends of reform to be achieved—equitable and sustainable access to high-quality health care as a social right of citizenship.

THE NUTS AND BOLTS OF THE EVOLVING NATIONAL SYSTEM OF HEALTH-CARE SYSTEM DELIVERY

The transition from a national health-care financing structure, predicated on an employment-based private insurance with a public insurance residual, to the two-tiered single-payer approach summarized in chapter 5 transfers enormous cost and quality control leverage to the federal government. To the provider and technology sectors of the health-care industry (leaving aside libertarian ideological objections), this is generally regarded as disastrous for the quality and sustainability of the nation's health-care system.

Indeed it would be, if the basic benefit package of the limited "Medicare for All" plan described in chapter 5 replicated traditional Medicare's fundamentally hands-off approach to the enormous (provider-driven) variability in average Medicare beneficiary expenditures in the absence of discernable health benefits (Fisher et al., 2009).

The nation cannot afford a uniform Medicare-like social insurance plan for health care in the absence of a national effective cost control strategy, nor do we want to achieve fiscal sustainability at the cost of reduced quality of care and less than optimal population health. So, aside from abandoning the notion of universal social insurance for health care altogether or turning to a public plan voucher approach that completely commodifies health care,[6] is there another alternative that ensures universal basic health insurance coverage while promoting fiscal sustainability? Indeed, there is such an alternative, one common to national health-care systems throughout the world that have achieved both universal coverage and fiscal sustainability—generally referred to as "global budgeting."

Defining Global Budgeting

In a nutshell, global budgeting refers to a process through which governments determine the totality of national publicly funded health-care expenditures in advance and allocate resources in accordance with budgetary limits (Shi & Singh, 2001). While this sounds very basic and reasonable given that budgeting public funds in accordance with public priorities and preferences is an essential function of good government, this has never been the approach taken in the United States, where health-care expenditures have multiple private and public payment sources in the absence of any particular government agency or structure providing overall oversight or control.[7] Even in the Medicare program, where there is complete federal responsibility and authority over the social insurance fund for hospital care, the primary function of the federal government has been to define benefits, pay claims, and forecast future expenditures and program solvency. Thus, we have a Medicare program that, while facing the prospect of financial insolvency in the absence of significant reforms, pays $14,165 per beneficiary each year in Miami, an amount that is over $5,000 in excess of the nation's median expenditure per demographically equivalent beneficiary[8] (Dartmouth Institute for Health Policy and Clinical Practice, 2012).

The Mechanics of Global Budgeting:
The Two-Tiered Global Budgeting Approach

Using global budgeting as a means of ensuring the sustainability of universal health insurance coverage has long been the practice in Canada and throughout much of Europe. The use of a global budgeting approach in the United States is not a new or original proposal but actually goes back to the early 1990s as the Clinton administration's Health Security Act was being designed and debated. The basic idea of global budgeting is a cap on overall spending while providing a high degree of local administrative autonomy to design and prioritize services and control costs (Hendrickson & Reinhart, 2010). While global budgeting is the typical approach to the management of a single-payer system where the government is the sole underwriter of health care, global budgeting can also be designed to accommodate a multipayer system (Long & Marquis, 1994). The approach suggested here is a two-tiered global budgeting approach, consistent with the two-tiered health insurance approach advanced in chapter 5. This would consist of a "hard" global budgeting process that places caps on basic social insurance fund expenditures for core services of health care and also government-subsidized investments in health-care infrastructure, as well as a "soft" global budgeting oversight of private-sector health-care expenditures that uses the government's taxing authority to restrain the growth of private health-care expenditures to a predefined share of overall national health expenditures. The rationale and basic details of both tiers of global budgeting are explained in more detail in the discussion that follows, beginning with the "hard" form of global budgeting that would be applied to the first-tier (Tier I) health insurance coverage provided through social insurance, and then elaborating on the specifics of the "soft" Tier II global budgeting approach that utilizes taxation as the enforcement mechanism.

Tier I global budgeting. The "hard" version of global budgeting is characterized by a process that allocates social insurance fund health-care expenditures in accordance with the population health and health-care priorities of a defined geographic unit, with a fixed cap on overall expenditures. While (as described before) the budgeting process grants a high degree of local administrative autonomy to design and prioritize services and control costs in accordance with the contingencies of local context (such as transportation infrastructure and prevalent population health risks), the basic array of local health services largely mirrors those of a national template of optimal "best practices" in health-care delivery of the core health-care services covered under the national social insurance fund for health care. There is, in the "hard" Tier I one version of global budgeting, the setting of health-care priorities, health-care delivery design, and dispersal of funds as a function of governance (both national and local), as opposed to health care in accordance with the vicissitudes of market forces and their relationship to embedded systems of social stratification.

Tier II global budgeting. As pointed by Long and Marquis (1994), if global budgeting were limited to the publicly funded health-care services with supplemental health insurance coverage available through an unrestrained private insurance market, it would both (1) exacerbate income-based inequalities since low socioeconomic status (SES) families would only be able to afford the basic core services in Tier I health care and (2) promote cost shifting between covered and uncovered services. In addition, to the extent that the more affluent segments of the population are able to purchase supplementary private insurance fashioned to their consumption preferences, they will be less inclined to support a sufficient package of core health-care services. On the other hand, consistent with arguments made in chapter 5, from the standpoint of political feasibility, an all-encompassing approach that would apply rigid cost controls and prioritized allocation of health resources to all health-care needs and services is unrealistic in a culturally heterogeneous and socially stratified society with a strong strain of libertarianism in its politics.

The two-tiered global budgeting approach provides a balance to these concerns by allowing the exercise of consumer preferences for supplementary insurance that would cover noncore health services or more convenient access to core health services. However, individual preferences for supplementary insurance would be exercised within (1) limits tied to accessibility and quality of core services for those reliant on Tier I services for the totality of their health care and (2) limits to the share of the nation's overall health expenditures consumed by noncore health-care services. Both of these limits to the private supplementary health insurance market are crucial obstacles to the evolvement of a two-tiered health-care system with large disparities between the rich and poor in the accessibility and quality of their health care. The question is, how could these limits be enforced?

In contrast to the direct budgetary control mechanisms in Tier I global budgeting as a function of government allocation and oversight of health service funds, enforcement mechanisms for Tier II health-care expenditures would entail federal taxation of supplementary health insurance coverage that is tied to indices of the accessibility and quality of Tier I core health-care services—in essence, federal taxation rate triggers that would make it more costly for health-care consumers to turn to private supplementary health insurance to the extent that the standard of health care for Tier I services is allowed to deteriorate.

The federal taxation rate trigger approach to Tier II health-care services would thus serve three functions. First, it would reduce the incentive of more affluent health-care consumers to substitute (both at the ballot box and in their personal health-care consumption choices) private supplementary health insurance coverage for inadequately funded public health-care coverage. Second, in tying the taxation rate of private supplementary insurance to measures of health-care accessibility and quality for Tier I services, it expands the numbers of stakeholders in the maintenance of high standards of care in Tier I core services to include the private insurance industry and providers of Tier II health services. Third, to the extent that the higher tax rates for supplementary insurance are triggered by less favorable indices of Tier I service accessibility and quality, tax revenues from supplementary (Tier II) coverage can be used to improve Tier I services.

For reasons explained in the discussion that follows on the optimal geographic boundaries for global budgeting, it is essential that the taxation triggers of Tier II supplementary health insurance be federally determined and the tax itself be federal. But we are still left to ponder not just the method or source of taxation of Tier II health insurance coverage but also the justification.

The Justification of Taxation as a Global Budget Enforcement Mechanism of Tier II Health Insurance Coverage

As noted by Nathan (2005), health care can be defined as both *a social right* and a *commodity*. In this book, I have defined the core health-care services listed in chapter 4 (table 4.1) as Tier I health-care provisions that are a social right, insomuch as they are crucial to the normal range of human functioning and therefore are essential to both the status and exercise of citizenship (Daniels, 2008). Tier II health care services, on the other hand, are defined as a *commodity* that, while they might be desirable and could enhance health and well-being, are not essential to the protection or restoration of the normal range of human functioning. Examples of such Tier II services include various forms of cosmetic medicines and surgery, medical procedures and medications that have a higher level of consumer demand that is not justified by evidence of efficacy, on-demand wait times for elective surgeries, and concierge primary care medicine. The central justification of taxation for Tier II services is that they are consumer goods rather than a public good, the latter defined as something that can be provided without reducing the availability of that good to others. Insomuch that it is not affordable for the nation to provide either concierge primary medicine or cosmetic surgery for all of its citizens, such Tier II health care services are treated as a taxable commodity.

There is also a second justification for the taxation of Tier II health services that is based on the social desirability of placing limits on the nation having a two-tiered health-care system, one for the rich and the other for the poor. Providing tax subsidies to a level of health care that is designed to exclude the poor and low income is as unacceptable as tax subsidies to private schools that exist to segregate students by race and social class. Thus, the elimination of tax subsidies for private supplementary health insurance is an easily defended justification.

On the other hand, the idea that for some may be more challenging to defend is the notion of an excise tax applied to Tier II health insurance coverage—broadly defined as a federal tax for nonessential consumer goods that would be applied to limit the share of the nation's health-care dollars going to Tier II services. However, to the extent that Tier II services allow more affluent health-care consumers to bypass inadequately funded Tier I core health-care services (the definition of a "hard" two-tiered health-care system as discussed in chapter 5), the justification for a Tier II health insurance equivalent of an excise tax becomes more evident. This, in fact, is precisely the kind of two-tiered health-care system that exists in Australia, where the public health insurance coverage provided to all Australians covers only about two-thirds of the nation's health expenditures and about 45 percent of Australians carry private health insurance that provides more rapid access to core health services as well as enhanced access to specialists (Foley, 2008; OECD, 2014a), thus promoting significant disparities in access to both hospital care and care from specialists based on the ability to afford private health insurance (Van Doorlaer et al., 2008).

The final points to be made on the justification of taxation as an enforcement mechanism for the global budgeting of Tier II health insurance coverage pertain to it needing to be a federal tax as opposed to a local tax. To begin with, the application of a federal excise tax on the purchase of nonessential consumer goods has long been accepted as a legitimate form of taxation by the public (although defining many forms of health care as "nonessential" consumer goods will certainly break new ground). Second, because reasonably equitable access to high-quality core health-care services for all Americans is defined (as in chapter 5) as a core national policy, its assessment and enforcement cannot be left to the varying degrees of local tolerance for high levels of inequality, as would be the case if it were left to the discretion of individual states to tax Tier II health insurance coverage. In this same vein, just as the ongoing assessment of the accessibility and quality of publicly financed Tier I health care relative to what can only be realized through the ability to purchase private Tier II health insurance coverage must be a function of the federal government, ceteris paribus, so must be the calibration of the excise taxation rate of private supplementary insurance in accordance with national benchmarks of relative equity in publicly funded health-care services.

Defining the Geographic Unit for Global Budgeting

While there is strong appeal for defining the geographic units for global budgeting in accordance with smaller, more coherent local health-care delivery systems like the health service areas defined by the National Center for Health Statistics (Makuc et al., 1991), this approach would all but eliminate the well-established and deeply entrenched role of the states in the regulation of local health insurance markets and health-care providers. This fact alone would likely preclude the political feasibility of the local health-care systems approach, but there is also the constitutional doctrine of federalism, which generally preserves for states a direct (if no longer a preeminent) role in the financing and delivery of publicly funded social and health services at the state level (Nathan, 2005). Aside from the constitutional basis of states maintaining a direct role in the financing and delivery of local health services (Madison, 1788a), there is also the argument that states function as crucial laboratories for a range of social policy innovations, including health-care reform (Nathan, 2005). Finally, there is the formidable health risk and health-care utilization data demands of global budgeting, which are better established at the state level than in smaller geographic units (Long & Marquis, 1994). In sum, as much as there is a high degree of within-state diversity in health-care access, quality, and cost that argues for a small area health-care market approach to global budgeting, the state-based approach is clearly the most feasible. So what should this look like in application?

Visualizing the Global Budgeting Structure for Tier I Core Services

Figure 6.1 represents the essential structure and functional components of the global budgeting of Tier I core health services, as would be suggested as optimal from the preceding discussion. There are two essential omnibus premises of the model of global budgeting depicted in figure 6.1, the

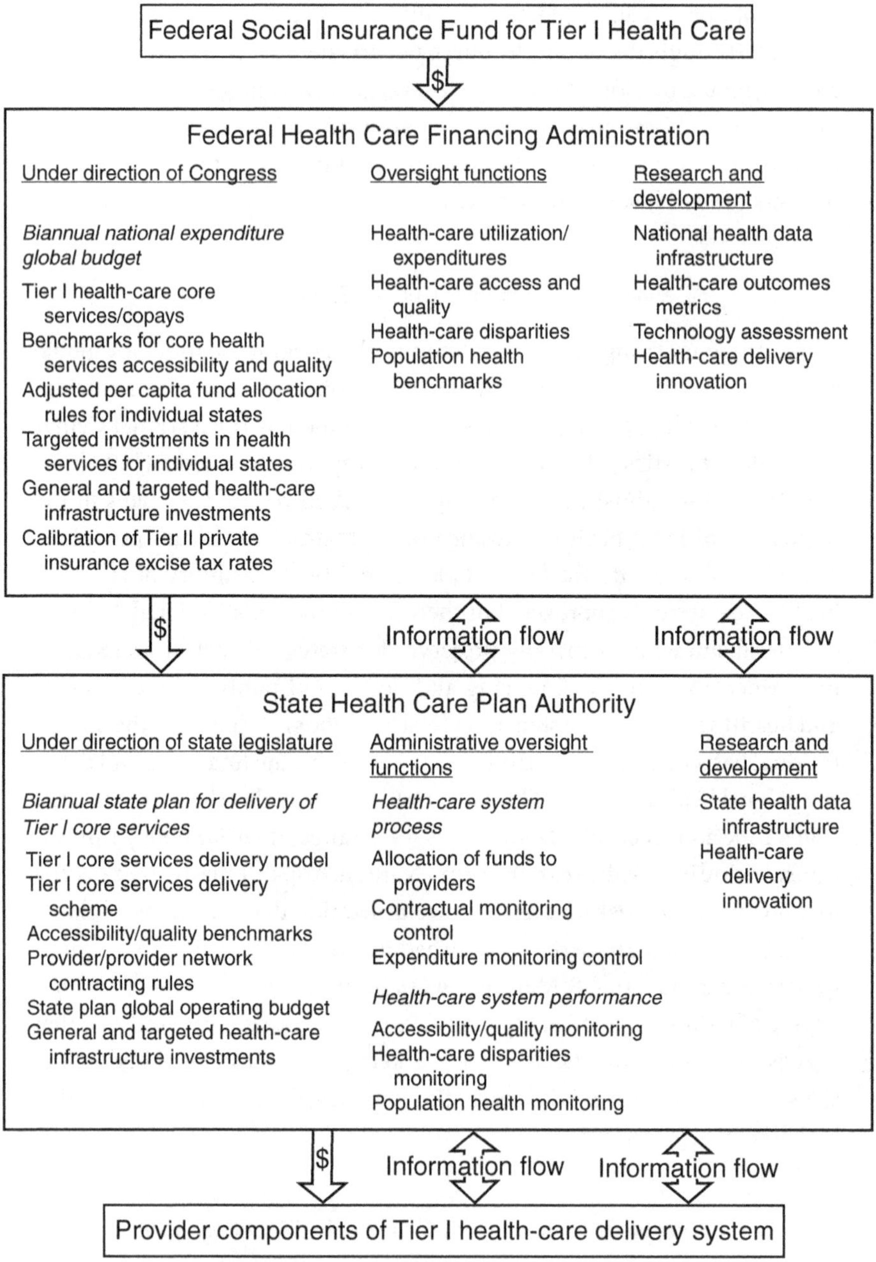

Federal Social Insurance Fund for Tier I Health Care

Federal Health Care Financing Administration

<u>Under direction of Congress</u>

Biannual national expenditure global budget

Tier I health-care core services/copays
Benchmarks for core health services accessibility and quality
Adjusted per capita fund allocation rules for individual states
Targeted investments in health services for individual states
General and targeted health-care infrastructure investments
Calibration of Tier II private insurance excise tax rates

<u>Oversight functions</u>

Health-care utilization/ expenditures
Health-care access and quality
Health-care disparities
Population health benchmarks

<u>Research and development</u>

National health data infrastructure
Health-care outcomes metrics
Technology assessment
Health-care delivery innovation

 Information flow   Information flow

State Health Care Plan Authority

<u>Under direction of state legislature</u>

Biannual state plan for delivery of Tier I core services

Tier I core services delivery model
Tier I core services delivery scheme
Accessibility/quality benchmarks
Provider/provider network contracting rules
State plan global operating budget
General and targeted health-care infrastructure investments

<u>Administrative oversight functions</u>

Health-care system process

Allocation of funds to providers
Contractual monitoring control
Expenditure monitoring control

Health-care system performance

Accessibility/quality monitoring
Health-care disparities monitoring
Population health monitoring

<u>Research and development</u>

State health data infrastructure
Health-care delivery innovation

Information flow   Information flow

Provider components of Tier I health-care delivery system

FIGURE 6.1. Global budgeting structure for Tier I health-care core services.

first pertaining to the authority and responsibilities of the federal government and the second pertaining to the authority and responsibilities allocated to the states.

The federal government has the authority and responsibility to do the following:

- Establish and collect revenues, disperse funds, and ensure the solvency of the national social insurance fund for Tier I health care in accordance with the substantive goals of a social right to basic health care for all citizens.
- Establish core health-care services.
- Set national benchmarks on the accessibility, quality, and equitability of core service health care.
- Define the national model for the delivery of care.
- Define health system population health priorities and outcomes.
- Determine national spending limits and allocations of global funds for operating and capital expenditures in each state.
- Set private insurance taxation rates in accordance with national criteria on the accessibility and quality of Tier I services and the limits of Tier II expenditures as a share of total national health expenditures.

The authority and responsibility allocated to the individual states are summarized as follows:

- The states have wide latitude and authority to work with communities and health-care delivery markets to design and implement local health-care delivery systems and to contract with health-care providers and provider networks in accordance with the achievement of national benchmarks of health-care accessibility, quality, and equitability.[9]
- The states represent the first line of provider and provider network accountability to national benchmarks of Tier I health-care accessibility and quality.
- Any state's allocation of national health-care funds will have three components: (a) an operating budget component for the delivery of core health services, (b) a capital budget allocation based on needed investments in health-care infrastructure that is based on national

infrastructure benchmarks (such as geographic proximity to tertiary care services), and (c) a capital budget allocation based on
investments in new technology that meet rigorous criteria for population health benefits relative to cost.

The Federal Levels of Global Budgeting

Moving beyond the basic premises of the global budgeting scheme represented in figure 6.1 to its specific structural components, we begin with
the Federal Social Insurance Fund for Tier I Health Care. As explained
in chapter 5, this social insurance fund for basic health care is financed
through progressive taxation of household income, in turn made feasible
by (1) the elimination of individual and employer contributions to
employment-based health insurance and Medicare Part A taxes on earnings and (2) the shifting of federal general fund revenues from Medicare
supplemental benefit subsidies and Medicaid to the Federal Social Insurance Fund for Tier I Health Care (Friedman, 2013). This is in essence the
equivalent of a "Medicare for All" trust fund, except that unlike the Medicare program, (1) its coverage of core services is folded into a single trust
fund (as opposed to Medicare's current structure of a trust fund for hospital care and subsidized supplemental benefit programs) and (2) the core
health services coverage is much more comprehensive and thus precludes
the necessity of private supplemental health insurance.

Moving downward on figure 6.1 to the Federal Health Care Financing
Administration (which replaces the current Centers for Medicare and
Medicaid Services, or CMS) are the three component structures for the
global budgeting and operational oversight of Tier I health care for all
Americans. The first component structure is the Biannual National Health
Expenditure Global Budget, which, as indicated, is developed by the Federal
Health Care Financing Administration under the direction of Congress as
part of the federal budgeting process.[10] As illuminated in figure 6.1, the main
elements of the Biannual National Health Expenditure Global Budget include the determination of the core health-care services covered and the
beneficiary copays, the biannual setting of target benchmarks of the accessibility and quality of core health-care services, the adjusted per-capita
Federal Social Insurance Fund allocations for each individual state (based on
such factors as the state's age distribution and a range of population health
metrics), targeted investments in health-care services and health-care
infrastructure for individual states that are critical to the amelioration of

health-care disparities, and the calibration of Tier II private health insurance federal excise tax rates in accordance to each state's balance between the accessibility and quality of Tier I services relative to the dollars spent on private health insurance. In sum, the Biannual National Health Expenditure Global Budget is the main process through which national health-care funds are allocated in accordance with both (1) the funding of core health services available to all Americans and (2) other national health-care priorities such as the amelioration of between-state and within-state disparities in health care and population health. Also, consistent with the national global budgeting requirements suggested by Long and Marquis (1994), there is a specific provision that places some degree of oversight and limits on expenditures for private supplementary health insurance.[11]

The next structural component of the Federal Health Care Financing Administration to be illuminated from figure 6.1 is the Oversight Functions, which represents the health expenditure monitoring and health system performance feedback mechanisms that are the accountability cornerstones to the global budgeting approach. As the structural diagram shows, this component of the Federal Health Care Financing Administration monitors, based on feedback health system performance data from states, both health-care utilization expenditures and the achievement of target benchmarks pertaining to health-care access, quality, and the amelioration of targeted health-care disparities. Because the penultimate goal of the Biannual National Health Expenditure Global Budget is not just to fund and deliver health care but rather to improve population health, the Oversight Functions of the Federal Health Care Financing Administration include the monitoring of crucial benchmarks of population health that would be identified in the biannual expenditure plan.

The third structural component of the Federal Health Care Financing Administration, Research and Development, consolidates and synthesizes the works of a number of federal agencies that comprise the highly fragmented and balkanized national health and health-care data infrastructure, such as the National Center for Health Statistics, the Census Bureau, the Department of Labor, the Agency for Healthcare Research and Quality, and many others. The first function of this structural component provides the platform for the development of a National Health Data Infrastructure envisioned over a decade ago by the National Center on Health Statistics for a unified national health database that would develop, capture, store, process, and disseminate data from a wide range of sources on population health and health-care delivery (National Committee on Vital and Health Statistics, 2001). Research and development on health-care outcomes metrics is an essential complement to the national health information database and envisioned to be a permanent function because innovation in health care is a continuous evolutionary process. The Technology Assessment function addresses what has been a significant deficit in the American health-care system: a depoliticized scientific evaluation of the clinical efficacy, cost-effectiveness, and net social benefits of current and emerging health-care technologies (Sullivan et al., 2009). The final function identified under Research and Development, Health Care Delivery Innovation, addresses the necessity of continuously identifying the optimal modes and models of health-care delivery as health-care technology and the societal context of health care evolve.

The State Level of Global Budgeting

In keeping with the premise that states should have wide latitude and authority to work with communities and health-care delivery markets to design and implement local health-care delivery systems in response to federal financing and health system performance parameters, shown at the state level of figure 6.1 is a State Health Care Plan Authority that largely mirrors the structure and functions of the Federal Health Care Financing Administration. As with the federal level of global budgeting, there is a biannual state plan for the allocation of funds and delivery of Tier I core health-care services. The distinct difference in the state biannual plan is that, instead of allocating funds in accordance with broad expenditure categories and general objectives, it allocates adjusted per-capita federal funds (in accordance with state-specific models and schemes of health-care delivery) through direct contracts with providers and provider networks. The state, in essence, acts as the purchasing agent and contractual monitor of federally funded health care for its resident citizens.[12]

   The first functional elements of the state Biannual State Plan for Delivery of Core Services are the Tier I Core Services Delivery Model and the Tier I Core Services Delivery Scheme. The Tier I Core Services Delivery Model refers to structure and functions of the optimal health-care delivery system at the patient encounter or clinical level, while the Tier I Core Services Delivery Scheme refers to the state plan for delivery of health services at the community level. The term *community level* is used broadly here to refer to either the small area geographic units within each state that are equivalent to the National Center for Health Statistics concept of a health service area (Makuc et al., 1991) or another geographic unit that may be selected by a given state that more coherently represents a community health-care system.

The point is that each state will have wide discretion over the form that its health-care delivery system takes at both the patient and the community levels, in keeping with principles of federalism and the capacity of local governments to adapt public services to local conditions. What is common to all states is the consistency of the core service accessibility and quality benchmarks at the state health plan level with those established at the federal level.

In keeping with this idea, the Provider/Provider Network Contracting Rules (PCRs) are a particularly crucial element of each state's Biannual Plan for the Delivery of Tier I Core Services. In essence, the PCRs address three kinds of contracting criteria. The first kind of broad contracting criteria address the necessary and sufficient conditions to be identified by the state as a qualified provider or provider organization. These "qualified provider" criteria include not only traditional criteria such as the credentialing of clinicians, a solid record of appropriate patient care, and the certification of facilities by such credentialing organizations as the Joint Commission on Accreditation of Healthcare Organizations (JCAHO) but also other elements of infrastructure that align with the capacity of the provider or provider organization to both monitor and meet benchmarks of high-quality patient care (e.g., timely access to providers and treatments, care that is responsive to patient preferences and appropriate to the needs of the patient population served). The second kind of broad criteria relate more directly not to provider infrastructure but to patient care performance benchmarks that measure the extent to which the individual provider or provider system is achieving the quality of care standards established for Tier I health care as a matter of social policy (these criteria and measures will be elaborated upon in chapter 7, which is devoted to the assessment of health system performance).

The third kind of contracting criteria are "pay-for-performance" criteria, sometimes referred to as P4P criteria, which pertain to the specific financial incentives for achieving the patient care performance benchmarks. The financial incentives entailed range from lowered provider payments for unsatisfactory performance to shared savings where the costs of providing care at the specified quality of care benchmarks are reduced through cost-efficient provider practices. While the evidence of the effectiveness of pay-for-performance approaches to health-care quality and cost reductions thus far has been mixed, it is widely believed among health-care policy experts that over time, the applications and methodologies of pay-for-performance provider contracts will yield significant net benefits in patient care outcomes and reductions in health-care cost (Galvin & McGlynn, 2003; Mehrotra et al., 2009). In this vein, it should be noted that the PCRs are a state-level version of the ACA's reform provisions for the Medicare program that foster the development of accountable care organizations as an alternative to the traditional fee-for-service payment system that has propelled the Medicare program toward bankruptcy.

The final two functional elements of the Biannual State Plan for Delivery of Core Services, the State Plan Global Operating Budget and the Health Care Infrastructure Investments, represent the specific operating fund and capital fund allocations made in accordance with the requirements and priorities of Tier I health-care benchmarks for both accessibility and quality. It is assumed that infrastructure investments fall into two categories: (1) ongoing general investments that address infrastructure depreciation and evolving technology and (2) targeted infrastructure investments that are essential to the amelioration of health-care disparities (such as capital funds directed toward the building of rural community care clinics).

The Administrative Oversight Functions of the State Health Care Plan Authority are divided into two broad categories (Health System Process and Health System Performance), and their titles are intended to be self-explanatory. What merits highlighting is the logical consistency between the Oversight Functions at the federal level of figure 6.1 and the Administrative Oversight Functions at the state level, as well as the bidirectional flows of health-care delivery expenditures and system performance information between the federal and state administrative functions. However, the term *administrative* is added to the oversight functions at the state level to denote the fact that at the state level, there is a direct governmental administrative role in the delivery of core health services through partnerships with specific providers. The final structural component of the State Health Care Plan Authority, Research and Development, largely mirrors the functions of the research and development component at the federal level, except that it defers to the federal government the functions of technology assessment and the development of health-outcomes metrics.

Visualizing the Provider Components of the Tier I
Health-Care Delivery System

The third level shown in figure 6.1 is essentially a placeholder for the provider components of the Tier I health-care delivery system under the national global budgeting structure advanced in this chapter. The general features of the provider component level are shown in figure 6.2.

As shown in figure 6.2, the centerpiece of provider components of the Tier I health-care delivery system is the Integrated Care Provider Organization (ICPO), which in most respects is conceptually synonymous with the accountable care organization (ACO) model advanced under the Medicare program reform provisions of the ACA. That is, the ICPO is a provider structure that integrates patient care management, patient data management systems, clinical case management models, and payment mechanisms across primary care, specialty care, acute hospital care, rehabilitation care, skilled nursing facility care, home health care, and behavioral health (Lieberman

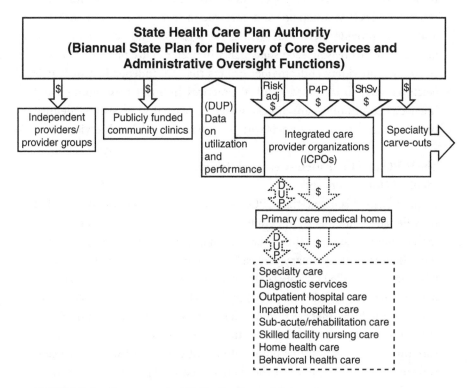

FIGURE 6.2. Provider components of the Tier I health-care delivery system.

& Bertko, 2011). The points of distinction between the ICPO and the ACO are that the ICPO is designed for a single-payer "Medicare for All" program that provides care to patients of all ages, the ICPO contracts with the health-care plans of the individual states rather than the federal government, and the ICPO model is predicated on a single primary care medical home rather than the multiple medical homes assumed in the ACO model (Council of Accountable Physician Practices, 2011). The "primary medical home" concept and linkages to the other provider categories in the ICPO structure will be discussed in more depth, following a general overview of the other non-ICPO provider components of the Tier I health-care delivery structure.

Although the Tier I health-care delivery model shown in figure 6.2 assumes that most state residents will be enrolled in the ICPO, there will be factors that will leave some patient populations outside of ICPO enroll-ment coverage—among them scarcity of the full range of health-care pro-viders in isolated rural areas and difficult-to-reach populations such as the chronically homeless, migrant workers, and undocumented immigrants.[13] In addition, some patient populations have health conditions and social characteristics that would be better serviced in specialized health-care pro-grams and provider networks, such as the seriously and persistently men-tally ill. For this reason, each state plan will need to have provider relation-ships with providers and provider groups that are independent of ICPOs (such as small unaffiliated medical practices in rural communities and inner-city community care clinics), as well as "specialty carve-outs," defined broadly as health-care contracts with providers of specialized services.

The ICPO and the Patient-Centered Primary Care
Medical Home Concept

As previously discussed, the ICPO, like the ACA's concept of an ACO, is a provider structure that (1) integrates patient care management, patient data management systems, clinical case management models, and payment mechanisms across primary care, specialty care, acute hospital care, reha-bilitation care, skilled nursing facility care, home health care, and behavioral health (Lieberman & Bertko, 2011) and (2) aligns the financial incentives and accountability metrics for providers across the full continuum of care (Rittenhouse et al., 2009). However, in contrast to the ACO provider struc-ture that envisions multiple points of patient care coordination, the cen-tral component of the ICPO is the "patient-centered primary care medical home," which is described by the Agency for Healthcare Research and

Quality (AHRQ) as encompassing five essential functions of primary care: comprehensive care, patient-centered care, coordinated care, accessible services, and patient care quality and safety (AHRQ, 2015). Although each of these five essential functions of primary care has multiple aspects, layers of conceptual complexity, and its own extensive literature, for the purposes of this discussion, each will be described only in broad terms based on the AHRQ's (2015) authoritative definitions.

The primary care function of *comprehensive care* means that the primary care medical home is accountable for meeting the large majority of each patient's physical and mental health care needs through its close linkages to the full range of providers along the care continuum. *Patient-centered care* refers to a "relationship-based" orientation to patient care that is holistic and characterized by a partnership between the patient and provider that is informed and respectful of the patient's unique needs, culture, values, and preferences. *Coordinated care* speaks to the primary care provider's role (and duty) of assuming responsibility for coordinating the patient's care by all other providers across the full continuum of care. The primary care function of *accessible services* means that the primary care provider ensures accessibility to primary care through limited wait times and twenty-four-hour availability for urgent care needs, as well as access through multiple modes of communication (such as e-mail, TTY transcription for the hearing impaired). Finally, the essential primary care function of *patient care quality and safety* encompasses evidence-based clinical practice, continuous quality improvement processes, and systems to assess and respond to patient experiences of care.

The argument for advancing the patient-centered primary care medical home as the preferred or optimal approach to accessing and delivering upon the substance of a social right to basic and comprehensive health care is twofold. First, from the standpoint of the substantive requirements of a social right to health care (as discussed in chapter 4), equitable access to the full range of preventative, curative, rehabilitative, and adaptive health-care services specific to individual needs is promoted through an access point to the health-care system that is organized around the unique health needs and preferences of the individual patient. That is, a high-performing patient-centered primary care medical home places every patient on equal footing with respect to access to high-quality comprehensive care based on the patient's individualized health needs, not the patient's social class, race, gender, or any other characteristic historically associated with health-care disparities. Second, from the standpoint of the fiscal sustainability of a social right to comprehensive health care, a growing body of evidence from a range of demonstration projects serving different populations (including Veterans Administration and Medicaid beneficiaries) suggests that the patient-centered primary care medical home approach to integrated comprehensive care can yield better patient care outcomes at lower cost (Arend et al., 2012).

That said, as noted by Rittenhouse et al. (2009), there are formidable challenges to the successful implementation of an integrated health-care system based on the patient-centered primary care medical home model, among them two in particular. First, although the patient-centered medical home model (advanced by the AHRQ, American Academy of Family Physicians, American Academy of Pediatrics, American College of Physicians, American Osteopathic Association, and a host of other provider organizations and health-care policy experts) "calls for primary care practices to take responsibility for providing, coordinating, and integrating care across the health care continuum, it provides no direct incentives to other providers to work collaboratively with primary care providers in achieving these goals and optimizing health outcomes" (p. 2301). Second, while the medical home approach to primary care has been shown to save costs to the health-care system as a whole, most primary care practices do not have arrangements with other providers or the health-care insurance sponsors that would allow them to share in cost savings (p. 2302).

The ICPO advanced here addresses these fundamental challenges in the following ways. First (as shown in figure 6.2), the payments made to the ICPO from the State Health Care Plan have three components: a per-enrollee risk-adjusted payment that is equivalent to the capitated financing approach in a health maintenance organization, a pay-for-performance (P4P) component that can either reduce or increase payments made to the ICPO based on both process and outcome quality of care metrics, and a shared-savings component (ShSv) that returns a share of the social insurance fund cost savings to the ICPO in accordance with preestablished benchmarks. Second, it assumed that the ICPO will align quality and cost incentives throughout the organization through provider employment and contracting arrangements that include pay-for-performance and shared-savings rewards. Third, in keeping with decades of evidence that shows health-care providers are motivated by the ability to provide high-quality care as well as money (Christianson et al., 2009), the ICPO's flow of data on patient care utilization and performance (shown in figure 6.2 as DUP) will move both upward and downward to facilitate transparency, accountability, and health-care innovation at all levels of the organization.

Visualizing Local Health-Care Markets and Related Challenges

As applied in this discussion, the term *health-care market* refers to a geographic unit defined by the referral patterns to tertiary care (that is, care for such high-intensity hospital procedures as cardiovascular surgery and neurosurgery), which is the same as the Hospital Referral Region (HRR) developed by the Dartmouth Atlas of Health Care project discussed earlier in this chapter (Dartmouth Institute for Health Policy and Clinical Practice, 2012). This captures the idea that a health-care market is defined by time and distance proximity to the full range of comprehensive health-care services and can be inclusive of both urban and rural communities. As also discussed earlier in the chapter, the optimal evolutionary progression for the nation's health-care delivery system would see local health-care markets gradually consolidate from the status quo (a fragmented patchwork of independent community providers seeking to promote utilization of their services among insured patients) to a small number of vertically integrated health-care networks that would compete for private and governmental health insurance plans on the basis of health-care cost and objective metrics of health-care quality (in both processes and outcomes). Under the proposal for health-care delivery reform advanced in this chapter is basically the vision of the future of health care for the 220 million Americans (68 percent of the national population) living in urban areas with a total population exceeding 100,000—except that private insurance would play a secondary role to government social insurance and the model of the vertically integrated health-care systems would be that of the ICPO as illuminated in figure 6.2 (U.S. Census Bureau, 2015).

However, for the 40 million Americans (13 percent of the national population) located in urban areas with smaller populations, it seems more likely that the population base will be sufficient for only one or two ICPOs, thus raising the concern that the state health-care plan authorities may be at a disadvantage with respect to bargaining power and holding the ICPO accountable for excess costs and problems in quality of care (Cutler & Morton, 2013; Dash & Meredith, 2010). In the absence of cost and quality-based competition between ICPOs, the incentives tied to pay-for-performance metrics and shared savings are therefore particularly crucial. Even with these incentives, it seems plausible if not likely that in local health-care markets with the equivalent of an ICPO monopoly, health-care costs will be higher than those in ICPO competitive markets.

For the 60 million Americans living in rural areas (19 percent of the national population), the state health-care authorities may need to contract directly with individual providers and specialized provider networks, in view of the presumed population density requirements of an ICPO infrastructure with the full range of comprehensive care. A plausible solution to this might be having a publicly funded local community-based care coordination structure in place, such as the "community health team" concept that had been proposed in the state of Vermont as a component of its strategic plan for a single-payer financing system (Slusky, 2011).

While myriad design and implementation challenges are specific to each local health-care market context, the premise of the state-based approached to health-care planning and budgeting is that health-care delivery system design is an iterative, continuous quality improvement process that is (1) informed by cost and quality metrics and (2) sustained by provider incentives directly tied to both cost and quality. There is nothing new or radical to this premise, in that it reflects decades of health services research and has already been embodied in Medicare program reform provisions in the 2010 Affordable Care Act. If there is anything radical here, it is the idea that under a federalized conception of social insurance, individual states might actually function as the optimal purchasing agent for the substantive provisions of a social right to health care as opposed to acting as an impediment.

THE STRUCTURAL COMPONENT OF GLOBAL BUDGETING: A SUMMARY OF THE KEY INVESTMENTS IN NATIONAL HEALTH-CARE INFRASTRUCTURE

As discussed at an earlier point in this chapter and as shown in figure 6.1, the biannual global budget for Tier I health-care services at both the federal and state levels will have two parts: an *operational budget* that is allocated to the ongoing delivery of health-care services and a *structural budget* for general and targeted investments in health-care infrastructure. As noted in the seminal study by Long and Marguis (1994) of the case for global budgeting in the U.S. health-care system, the primary rationale for a separate global budget for capital investments in health-care infrastructure is the role that innovations in health-care technology play as a major factor in the historical growth of the nation's health-care expenditures. While many innovations in health-care technology have yielded dramatic cost savings or contributed immensely to gains in life expectancy, on balance, technological innovations in health care and related improvements in health-care infrastructure have fueled the growth in national health-care expenditures with increasingly limited returns on population health (Newhouse, 1993). Simply put, to secure the fiscal sustainability to a robust social right to health care, choices in technology and other health-care infrastructure investments must be made in accordance with explicit national and local population health and health-care priorities—among them the amelioration of health and health-care disparities.

With this justification in mind, four categories of key investments in health-care infrastructure need to be considered: the health-care labor force, health-care facilities, health and health-care data infrastructure, and clinical technology.

Health-Care Labor Force Investments

While it is beyond the purpose and scope of this book to fully delineate all of the health-care labor force investments that are necessary for the fulfillment of a social right to comprehensive health care through the life course, at least the most crucial labor force needs can be highlighted—beginning with the adequacy of the primary care physician labor force. As pointed out at the beginning of this chapter, despite primary care being the cornerstone of access to comprehensive health care, there are 6,100 areas of the country that the Health Resources and Services Administration has identified as primary care shortage areas, meaning that the ratio of PCPs to the local population is inadequate to provide for population health needs (HRSA, 2015). The shortages are also particularly prevalent in urban and rural communities characterized by poverty and disparities in health (Cunningham, 2011). Even should the current national policy of using medical education and Medicaid payment incentives prove helpful to the mitigation of PCP shortages among some disadvantaged communities and populations, there is a significant shortage of PCPs nationally that will grow worse in response to both the aging of the population and the extent that the primary care medical home model is more widely adopted—by some estimates, as many as 44,000 adult care PCPs by 2025 (Carrier et al., 2011).[14]

In contrast to the national supply of PCPs, the supply of registered nurses (RNs) and licensed practical nurses (LPNs) is expected to meet if not actually outpace demand through 2025 (National Center for Health Workforce Analysis, 2014).

That said, there are significant disparities between states in the adequacy of the RN/LPN labor force relative to current and future demand. Because the nursing component of health care is so crucial to patient care process and outcomes, the mitigation of local shortages in the nursing labor force is a clear priority for the "targeted investment" of global budgeting funding streams depicted in figure 6.1 at both the national and state levels. Hypothetically if not practically, at the national level, funds could be allocated for tuition subsidies for nursing students in selected states, while at the state level, targeted infrastructure investments might be allocated to capacity building in college and university nursing programs.

The Social and Behavioral Health Component of the National Health-Care Labor Force

As noted by eminent health economist Victor Fuchs thirty years ago, the dollars invested in health care are only a minor component to health relative to the social context of health and individual behavioral choices (Fuchs, 1986). While behavioral health practitioners (psychiatrists, psychologists, psychosocial nurse practitioners, and social workers) cannot address the structural causes of disease and disablement, they can be highly effective at helping patients cope with the proximate causes of disease-producing stress, make behavioral changes to enhance health, and adhere to treatment essentially to disease prevention and recovery. Needless to say, behavioral health practitioners are also a crucial component of such specialized health services as addiction treatment, mental health, and end-of-life care. In a recent comprehensive appraisal of the adequacy of the behavioral health workforce relative to demand, sponsored by the Substance Abuse and Mental Health Services Administration (SAMSHA), it was noted that the current behavioral health labor force is insufficiently staffed in all core disciplines for even current demands, behavioral practitioners have limited access to effective and appropriate training, and provider organizations have difficulties in the recruitment and retention of specialists in behavioral health (Dilandardo, 2011).

The Low-Wage Caregiving Component of the National Health-Care Labor Force

The term *low-wage* caregiving labor force encompasses the nursing assistants, home care aides, homemakers, and in-home companions who are essential to the long-term and end-of-life care components of health-care services. "Low wage" does not necessarily imply low skill or low-value work; in fact, low-wage caregivers are among the most empathetic, intuitively skilled, and most essential of all health-care workers. They are typically paid poorly, lack even meager employment benefits, and work without the protections afforded to almost all other classes of workers under the federal Fair Labor Standards Act. This is not because the work of low-wage caregivers is of limited value to society; rather, it is because low-wage caregivers are drawn from the least advantaged segments of society, and caregiving work is often regarded as the quasi-obligatory function of women as opposed to productive labor that is crucial to national prosperity (Nakano-Glenn, 2010).

There are two budgetary challenges entailed in the state of the low-wage caregiving labor force infrastructure, the first having to do with investments in human capital in the form of training programs for paid caregivers, adequate wages, and the full range of employment protections afforded to other classes of workers. The second challenge has to do with growth in the paid caregiving labor force that will be needed to match the caregiving demands of an aging population. While the expanded training programs for caregivers relate to the capital component of global budgeting, adequate labor protections and compensation as well as the needed growth in labor supply will be represented in increased operational global budget expenditures.

Health-Care Facility Investments

The health-care facility component of the nation's health-care system encompasses general and specialty hospitals, ambulatory care clinics, outpatient diagnostic and surgical centers, community care clinics, mental health centers, nursing homes, inpatient hospices, and buildings housing community-based long-term care programs. The facility component of the health-care system, like the health-care system as a whole, has been built upon over many decades in a piecemeal basis in response to both social policy and market forces, with the heaviest public and private investments in health-care facility infrastructure favoring well-insured populations (Carrier et al., 2012; Starr, 1982). As a result, there are two kinds of mismatch between the health-care needs of the national population and the adequacy of the facility component of health-care services. The first pertains to the spatial maldistribution of health-care facilities for underresourced poor populations and poor communities (Institute of Medicine, 2000). A prime example of this kind of spatial mismatch is the disproportionate share of hospital expansion and modernization investments between African American neighborhoods and white neighborhoods, thus in effect sustaining a racially segregated health-care system (Barton, 2005; Berggren, 2005). The second kind of health-care facility mismatch arises from the legacies of social policies that have created physical infrastructures in health care that are ill-suited to contemporary health-care needs and optimal health-care solutions. An example of this form of mismatch is in the magnitude of the social investments sunk into the nation's 15,600-facility nursing home industry that operates at an annual cost of $135 billion per year, an expenditure that in large part is sustained by the legacies of 1960s era social policies favoring institutional solutions to long-term care needs over community-based approaches such as adult day health-care facilities (IBISWorld, 2015; Kane et al., 1998).

Both forms of facility infrastructure mismatch can be addressed over time by the targeted investments of capital at both the state and national levels. In the case example of the nursing home industry, which is dominated by for-profit corporations reliant on Medicaid and Medicare funds, an optimal balance of institutional versus community-based long-term care programs can be realized through a combination of both targeted capital investments and de-investments in long-term care facilities and long-term care payment incentives from the operational component of global budgets. Spatial mismatches in facility infrastructure, represented by such examples as the well-documented crumbling safety net hospital infrastructure in poor inner-city neighborhoods and the lack of accessible health-care clinics in many tribal reservations (Institute of Medicine, 2000; Needlenan & Ko, 2012; United States Senate Committee on Indian Affairs, 2010), represent crucial targeted investments from the capital component of state and national global budgets.

Investments in Health and Health-Care Data Infrastructure

When Long and Marquis published their seminal RAND Corporation paper on global budgeting and health system reform in 1994, they described in detail the kinds of investments and innovations in health information technology and integrated health information systems that would be foundational to the achievement of that policy goal (Long & Marquis, 1994)—that is, information on health utilization, costs, payments, and quality of care that would be patient, payer, and provider specific and aggregated at all health system levels (provider organizations, community health systems, and at the state, regional, and national health system levels). In the first decade since Long and Marquis outlined the general requirements for a national health information infrastructure, the development of health information technology and infrastructure at the provider organization level had been fostered with only limited success by incentives tied to performance bonuses from private-sector health insurance plans, policy initiatives at the state and national levels that have made provider organization performance data available to the public, and mandated external quality review (EQR) requirements for Medicaid and Medicare participation (Casalino et al., 2003). However, the more recent post-2010 ACA Medicare reform provisions that align provider payments with both cost efficiency and quality of care outcomes hold great promise for speeding up the pace of health information technology and infrastructure at the provider organization level.

At the national health information infrastructure level, the key milestone has been the George W. Bush administration's 2004 executive order establishing the Office of National Health Information Technology Coordinator (ONC), which was later legislatively institutionalized by Congress through the Health Information Technology for Economic and Clinical Health Act (HITECH Act) of 2009. In a nutshell, the ONC is the principal federal entity charged with coordination of nationwide efforts to implement and use the most advanced health information technology and the electronic exchange of health information that would guide all stakeholders in the health-care system (patients, provider organizations, and private and public health insurance payers) toward a health-care system that yields better health outcomes at lower cost. While the ideological foundations of the ONC initiative were based on a free-market consumer-oriented health-care system, the coherent national health information infrastructure it proposes to foster is fundamentally consistent with the kind of health information infrastructure that would be necessary for a health-care delivery system predicated on universal social insurance for health care and global budgeting.

In sum, over the first two decades of the current century, the nation has made significant strides toward the development of a health and health-care information infrastructure that is capable of better aligning individual and collective expenditures on health care with better health-care outcomes at hopefully a more sustainable cost.

This effort in many respects is analogous to the development of the nation's superhighway transportation infrastructure during the 1950s and 1960s, a public good with transformative long-term benefits that required a clear public policy vision of the possible, an enormous initial investment to achieve it, and continuous ongoing investment to sustain what has been achieved. The assumption is that the ongoing investments in health and health-care information infrastructure will be more than offset by reduced expenditures in high-cost/low-benefit health care.

Investments in Clinical Technology

In the United States, national investments in clinical technology have been dominated by an orientation toward health care as a commodity, as opposed to health care as a public good and social right to be allocated in accordance with shared principles of distributive justice. One manifestation of this commodification of health-care orientation has been aptly named the "medical arms race" between hospital systems seeking to preserve and expand their market share of well-insured patients through the acquisition of the latest innovations in health-care technology, irrespective of individual patient and population health benefits relative to other kinds of investments (Robinson, 2008). For example, in the United States, there are 31.5 multimillion dollar magnetic resonance imaging (MRI) units per million persons, relative to an average of only 13.3 MRI units per million in other OECD countries (OECD, 2014a).

Another manifestation of this commodification orientation, closely tied to the so-called medical arms race, is the weak and fragmented medical technology assessment process in the United States relative to that prevalent in other modern democracies with advanced health-care systems, despite the fact that the United States was an early innovator of the health technology assessment process as a tool of public policy (Sullivan et al., 2009). The health technology assessment process, which examines new innovations in medical technology (ranging from new pharmaceuticals to surgical robotics) for impacts on health system cost, clinical efficacy, ben-

efits relative to other social investments, and social/ethical/legal ramifications, was actively carried out by the nonpartisan congressional Office
of Technology Assessment (OTA) from its establishment in 1972 until it
was defunded by Congress in 1995. While the 1995 defunding of the OTA was
rationalized by its opponents as a cost-cutting measure, the inherent conflict between OTA's evidence-based cost-benefit approach to public investments in medical technology and the interests of the politically powerful
health-care technology industry is the primary reason for its demise. Subsequent to the defunding of the OTA, what new health technologies are
either covered or not covered by health insurance is determined by a fragmented payer-specific process that is heavily influenced by the monetary
and political clout of the medical technology industry as opposed to objective scientific evidence.

While it might be argued that the investments in health technology
will become more rationalized and consistent with the public interest to the
extent there is better alignment between health-care provider incentives and
patient care outcomes, other countries that provide health care as a social
right of citizenship have found that investments in health technology must
be guided by population health outcomes relative to costs and represent
important trade-offs between competing social priorities. Thus, outside of
the United States, health technology assessment is commonly regarded as
a crucial function of governance as opposed to the health-care market. This
perspective applies not only to countries like Sweden with a social insurance fund that pays for almost all health-care expenditures but also to
countries like Australia where over 30 percent all health-care expenditures
are paid for by private health insurance or out of pocket (Australian Institute of Health and Welfare, 2013). As briefly touched upon earlier in the
chapter and as shown in figure 6.1, health technology assessment is proposed as a Research and Development function of the Federal Health Care
Financing Administration.

CONCLUDING REMARKS: APPRAISING EQUITY, SUSTAINABILITY, AND POLITICAL FEASIBILITY

To recap on remarks made in this chapter's introduction, the task of this
chapter is to establish the general features of health-care delivery reforms
that will both fulfill the core criteria of equitability, sustainability, and feasibility and be adaptable to the two-tiered health-care financing structure

described in chapter 5. Equity refers to the extent to which any particular health-care system delivery reform achieves a fair balance between the competing interests of different segments of the patient population and society at large. Sustainability refers to the extent to which a health-care system delivery reform initiative yields favorable impacts on population health while realizing large reductions in immediate and future health-care costs. Finally, political feasibility refers to the likelihood of a given health-care system delivery reform in view of the competing interests of different stakeholder groups affected.

Prospects for Realizing Equity in a Social Right to Health Care

As discussed in chapter 4, a social right to health care is defined as universal comprehensive health insurance coverage, with adequate and equal risk protection, for those health-care needs that are essential to the optimal realization and preservation of the normal range of functioning and fair equality of opportunity. In substantive terms, this social right to health care is defined as universal and equitable access to Tier I health-care services. A social right to health care is not defined as a subsidized right to the Tier II health-care services classified as a commodity, meaning that there will always be disequities in the level of access and access to the full range of health-care services available in the nation's health-care system based at least on income.

With this bounded definition of a social right to health care in mind, to what extent does the blueprint for the delivery of Tier I health-care services promise to achieve equity of access and quality? The argument here is that it largely if not wholly does so, based on the following observations.

First, because a social insurance fund for Tier I health-care services cuts altogether the ties between employment and labor market stratification, it eliminates also the primary proximate source of disequities in health-care access and quality: the employment-based health insurance system. Disparities in health care by class, race, and gender are all substantially mediated through employment-based insurance. Second, social insurance for Tier I health-care services eliminates the well-documented disparities in health care that are tied to means-tested health insurance coverage.

Third, at both the state and federal levels, the global budgeting and related strategic plans for the delivery of Tier I services are predicated on the advancement of equity of access and quality in accordance with explicit and transparent benchmarks and a continuous quality improvement process. Fourth, the global budgeting process proposed in this chapter incorporates targeted investments in health-care services and health system infrastructure at both the federal and state levels that are based on the advancement of equitable access to high-quality health care.

Prospects for Sustainability

The primary advantage of basing the design of the nation's Tier I health-care delivery system on the global budgeting model, from the standpoint of sustainability, is the capacity to define the baseline of overall and selected domains of health-care expenditures and then specify a sustainable level of expenditure growth (Long & Marquis, 1994). There are no illusions this will be a wholly rational and depoliticized process at the federal or the state level. In fact, the most realistic assumption is that the allocation of ongoing Tier I health system expenditures and infrastructure investments will be a continuous battle among stakeholders throughout the health-care system (as exampled by competing interests among the health professions over the scope of practice and reimbursement, pharmaceutical manufacturers seeking to influence both investments in innovation and Tier I prescription coverage formularies, and regional health networks battling over infrastructure investments). It is more that these battles will be framed within a rational planning process with explicit goals consistent with the public interest, not immune to corruption and influence peddling but at least more resistant than the purely legislative approach to resource allocation.

This is the first way in which the fiscal sustainability of Tier I health care is advanced. It is also advanced by the social insurance trust fund structure of Tier I health-care coverage. Unlike health-care expenditures from private insurance plans and general revenue public funds, the principles of trust fund management are completely predicated on long-term solvency and sustainability. In practice, the revenues, expenditures, and fund balance forecasts from the Tier I social insurance fund will continuously and objectively define the parameters for sustainable health-care expenditures as opposed to expenditure forecasts based on health-care utilization and pricing trends.

Although fiscal sustainability is of primary concern, there is a political dimension to sustainability that should be considered as well. That is, should it ever be achieved, the demise of a universal social insurance entitlement to comprehensive health care could come in two forms. The first is an outright repeal of the social insurance entitlement legislation in favor of other approaches (such as the subsidized health insurance voucher approach that has been advanced as an alternative to the current Medicare program). The second is through the gradual decay of Tier I health insurance coverage in favor of private insurance supplemental Tier II coverage that will represent both a substantial retreat from an adequate and equitable social right to health care and a hardening of the layers of the two-tiered health-care system—one for the well insured and the other for the poor. The primary safeguard against both forms of demise is achievement and preservation of a perception among both the broad public and health care providers that Tier I health insurance coverage provides both adequate access to necessary health care and sufficient protection against "unaffordable" (not just catastrophic) health-care expenditures. It is this perception that has been pivotal to the political base of the Medicare program over decades of social welfare retrenchment, ironically despite the fact that the expenditure protection under the Medicare program has actually become significantly weaker over time (Cubanski et al., 2014). This suggests that both the true adequacy of Tier I benefits and the politics of perception of adequacy are also critical to the sustainability of the vision of a social right to health care advanced in this chapter.

Political Feasibility

The term *political feasibility* encompasses not only the possibility of some desired political outcome but also the likelihood of its being achieved. From the standpoint of the merely possible, the conclusion of a robust social right to health care financed by a national social insurance fund along the lines proposed in this chapter is readily defensible. Here are some compelling reasons. First, the partnership between the medical profession and the health insurance industry that orchestrated the demise of the Truman administration's single-payer plan, despite having overwhelming public support (see chapter 1), has long been dissolved in acrimony and divergent interests. The bureaucracy and controls over medical practice that the AMA had for decades claimed would be the essence of national health insurance have characterized the essence of private health insurance health-care financing since the advent of managed care in the 1980s. Second, the "medical free enterprise" model and ideology that for the better part of the past century had unified the medical profession against social insurance for health care is well on the road to extinction in favor of the dominance of multihospital corporations with either salaried or contractual control of physicians, just as sociologist Paul Starr had predicted three decades ago in his prescient *Social Transformation of American Medicine* (1982). Third, at some point during the first decade of the current century, the opinion in the medical profession on the financing of health care shifted from opposition to national health insurance to substantial majority support for national health insurance, a shift that is in line with the views of the American public (Carroll & Ackerman, 2008; CBS/*New York Times* Poll, 2009). This is not the claim of some left-wing blog or a proponent organization of national health insurance (such as the Physicians for a National Health Program) but rather the conclusion from two rigorous physician opinion investigations published in the *Annals of Internal Medicine* (Ackermann & Carroll, 2003; Carroll & Ackerman, 2008). Finally, there are the merits of a single-payer social insurance approach to health care from the standpoint of prioritizing national health expenditures and fiscal sustainability (Glied, 2009), in contrast to the status quo of employment-based insurance with a public funding residual that has produced the most expensive health-care system in the world.

However, the political feasibility of the nation's adopting a single-payer health-care health insurance entitlement from the standpoint of *high likelihood* is a murkier proposition. For those who believe that the single-payer approach merits will eventually triumph over the status quo, there are articles like the one published in *Forbes*, two years after the passage of the ACA, that assert in no uncertain terms that the nation's adoption of a single-payer national health insurance plan is inevitable. The reasons highlighted are the demise of the for-profit insurance industry in the wake of ACA health insurance market reforms, the share of the public that either views health care as a basic human right or believes that the deeply fragmented health-care system is not working, and the unsustainable costs associated with a multipayer finance system with its enormous administrative costs and insurance industry profits (Ungar, 2012). There is also the shift in public opinion toward a single-payer system (as discussed in chapter 5) that moved from 36 to 42 percent of active voters in favor of a single-payer system to somewhere between 54 and 65 percent of the public (AP/YAHOO Poll, 2008; Blendon et al., 2006), which is joined by the aforementioned parallel shifts toward majority support of a national health insurance plan within the medical profession documented by Carroll and Ackerman (2008). Finally, single-payer proponents can point to post-ACA robust single-payer popular movements gaining ground at the state level, including Vermont, Hawaii, Oregon, New York, Washington, California, Colorado, and Maryland, with both Vermont and Hawaii having won majority legislative support (Harrop, 2014).

For those who are inclined to be skeptical about the prospects for the political viability of a single-payer system in the United States, there are also numerous strong arguments available, among them (1) weakened faith in government/Congress, manifested in and propelled by the resurgence of libertarian ideology, (2) the fiscal resources and monetary political clout of the health insurance industry, coupled with the convergence of the health insurance industry's interest in conservative market-based solutions to social problems, (3) the potential success of the ACA as an accommodation to a limited social right to health care to most Americans that contains the "crisis in health care" to the most disadvantaged and politically powerless segments of society, and (4) the political demise of state-level single-payer initiatives in states like Vermont and Hawaii where widespread legislative support had at one point been won. Skeptics can also point out that the so-called majority preference for a single-payer system among likely voters includes a substantial share that want to retain the choice to enroll in either a private health insurance plan or a single-payer plan as their primary insurance coverage (GBA Strategies, 2015),[15] a preference that is categorically incompatible with the financial viability of a single-payer financing model.

The merits of all of these pro and con arguments notwithstanding, there are two reasons why the prospects for the eventual transition to a health-care system financed primarily through a universal social insurance fund (aka single payer) are far more favorable than not. The first is that restraint in the growth of national health expenditures while achieving inroads in the amelioration of health-care disparities is advanced only to the extent that the financing and delivery of health care become less fragmented and more rationalized in line with these policy goals. These are national health policy goals that have been formally legislated in the provisions of the ACA and are unlikely to be abandoned as national health-care policy continues its evolutionary progress. The second reason is that new generations of voters will, based on a collective embracement of health care as a basic necessity and right of citizenship, ultimately reject both the employment-based insurance model and the manifest unfairness of social insurance for health care as a privilege of only older Americans rather than all generations of Americans. There are multiple plausible paths to this outcome, including an innovation and diffusion process of state-level single-payer plans that leads to a national consensus, a public option plan at the federal level that over time enrolls an ever increasing share of the population, the demise of the ACA's expanded health-care entitlements and private insurance subsidies in the face of resurgent health-care inflation and its replacement by a single-payer plan as a matter of fiscal and political necessity, or a radical response to an as yet unanticipated but historically plausible national economic crisis. The current system of health-care financing is neither loved by Americans nor adequate to the needs of future generations. Rather, it is the legacy of the unfortunate marriage of convenience between nineteenth-century medical free enterprise and Cold War politics that occurred a lifetime ago. It is also not our national fate to endure.

Chapter Seven

ASSESSING HEALTH-CARE SYSTEM PERFORMANCE AGAINST THE FOUR CORE AIMS OF HEALTH-CARE POLICY

Up until now, this book has been about the justifications of a social right to health care in light of the requirements of citizenship in a democratic society, the core health-care policy aims that are essential to the substantive realization of an adequate social right to health care, and the general features of a health-care system redesigned to achieve those core health policy aims. This chapter is about assessing the success of that redesigned health-care system. The question that this chapter addresses is the following: What are the measures and benchmarks of success that should be used that are specific to the core policy aims the health-care system has been redesigned to achieve?

Before delving deeply into the response to this question, there are two caveats that need to be brought to light. The first pertains to the general requisites of policy success as described in chapter 2. That is, successful social policy requires that a social policy be implemented as designed, that its basic aims are achieved, and that its unintended consequences must not be so detrimental as to outweigh its intended benefits (Almgren, 2013). In the discussion of optimal health-care system performance measures and benchmarks of success that follows, it is acknowledged that the measures of health-care system performance proposed are primarily outcome focused—when outcomes fall short of their benchmarks, the shortcomings can be in policy implementation, policy design, or some combination of both. They also do not address what are sure to be at least some unintended policy consequences. While the proposed measures and benchmarks will provide us with crucial evidence with respect to progress toward the achievement of core policy aims, in historical reality, massive institutional reforms are never implemented as initially designed, nor are they unaccompanied by unanticipated and unintended policy consequences. Rather, fundamental institutional reforms take shape in an iterative and deeply politicized process (Skocpol, 2010).

The second caveat pertains to the proposed benchmarks of performance. In the case of some performance benchmarks, they have been selected on the basis of a substantial literature on the specific measure of performance and the value on the measure that represents optimal achievement. In other benchmarks, where there is not a research literature on the optimally achievable metric, a value on the benchmark is proposed based on desired ends and reasoned consideration of the achievable given the limited evidence available. In both cases, it is assumed that the desirable and achievable performance benchmarks will continue to evolve over time in an ongoing exchange between the desired ends to be achieved, the state of knowledge on effective and cost-efficient health-care delivery, and allocation of resources in accordance with competing social priorities.

The balance of this chapter now devotes itself to the illumination of major dimensions and measures of health-care system performance that are specific to the core policy aims the health-care system has been redesigned to achieve, as well as their target benchmarks. The measures of health-care system performance presented in the discussion that follows are not argued to be either exhaustive or even ideal so much as they are represented to be fairly comprehensive with respective to core policy aims and well grounded in the health-care system performance literature.

POLICY AIM 1: UNIVERSAL COMPREHENSIVE HEALTH INSURANCE COVERAGE WITH ADEQUATE AND EQUAL RISK PROTECTION

The assessment of this first core policy aim is framed by the assumption that the Tier I health-care entitlements, as defined in chapter 5, fully represent comprehensive health-care coverage, in that they encompass preventative, curative, rehabilitative, and adaptive health services, technologies, and products that are deemed essential to the realization and preservation of the normal range of functioning. This critical assumption reduces the necessary health system performance metrics for this first core health-care policy aim to two evaluative criteria: universal insurance enrollment and adequate and equal risk protection.

Defining and Measuring Universal Health Insurance Enrollment

Strictly speaking, the accomplishment of universal insurance enrollment would require that all insurance-eligible individuals who fit the criteria for inclusion would be enrolled as participants in the Tier I social insurance benefits. This would include U.S. citizens, permanent legal residents residing in the United States for five or more years, and (as later discussed in chapter 8) undocumented workers who either are taxed for or make voluntary contributions to social insurance for health care for themselves and their dependents. The measure employed to assess enrollment in the social insurance fund for Tier I health care, conventionally known as the take-up rate, is defined as the percentage of persons who are eligible for and enrolled to receive various kinds of compensation, benefits, or social entitlements. While a take-up rate benchmark of 100 percent enrollment is feasible for citizens and permanent legal residents,[1] it is not for undocumented workers and their dependents. What follows is the explanation as to why, as well as a proposal for an alternative take-up benchmark for the undocumented worker segment of the national population.

Although low take-up rates are typically a problem for means-tested programs, the low take-up problem can occur in non-means-tested social entitlement programs where enrollment requires knowledge about the enrollment process and specific actions to enroll, and there are transaction costs associated with the enrollment process (such as complicated forms and extensive time devoted to eligibility documentation) (Currie, 2004). For this reason, automatic or default enrollment in the social insurance fund for Tier I benefits is optimal where feasible, as it could be for citizens and permanent legal residents as a part of birth registration or through the U.S. Citizenship and Immigration Services process for becoming a naturalized citizen or permanent legal resident. For undocumented workers and their dependents living in the shadows and under the threat of deportation, another enrollment process is required that allows contributions to social insurance while not putting the undocumented worker at particular risk for deportation.

205

ASSESSING HEALTH-CARE SYSTEM PERFORMANCE

The suggested mechanism for this is the 1996 Internal Revenue Service provision that allows undocumented workers and their dependents to file an income tax return and any owed income taxes and Social Security contributions under an Individual Taxpayer Identification Number (ITIN). In brief, undocumented workers may obtain an ITIN by filing an application along with documentation of their identification and foreign status by mail or in person through a designated IRS taxpayer assistance center under Internal Revenue Code Section 6103. The IRS is generally prohibited from disclosing taxpayer information to other federal agencies, including U.S. Immigration and Customs Enforcement. A significant share of undocumented workers already file IRS returns under the ITIN option for a variety of reasons, including establishing a record of working and paying taxes in the event that a path to citizenship becomes possible, establishing eligibility for such subsidies and the Child Tax Credit, and claiming premium tax credits for those dependents who are citizens and thus eligible for health-care coverage under the ACA (National Immigration Law Center, 2014). According to an IRS audit of the 3.2 million ITIN tax returns filed in 2010, 72 percent were eligible for tax credits, amounting to $4.2 billion in refunds (Treasury Inspector General for Tax Administration, 2011), so the ITIN provides a path to Tier I health insurance enrollment that is well known and credible to undocumented workers and their advocates. The question is, what would be a reasonably feasible take-up rate for ITIN health insurance enrollment for undocumented workers and those of their dependents who are not enrolled through birth registration as U.S. citizens?

Unfortunately, because undocumented workers have been excluded from almost all means-tested programs and social insurance entitlements as well, there is no research available on comparable take-up rates that would provide a sound basis for answering this question. However, research conducted by the USAID among informal economy sector workers (such as street vendors and independent day laborers) in Nicaragua showed that the elimination of monetary cost and time barriers to health insurance enrollment achieved a 70 percent take-up rate for eligible informal economy workers (Hatt et al., 2009). This is consistent with the cost and convenience of the ITIN enrollment mechanism proposed here, since (1) undocumented workers who report income under the ITIN process are already subject to social insurance taxes and (2) the enrollment action could easily be linked to the ITIN filing process. Although a range of unknown immigration policy changes might affect the take-up rate for better or worse, a 70 percent take-up seems like a reasonably feasible initial benchmark, pending more experience with the health insurance coverage policy proposed.

Defining and Measuring Adequate and Equal Risk Protection

As discussed in chapter 4, to the extent that individuals possessing citizenship status are placed at risk for financially catastrophic health-care expenditures, that aspect of citizenship status pertaining to a basic modicum of material security is undermined. Second, to the extent that there are significant disparities in the economic protections against the financial burdens of illness and health-care needs, equity in citizenship status is also jeopardized. Considered together, these two risks to the full realization of citizenship status create the necessity of adequate and comprehensive health insurance coverage as a social right of citizenship. The term *adequate risk protection* refers to a level of risk protection against the out-of-pocket health expenditures for Tier I health care that is essential to *financial security*, meaning that the costs associated with health care are not a threat or impediment to the realization of a decent standard of living commensurate within the prevailing social norms. The concept of *equal risk protection* requires that no individuals or segments of society are at *disproportionate risk* for out-of-pocket Tier I health expenditures that threaten the loss of financial security.

Personal health-care expenditures that are (in the above sense) either catastrophic or impose a significant hardship to financial security affect individuals and households in three related but distinct ways. The most financially devastating and sadly too prevalent in American society is the phenomenon of medical bankruptcy, in essence accumulating a burden of debt for health-care costs that is unpayable in light of income and assets. Although bankruptcy due to health-care expenditures is typically confounded with other factors, such as the burden of nonmedical debt relative to income and the loss of income associated with the illness/injury that caused the cumulative medical debt, the methodological challenges to a valid measurement of the prevalence of the medical bankruptcy are not insurmountable (Dranove & Millenson, 2006). A second way that the financial burden of health-care expenditures is revealed is in the share of health-care spending for essential health care relative to discretionary household income, the latter defined as the income left over after paying for basic household expenses such as rent, food, utilities, clothing, childcare, and transportation to work or school. That is, discretionary household income measures the share of household income that can be used for vacations, entertainment, college educations, and savings (Landefeld et al., 2010). Health-care expenditures that consume household resources that allow for family vacations, investments in college education, and savings are not necessarily catastrophic, but they nonetheless function as a significant impediment to a standard of living consistent with prevailing social norms and also the future prospects of children. A third way burdensome health-care expenditures reflect financial hardship is when they impose a significant impediment to seeking necessary health care. In the most dramatic way, this can show up in the choice to spend one's limited money on either prescribed medication or food, but financial hardship can also be revealed in more mundane decisions to delay or avoid necessary health care to invest in modest savings, help a teenager afford a high school prom night, or travel home every few years to visit aging parents.

Taken together, these three measures of the financial burden of out-of-pocket health-care expenditures (the prevalence of medical bankruptcies, health-care expenditures as a share of discretionary household income, and the incidence of avoiding or delaying necessary health care due to financial cost/affordability) encompass the full range of financial hardship that should be seen as the object of *adequate risk protection* (Mioreno-Serra et al., 2013). While the specific health-care system performance benchmarks for each of these indicators should be determined and then periodically reevaluated in light of other societal priorities (such as the public dollar investments needed to achieve basic education benchmarks), the benchmarks that follow are at least a plausible starting place.

With respect to the prevalence of medical bankruptcy, it seems reasonable to fix the U.S. benchmark to a threshold of 16 percent, the maximum rate observed among Canadian adults in the high health-care consumption age range of fifty-five and older (Redish et al., 2006). This is proposed as a starting benchmark because economically and in many ways politically, Canada is as much like the United States as anywhere in the world, with the very large difference of having a single-payer health-care system.

The determination of a reasonable benchmark for the proportion of discretionary spending consumed by out-of-pocket health-care expenditures is a bit more complex. According to an in-depth analysis of U.S. health-care expenditures for a typical middle-income family of four with comprehensive health insurance coverage, as of 2009, $235 per month went to out-of-pocket medical expenditures (Auerbach & Kellerman, 2011). Compared to the research on discretionary spending by income level that suggests that this average case family would have $1,200 per month in discretionary income (Experian Simmons, 2011), it can be said that the average American family (with health insurance) spends about 20 percent of their discretionary income on health care.[2] This seems like a reasonable beginning benchmark to set as the *maximum* threshold for the typical household under the redesigned health-care system that might be readjusted gradually downward as a national goal. However, because lower-income households spend more of their limited income on health expenditures than high-income households, the literature on the risk protection aspect of health-care system performance also suggests that the target maximum threshold of discretionary spending on essential medical expenditures should be calibrated by household income level (Mioreno-Serra et al., 2013).

The final measure of the adequacy of risk protection to be illuminated is the incidence of avoiding or delaying necessary health care due to financial cost/affordability. While this measure in its various versions is most often used as an indicator of financial impediments to health-care access, it also works as a valid measure of the adequacy of health insurance coverage for insured populations—with an important caveat pertaining to the role that out-of-pocket costs plays as an impediment to health care at all levels of income. That is, even among high-income health-care consumers, many will report that they avoided or delayed needed care due to perceived affordability. For example, in the Medical Expenditure Panel Survey (MEPS) of a representative sample of adults, among those of high income, 27 percent (standard error = 4.1) reported that they were "unable or delayed in receiving needed medical care" because they "couldn't" afford it (AHRQ, 2012a). Since all but a very small fraction of high-income adults lack health insurance (DeNavas-Walt et al., 2013), the subjective qualities of both "needed care" and "affordability" must be taken into account in the interpretation of this measure and the establishment of a reasonable benchmark. In recognition that the needed health care referenced in the measures of insurance risk protection will be Tier I services (as opposed to Tier II services such as cosmetic surgery), it is proposed that an incidence of no more than 20 percent of adults eighteen and older reporting delayed or avoided care due to cost be used as a reasonable benchmark for adequate risk protection. This would be a substantial reduction in the incidence of avoiding/delaying health care due to cost for all but the highest income level,[3] and it takes into account (1) some proportion of respondents at all income levels who might view some kinds of optional care as "needed" and (2) differing perceptions of "affordability." To capture the equity dimension of adequate risk protection, the 20 percent benchmark would apply to all household income levels. Expressed in another way, equity in this insurance risk protection measure requires that household income does not predict the probability of experiencing delayed or avoided care due to affordability.

POLICY AIM 2: THE AMELIORATION OF DISPARITIES IN HEALTH-CARE ACCESS AND QUALITY

The Conceptualization and Measurement of Health-Care Access, Equity of Health-Care Access, and Disparities in Health-Care Access

Although a voluminous literature on health-care access abounds with competing definitions of the concept and the optimal means of measuring its multiple dimensions, the definition of health-care access that is used in this book is the ability to obtain needed, affordable, convenient, acceptable, and optimally effective personal health care in a timely manner (Shi & Singh, 2001, p. 493).[4] Equitable access to health care is defined as equal access to health care based on equal medical need, irrespective of other individual characteristics, such as income, race, gender, age, or place of residence (Hernandez-Quevedo & Papanicolas, 2013, p. 202). This then is logically extended to the definition of disparities in access to health care, which are disequities in access to health care that are not attributable differences in the need for health care (Dehlendorf et al., 2011). With that in mind, in the discussion that follows, the terms *disequities in health-care access* and *disparities in health-care access* will be used interchangeably.

Measures of health-care access and also disequities in health-care access stem in one way or another from medical sociologist Ron Andersen's model of health-care utilization, which makes the crucial distinction between *potential* access to health care (the opportunity to use health care) and *realized* access to health care (actual health care utilization) (Andersen, 1968, 1995). The opportunity to use health care is dependent on enabling factors that take place at both the health-care system and the individual levels. At the health-care system level, there is not only affordable health insurance but also the availability of health services personnel and facilities where people live and work. At the individual level, there is knowledge about when and where to seek health care, personal impediments to accessing health care such as childcare and the ability to take time away from work, and the beliefs about the health-care provider's sensitivity to their needs, preferences, and ability to provide effective treatment (Andersen, 1995). Measures of disequities in health-care access that capture the enabling factors therefore include such factors as the availability of a usual source of primary care and the various impediments to obtaining needed health care, such as unaffordable out-of-pocket expenditures, the inability to take time off from work or obtain childcare, the provider's use of a different language, and the provider's limited availability. On the other hand, measures of health-care access that capture disequities in the *realized* dimension of access to health care involve differences in health-care utilization by such characteristics as income, education, race, and gender that are not explained by differences in health needs—or, as conversely stated by Anderson (1995, p. 4), equitable *realized* access is occurring where both demographic variables and need variables largely if not wholly account for the variation in health-care utilization.

With all of this in mind, figure 7.1 presents a schematic for the measurement of disparities in health-care access that considers the health-care system preconditions to access, the enablers and impediments to health-care access that are experienced at the household level (through the reported experiences of individuals or members of the individual's household), and manifestations of disparities in realized health-care access through observed disequities in the major domains of health-care utilization that are crucial to health outcomes. While the measures proposed do not exhaustively consider all the factors that influence disparities in health-care access or, for that matter, the complete array of health-care access measures in national and international health system databases, taken together, they do offer a theoretically coherent and feasible approach to a straightforward assessment of the "access to care" dimension of health system performance. The measures selected are drawn from the well-established MEPS's health-care access section, which are closely comparable to access measures from multicountry surveys on health and health care, and the extensive literature on the measurement of health-care access in comparative analysis of health systems' performance.[5]

As shown in figure 7.1, four system-level (precondition) access measures conceptually precede and set the context for the experience of health-care access at the household level. The term *precondition* refers to the measurement of those structural arrangements that are essential to the *possibility of access* to health care (Hernandez-Quevedo & Papanicolas, 2013). These structural arrangements include enrollment into the insurance coverage provided for the affordability of health care, enrollment into a health-care provider system that provides the connection to a comprehensive array of health services, and two measures of health-care resource deprivation: the relative risk (given such social characteristics as income, race, ethnicity, and geographic location) of living in a poorly resourced community (medically underserved area) and the relative risk of being a member of a poorly resourced population (medically underserved population).[6] All four measures reflect the extent to which the health-care system's redesign is effective in reshaping the structural preconditions of disparities in health-care access. For example, the adjusted odds ratios[7] by race for residing in a medically

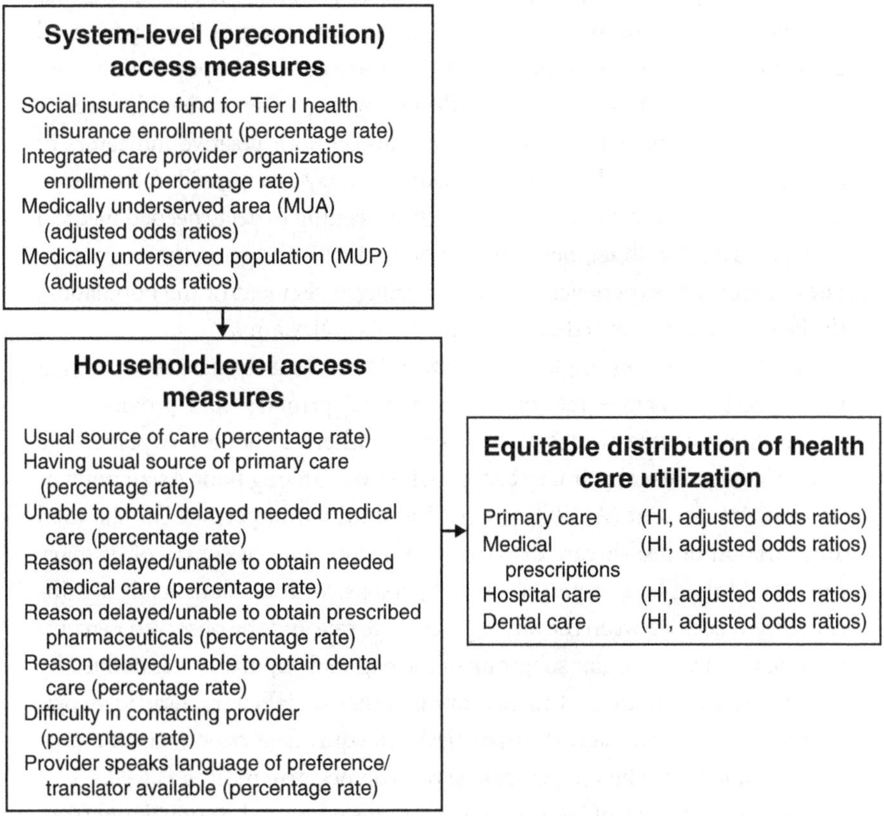

System-level (precondition) access measures

Social insurance fund for Tier I health insurance enrollment (percentage rate)
Integrated care provider organizations enrollment (percentage rate)
Medically underserved area (MUA) (adjusted odds ratios)
Medically underserved population (MUP) (adjusted odds ratios)

Household-level access measures

Usual source of care (percentage rate)
Having usual source of primary care (percentage rate)
Unable to obtain/delayed needed medical care (percentage rate)
Reason delayed/unable to obtain needed medical care (percentage rate)
Reason delayed/unable to obtain prescribed pharmaceuticals (percentage rate)
Reason delayed/unable to obtain dental care (percentage rate)
Difficulty in contacting provider (percentage rate)
Provider speaks language of preference/ translator available (percentage rate)

Equitable distribution of health care utilization

Primary care   (HI, adjusted odds ratios)
Medical   (HI, adjusted odds ratios)
  prescriptions
Hospital care   (HI, adjusted odds ratios)
Dental care   (HI, adjusted odds ratios)

FIGURE 7.1. Measurement of disparities in health-care access.

underserved area capture whether targeted investments in the health-care infrastructure of medically underserved areas are effective in reducing the disproportionate risk of African Americans residing in medically under-served areas relative to other racial groups (Williams & Jackson, 2005).

The household-level access measures shown in figure 7.1 collectively en-compass what the U.S. Department of Health and Human Services describes in its HealthyPeople 2020 strategic plan as the three steps necessary to achiev-ing health-care access: gaining entry into the health-care system, accessing a health-care location where needed services are provided, and finding a health-care provider with whom the patient can communicate and trust (HealthyPeople 2020, 2015). They address the relative percentage rates (by se-lected demographic characteristics associated with health disparities) of hav-ing a usual source of health care, a usual primary care provider, being unable to obtain or having to delay needed health care and the specific reasons why, and having a provider that either shares the language of the reference group or makes a translator available. Simply stated, they capture the experienced capacities to access the health-care system across the subpopulations and communities that have been most affected by disparities in health-care ac-cess. To the extent that the percentage rates on both positive indicators of health-care access (such as having a usual primary care provider) and nega-tive indicators of health-care access (such as needing to delay needed medical or dental care) for all segments of the population converge on the percentage rates historically experienced by the advantaged segment of the population, the health-care system redesign is realizing its policy aims.

To cite a specific example, as of 2012, the MEPS survey data revealed that the highest percentage rate of having a usual primary care provider was among high-income whites at 83.2 percent, whereas the lowest percentage rate of having a usual primary care provider was among poor Asian popula-tions at 62.1 percent (AHRQ, 2012b). The minimal target rate for the total amelioration of health-care disparities in having a usual source of primary care would then be 83.2 percent for all persons, with no statistically signifi-cant differences between the target percentage rate and the observed percent-age rate for any particular subgroup of the national population (as defined by income, education, race, ethnicity, or any other social characteristic associ-ated with health-care access disparities). An equivalent benchmarking pro-cedure could be applied to percentage rates on negative indices as well.

The final category of health-care access measures to be considered from figure 7.1 pertains to the major domains of health-care utilization (primary care, prescribed pharmaceuticals, hospital care, and dental care). As stated by Andersen (1968, 1995), health-care utilization represents *realized* access to health-care access. Equity in realized access to health care would mean that the summed total of all health care provided (whether in dollars of cost, clinic visits, hours of care, etc.) would be used equally across all persons of equal health-care need. We know this not to be true in the United States as well as elsewhere, due to barriers in access to care that are associated with such factors as income, education, race, gender, and the geographic distribution of accessible health-care services. While disequities in health-care utilization are often measured in differences in rates of health-care service use, more recent work in the analysis of health system performance advocates the distributional approach taken to the measurement of disequities in health-care utilization that provides a more encompassing summary index of health-care utilization by level of need (Hernandez-Quevedo & Papanicolas, 2013). That is also the approach that is advanced in this chapter, referred to by its developers as the Index of Horizontal Inequity or HI (van Doorslaer et al., 2006).

The Index of Horizontal Inequity

The term *horizontal inequity* is based on the concept of horizontal equity, meaning equal treatment of equals (Hernandez-Quevedo & Papanicolas, 2013). In the case of the utilization of primary care, this might be represented in the equal distribution of all episodes of care from a "usual primary care provider" for persons who are equal with respect to health-care needs, irrespective of income. The specification of a usual primary care source is applied in this example to make a distinction between episodic care from several different primary care providers (such as a low-income person who relies on a combination of care from community clinics and hospital emergency departments) and an individual well connected to a usual source of primary care better positioned to treat the patient holistically (Xu, 2002). This is represented in the diagonal line of figure 7.2, where the cumulative percentage of all episodes of care from a usual primary care provider coincides with the cumulative percentage of income, with the momentary caveat that all persons are equal with respect to health needs irrespective of income. However, the curve that lies below the diagonal (referred to as the unadjusted Lorenz curve of inequity)[8] represents the situation where the utilization of care from a usual source of primary care is more concentrated among persons of higher income—analogous to the

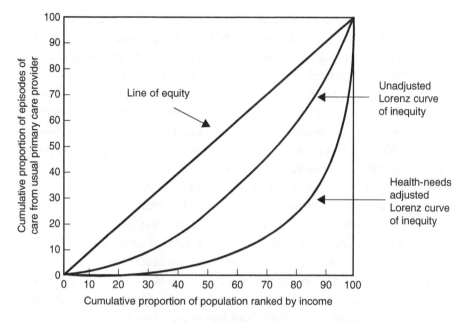

FIGURE 7.2. Sample Lorenz curve of primary care utilization by income.

well-known Lorenz curve of income inequality that is the basis of the Gini coefficient of income inequality.

The HI is an elaboration of this approach that determines a Lorenz curve of observed inequity that is adjusted for predictors of health-care need.[9] This is illustrated further to the right of the Lorenz curve in figure 7.2. Also analogous to the Gini coefficient of income inequality, the area between the diagonal and the dotted Lorenz curve represents the proportion of the cumulative total episodes of primary care that would need to be redistributed to achieve perfect equity.

As an example application of the HI, in a comparative analysis of inequities in access to medical care by income among developed countries, van Doorslaer et al. (2006) used age, sex, self-reported general health, and the presence and degree of limitation due to chronic physical and mental health conditions as their predictors of health need, finding that among most of the twenty-one developed countries sampled, primary care visits were equitably distributed among all income groups (indicated by an HI≈0, with the "≈" representing a value that is not statistically different from zero). As might be expected based on its fragmented and exclusionary approach to health insurance coverage, the United States was not among them.

Since income plays such a determinant role of health-care utilization (realized access) among all segments of society, the approach to measuring the amelioration of disparities in utilization advanced in this chapter would be to apply the HI to the utilization of primary care, prescribed pharmaceuticals, hospital care, and dental care. The complete amelioration of disparities in health-care utilization (realized access) by level of income would thus be represented as HI$c \approx$ 0, where c=all the major categories of health care shown in the right-hand box of figure 7.1. However, this still leaves the problem of how to measure disparities in the utilization of health care by race, ethnicity, geographic location, and other demographic characteristics associated with disparities in health care.

While the conventional technique for the measurement of inequities between different segments of the population in health-care utilization is a simple comparison of group differences in rates, crude differences in rates of utilization do not necessarily represent disequities, in that they do not account for differences in health needs. To account for group differences in health-care utilization that are adjusted for differences in level of need, regression methods are employed such as adjusted odds ratios and the just described HI (Hernandez-Quevedo & Papanicolas, 2013). In the case of group differences in health-care utilization that are measured at the nominal level such as race, ethnicity, and geographic location, the logistic regression technique is the most widely applicable to the detailed individual-level data produced from national surveys of health and health-care utilization (such as the National Health Interview Survey). This is because logistic regression produces robust estimates of the specific effects of selected demographic characteristics on an individual's probability of using different types of health care adjusted for differences in health-care needs. In general form, the logistic regression model for an individual's probability of experiencing a health-care utilization event (such as a visit in the past thirty days with a primary care provider) would be defined in the following equation as p, whereas the individual's probability of not experiencing the health-care utilization event would be defined as 1-p.

$$\ln\left(\frac{p}{1-p}\right) = \beta_0 + \beta_c + \beta_h$$

The symbol ln refers to a natural logarithm, with β_0 representing the parameter estimate for the intercept of the regression line, β_c the parameter estimate for the net effect of the demographic categorical variable on the log odds of the health utilization event, and βh the parameter estimate for the net effect of health needs on the log odds of the health utilization event. Analogous with the HI discussed previously, perfect equity in health-care utilization net of differences in health needs would be represented as $\beta c \approx 0$, meaning that the demographic categorical variable fails to have a net effect on the probability of the health utilization event occurring or not occurring. An observed $\beta c \approx 0$ is therefore the ultimate health-care policy aim of the redesigned health-care system, whether c refers to a category of race, ethnicity, location in an underresourced community, or any other demographic characteristic associated with disparities in health-care utilization that are not attributable to differences in health-care needs.

The same approach to the measurement of disparities in utilization could also be applied at higher levels of aggregation, such as communities, with the dependent variable being utilization rates rather than individual-level events using ordinary least squares (OLS) techniques, with the OLS equivalent of $\beta c \approx 0$ serving as a benchmark representation of perfect equity. It should also be pointed out that regression-based measures of equity in health-care utilization have the advantage, where disparities in health-care utilization do exist, of extending the analysis of observed disequities in health-care utilization to the relative contributions of such confounding factors as income, education, and the household-level access barriers that are highlighted in figure 7.1.

Setting the Target Performance Benchmarks for the Amelioration of Disparities in Health-Care Access

Up until now, the discussion on the measures of health-care access have been primarily conceptual, and not as much has been said about rationale behind the target performance benchmarks selected for each measure. As a general point, the target performance benchmarks are the values on each measure that are viewed as desirable and achievable *as a long-range goal*, which is consistent with the approach to health system performance benchmarking advanced by the Commonwealth Fund's *Path to a High Performance U.S. Health System: A 2020 Vision and the Policies to Pave the Way* (The Commonwealth Fund Commission on a High Performance Health System, 2009). It is assumed that the redesigned health-care system is meeting its performance objectives to the extent that at each stage of its implementation and evolution, the values on each measure are moving toward the target performance benchmark and that incremental performance benchmarks will be progressively recalibrated as a part of the global budgeting process. The relationship between the selected health system performance measures, the core policy aims they represent, and the target values for each performance benchmark is shown in table 7.1. Although the discussion that follows will be concerned primarily with the target performance benchmarks for measures of health-care access, it will be seen that table 7.1 also illustrates the relationships between the core policy aim of universal comprehensive health insurance with adequate and equal risk protection, and its performance measures and target benchmarks (as discussed in the previous section of this chapter).

As shown in table 7.1, the first two target performance benchmarks for equitable *system-level access* are the same as those for the health insurance enrollment measures pertaining to adequate and equal risk protection (core health-care policy aim 1). That's because health insurance serves the dual functions of both risk protection and access into the health-care system. The third and fourth target benchmarks for equitable system-level access are the logistic regression parameter values that reflect the realization of equity in the probability of living in a medically underserved area or being a member of a medically underserved population. That is, there is equal shared risk of living in a medically underserved area or being a member of medically underserved population irrespective of individual characteristics that have long been associated with disparities in access to health care.

The most difficult target benchmark for system-level access is the third, pertaining to the desired and achievable rate of enrollment in Integrated Care Provider Organizations (ICPOs). While universal ICPO enrollment might be desirable as a way of promoting a high standard of care for all Tier I health-care beneficiaries, the maximum achievable enrollment in ICPOs is subject to two limiting factors. The first is the prevalence of individual-level social and health/mental health conditions that would either pose a significant barrier to stable ICPO enrollment or would be better treated through specialized providers (as specified in the provider components of the Tier I health-care delivery system depicted in figure 6.2 of the preceding chapter). The second limiting factor is the geographic distribution of the national population, which locates about 15 percent of the population in rural areas that lack the population density essential to the economic

TABLE 7.1
Core Health-Care Policy Aims 1 and 2 and Health-Care System Performance Benchmarks

Core health-care policy aim	Health-care system performance measures	Target performance benchmarks
1. Universal comprehensive health insurance with adequate and equal risk protection		
Universal Tier I health insurance enrollment	Enrollment of U.S. citizens (percentage rate)	100 percent
	Enrollment of permanent legal residents (percentage rate)	100 percent
	Enrollment of undocumented workers and dependents on ITIN IRS tax returns (percentage rate)	70 percent
Adequate and equal risk protection	Proportion of bankruptcies/home foreclosures attributable to health-care expenditures (percentage rate)	≤ 16 percent
	Share of discretionary household income to Tier I out-of-pocket expenditures (percentage)	≤ 20 percent, adjusted to household income level
	Incidence of delayed necessary health care due to cost, adjusted to discretionary household income (percentage rate)	≤ 20 percent at all household income levels
2. Amelioration of disparities in health-care access and quality		
System-level access	Social insurance fund for Tier I health insurance enrollment (percentage rate)	100 percent U.S. citizens/permanent legal residents, 70 percent undocumented workers/ dependents
	Integrated care provider organizations enrollment (percentage rate)	80 percent of Tier I health insurance enrollees
	Medically underserved area (MUA), logistic regression coefficient	$\beta c \approx 0$, c=race, ethnicity, low income, or other demographic characteristic associated with disparities
	Medically underserved population (MUP), logistic regression coefficient	$\beta c \approx 0$, c=race, ethnicity, low income, or other demographic characteristic associated with disparities
Household-level access	Usual source of care (percentage rate)	$\mu benchmark\ value=\mu c_1=\mu c_2=\ldots \mu c_i$
	Having usual source of primary care (percentage rate)	$\mu benchmark\ value=\mu c_1=\mu c_2=\ldots \mu c_i$
	Unable to obtain/delayed needed medical care (percentage rate)	$\mu benchmark\ value=\mu c_1=\mu c_2=\ldots \mu c_i$
	Reason delayed/unable to obtain needed medical care (percentage rate)	$\mu benchmark\ value=\mu c_1=\mu c_2=\ldots \mu c_i$
	Difficulty in contacting provider (percentage rate)	$\mu benchmark\ value=\mu c_1=\mu c_2=\ldots \mu c_i$
	Provider speaks language of preference/translator available (percentage rate)	$\mu benchmark\ value=\mu c_1=\mu c_2=\ldots \mu c_i$
Realization of access (health-care utilization)	Primary care (HI, logistic regression coefficient)	$HI. \approx 0$: $\beta c \approx 0$, c=race, ethnicity, low income, or other demographic characteristic associated with disparities

Core health-care policy aim	Health-care system performance measures	Target performance benchmarks
	Pharmaceutical care/Rx (HI, logistic regression coefficient)	$HI \approx 0$: $\beta c \approx 0$, c=race, ethnicity, low income, or other demographic characteristic associated with disparities
	Hospital care (HI, logistic regression coefficient)	$HI \approx 0$: $\beta c \approx 0$, c=race, ethnicity, low income, or other demographic characteristic associated with disparities
	Dental care (HI, logistic regression coefficient)	$HI \approx 0$: $\beta c \approx 0$, c=race, ethnicity, low income, or other demographic characteristic associated with disparities
Quality of care	Effectiveness (measurement domain)	$\mu benchmark\ value = \mu c_1 = \mu c_2 = \ldots \mu c_i$
	Safety (measurement domain)	$\mu benchmark\ value = \mu c_1 = \mu c_2 = \ldots \mu c_i$
	Timeliness (measurement domain)	$\mu benchmark\ value = \mu c_1 = \mu c_2 = \ldots \mu c_i$
	Patient centeredness (measurement domain)	$\mu benchmark\ value = \mu c_1 = \mu c_2 = \ldots \mu c_i$
	Care coordination (measurement domain)	$\mu benchmark\ value = \mu c_1 = \mu c_2 = \ldots \mu c_i$
	Efficiency (measurement domain)	$\mu benchmark\ value = \mu c_1 = \mu c_2 = \ldots \mu c_i$
	Adequacy of infrastructure (measurement domain)	$\mu benchmark\ value = \mu c_1 = \mu c_2 = \ldots \mu c_i$

sustainability of a fully developed ICPO (Cromartie, 2013). Given these considerations, the hypothetical target value for ICPO enrollment of 80 percent among Tier I health-care beneficiaries is but an educated guess that endeavors to balance the social desirability of nearly universal ICPO enrollment with the uncertain limits to that enrollment.

The household-level access measures shown in figure 7.1 are taken from the MEPS discussed earlier in the chapter. To recap, MEPS is an ongoing survey of families and individuals, their medical providers (doctors, hospitals, pharmacies, etc.), and employers across the United States that is administered by the Agency for Healthcare Research and Quality. The MEPS measures and data have three distinctive advantages that make them highly adaptable to the ongoing performance evaluation of the nation's health-care system. The first is that the household measures of health system access are theoretically consistent with the core determinants of health-care access established in the extensive literature on health-care access. The second is that the MEPS surveys are conducted annually, thus allowing for an ongoing assessment of the health-care system's progress toward the achievement of its core policy aims. The third is that MEPS measures of health-care access align very closely with the individual- and household-level health-care access measures used in the European Union Statistics on In-come and Living Conditions (EU-SILC), the Commonwealth Fund Inter-national Health Policy Survey, and the European Social Survey (ESS) (Hernandez-Quevedo & Papanicolas, 2013).

As also touched upon previously, the target performance benchmarks for the household measures of health-care access represent the realization of perfect equity in accordance to what at any point in time is optimal health-care access.[10] To revisit the illustrative example of this approach to benchmarking optimal health system performance, as of 2012, the MEPS survey data revealed that the highest percentage rate of having a usual primary care provider was among high-income whites at 83.2 percent, whereas the lowest percentage rate of having a usual primary care provider was among poor Asian populations at 62.1 percent (AHRQ, 2012b). The minimal target rate for the total amelioration of health-care disparities in having a usual source of primary care would thus be 83.2 percent for persons, with no statistically significant differences between the target percentage rate and the observed percentage rate for any particular sub-group of the national population. Statistically, this is represented as $\mu benchmark\ value = \mu c_1 = \mu c_2 = \ldots \mu c_i$, with $\mu benchmark\ value$ in this ex-ample equal to 83.2 percent and $\mu c_1 = \mu c_2 = \ldots \mu c_i$ representing the observed percentage rates for different segments of the population historically at risk for disparities in access to health care.[11] As shown in table 7.1, this approach to benchmarking the optimal value on household-level access measures and defining perfect equity is applied to all of the household-level access measures.

The final performance benchmarks to be considered are those pertain-ing to the major domains of health-care utilization (or as defined by Ander-sen, 1995, the *realization* of health-care access). Consistent with the earlier discussion on the use of regression methods and indices disequities in ac-cess to health care, the target performance benchmarks for perfect equity of utilization are represented as an HI value of 0 and a logistic regression coefficient (βc) of 0 across all categories of race, ethnicity, and other char-acteristics associated with disparities (as shown in table 7.1). The HI benchmark is targeted at the disequities in health-care access by income, while the $\beta c \approx 0$ criterion is applied to categorical differences associated with health-care access disparities. For both HI and βc, progress toward the amelioration of disparities in health-care utilization (as *realized* access) is represented in ever smaller values of HI and βc as the redesigned health-care system is implemented and evolves over time.

The Conceptualization and Measurement of Health-Care Quality,
Equity of Quality, and Disparities in Quality

The Institute of Medicine (IOM) has defined quality as "the degree to which health services for individuals and populations increase the likelihood of desired health outcomes and are consistent with current professional knowledge" (McGlynn, 1997, p. 7). While there are several implications to this definition of health-care quality, the most important one from the standpoint of this chapter is that measures of health-care quality, and therefore disparities in health-care quality, must address the processes of care and related health outcomes at the individual and population health levels. Toward that end, beginning in 2003, the Agency for Healthcare Research and Quality (AHRQ) has published a series of annual reports on progress toward the improvement of health-care quality and reducing health-care disparities. The domains of health-care quality that have been covered in the National Healthcare Quality (NHQR) reports have included effectiveness, safety, timeliness, patient centeredness, care coordination, efficiency, and the adequacy of health system infrastructure—thus, many of the NHQR health quality measures and much of the data on recent health system performance can and should be used as the baseline for the evaluation of the redesigned health-care system's effectiveness in improving health-care quality. It is also important to note that the health-care quality constructs and measures that have provided the framework for the NHRQ reports largely represent the state of the science in health-care quality assessment and reflect the priorities advanced in the *National Strategy for Quality Improvement in Health Care* that was mandated as a part of the ACA (specifically Section 311). In sum, there is no need to reinvent a new approach to the quality of care component of the redesigned health-care system's performance so much as to briefly highlight the AHRQ's approach that should be extended into the future as the nation's health-care system evolves to a form that will be superior.

The first aspect of the AHRQ approach worthy of highlighting is that both the domains of health-care quality and the measures specific to each domain are the outcome of an ongoing collaborative process that involves health data experts from key health and health-care agencies such as the National Center for Health Statistics (NCHS), the Centers for Medicare and Medicaid Services (CMS), the Substance Abuse and Mental Health Services Administration (SAMHSA), and the Centers for Disease Control and Prevention (CDC), as well as nongovernmental health-care quality experts from various branches of medicine and the health and social sciences.

That is, the AHRQ functions as the lead agency on an ongoing national effort to assess and improve health-care quality and reduce health-care disparities. The second aspect of the AHRQ's process for the evaluation and improvement of health-care quality is that, while the domains of health-care quality assessment and improvement provide a stable framework for the analysis of health-care quality, the specific measures themselves change over time in response to such factors as changing standards of clinical practice in response to research findings and innovations in health-care technology, changes in population health and newly emergent risk factors, innovations in quality measurement, and new forms of health disparities. The dynamic nature of health-care quality measures and the huge health data infrastructure investments entailed in fact create a difficult policy dilemma for the AHRQ and other governmental agencies involved in health-care quality assessment and improvement, a policy problem to be revisited in more depth in a forthcoming discussion.

The final aspect of the AHRQ health-care quality assessment and improvement approach highlighted is its main methodology for the measurement and tracking of the amelioration of disparities in the quality of health care. In essence, disparities in health-care quality are typically operationalized as statistically significant differences on the measures of health-care quality between different subgroups of the population representing the range from the most to least advantaged with respect to health care—on most health-care quality measures, this is a difference between subgroups in percentage rates of something good or bad occurring from the standpoint of health-care quality (as in subgroup rates of age-appropriate mammography screening for breast cancer versus subgroup rates for diagnosis of advanced state breast cancer). The subgroup categories of course encompass all of the major dimensions of health and health-care disparities inclusive of age, sex, socioeconomic status, race, ethnicity, and also geographic location. Disparities are also typically expressed as differences on a given measure of quality between the most advantaged group on that measure (termed the reference group) and the comparison group.[12] In addition, since 2010, the AHRQ approach to the measurement and tracking of disparities in health-care quality has incorporated a benchmarking methodology that defines the benchmark for a given measure of quality as the average value for the 10 percent of states that had the best performance on that quality measure (AHRQ, 2014b, pp. 31–32). The premise is that the standards of health system performance should not differ across population groups and that all population groups should be moving toward this health-care system performance benchmark over time.

In keeping with this equity premise, the AHRQ annual health disparities reports include findings from an expected time-to-achieve benchmark for different subgroups of the population. Finally, the AHRQ methodology for tracking the amelioration of observed disparities between population subgroups on health-care quality measures defines progress toward the amelioration of disparities as an average annual rate of change of greater than 1 percent in the desired direction (AHRQ, 2014b).

The Selection of Specific Measures of Health-Care Quality

The AHRQ's methodological framework for ongoing assessment of health-care quality and related health-care disparities provides the essential foundation for the performance evaluation of the health-care system of the future. However, there remains a significant policy challenge with respect to the selection of the specific measures of health-care quality over time as the social and economic context of population health changes and the health-care system itself continue to evolve. Each new iteration in the measures used to capture various aspects of health-care quality entails significant direct costs in data infrastructure investments and difficult trade-offs between optimal validity, logistical feasibility, and competing priorities on the most valuable aspects of health-care quality to assess. Moreover, there are simply too many measures of health-care quality to choose from. As of 2014, the Department of Health and Human Services National Quality Measures Clearinghouse identified some 2,100 measures of health-care quality. Even among the National Healthcare Quality and Disparities Reports published between 2003 and 2013 (where there was authoritative consensus on which measures of health-care quality were most valid and policy relevant), there were 250 different measures of health-care quality (Meltzer & Chung, 2014). Although each of these hundreds of measures has been scientifically validated as an indicator of some specific aspect of health care deemed to represent quality, by what criteria other than validity should particular measures of health-care quality be chosen?

The argument here is that the optimal measures of health-care quality (being equal with respect to validity) are those most associated with *allocative efficiency*, defined in this context as the extent to which limited resources are directed toward producing the correct mix of health-care system outputs in line with the core aims of national health-care policy (Cylus & Smith,

2013, p. 284).[13] Based on this allocative efficiency approach, Meltzer and Chung (2014) have suggested that the criterion for the selection of health-care quality measures should be those that measure health system outputs that yield the highest *net health benefits*—in essence, the greatest improvements in population health and the greatest reductions in health disparities net of the costs that result from using a specific quality measure (p. 133). Meltzer and Chung demonstrated the utility of this approach through their use of quality-adjusted life years (QALYs) as the metric for health benefits and then testing this criterion against the population health data relevant to thirteen measures used in the AHRQ National Health Care Quality Reports. Interestingly, of the thirteen quality of care measures they examined, seven measures produced 93 percent of the yield in estimated population health benefits, while the bottom six accounted for only 7 percent of possible improvements in population health.[14] Based on logic and the evidence, the net health benefit criterion is therefore advanced as the primary selection method for the measures of health-care quality.

That being said, some other selection criteria will also remain essential, such as relative validity, the coverage of all domains of health-care quality, and patient preferences for aspects of quality of care that (while not directly tied to population health outcomes) reflect cultural values.

Defining the Core Quality of Care Measurement Domains

Revisiting table 7.1, it can be seen that with respect to quality of health-care measures, quality of care domains are substituted for a listing of the specific measures of quality of care, which are too numerous to list but would be subject to the selection criteria just discussed. These quality of care domains, which are taken directly from the AHRQ quality of care framework, include effectiveness, safety, timeliness, patient centeredness, care coordination, efficiency, and the adequacy of the health system infrastructure. Briefly stated, *effectiveness* is defined as the extent to which a health-care benefit yields health benefits, *safety* refers to patient safety or the incidence of accidental injuries due to medical care or medical errors, and *timeliness* refers to the system's capacity to provide care quickly after a need is recognized (AHRQ, 2014b). *Patient centeredness* is a more encompassing construct, which is defined by the Institute of Medicine as "health care that establishes a partnership among practitioners, patients, and their families (when appropriate) to ensure that decisions respect patients' wants, needs, and preferences and that patients have the education and support they need to make decisions and participate in their own care" (AHRQ, 2014b, p. 167).

Broadly defined, *care coordination* is the extent to which health-care providers collaborate effectively with one another to facilitate the appropriate delivery of health-care services (Shojania et al., 2007). Health-care "efficiency" has two related but distinct conceptualizations; the first is the net health benefits in relation to the costs of health care (Shi & Singh, 2001), and the second is the extent to which waste, overuse, and misuse of health care are eliminated (AHRQ, 2014b). Finally, the adequacy of the health system infrastructure is a very broad domain of health-care quality that includes the health-care workforce, information systems, diagnostic and treatment technologies, physical facilities, and other structural and organizational components essential to the delivery of emerging and high-quality health care (AHRQ, 2014b).

Although the specific measures of health-care quality that reflect each quality of care domain are not identified in table 7.1, most of the quality of care measures that have thus far been developed in national health-care databases have been expressed as percentages or incidence rates, which conform to analyses of quality of care disparities based on differences between group means. Thus, the third column of table 7.1 shows that the target health system performance benchmark for the total amelioration of disparities in quality of care would be stated as $\mu benchmark\ value = \mu c_1 = \mu c_2 = \ldots \mu c_i$, with $\mu benchmark\ value$ equal to the mean value for the subgroup of the population receiving the *highest* level of health-care quality on the particular measure used. This is consistent with the most recent approach to the measurement and benchmarking of disparities in health-care quality used by the AHRQ and also the approach used for the other means-based measures of health-care disparities shown in table 7.1.

POLICY AIM 3: THE EQUITABLE DISTRIBUTION OF PREVENTATIVE, CURATIVE, REHABILITATIVE, AND ADAPTIVE HEALTH-CARE SERVICES/TECHNOLOGIES SPECIFIC TO HEALTH NEEDS, AND PUBLIC HEALTH INVESTMENTS AND MEASURES

Assessing the Equitable Distribution of Services

As discussed in chapter 4, the health-care provisions encompassed in core policy aim 3 represent the essential substance of a social right to health

care. While the provisions in core health-care policy aim 2 pertain to amelioration of distributive injustices in whatever the corpus of a social right
to health care has been defined to encompass, core health-care policy aim
3 delineates the health-care provisions that every citizen is entitled to a fair
and equal share in. As also discussed in chapter 4, the health-care provisions
included under core health-care policy aim 3 are those deemed necessary
to the development and preservation of the capacities that are essential to
the normal range of human functioning, both at the individual level and
at the population level. They thus include (a) the preventative, curative,
rehabilitative, and adaptive health-care services/technologies specific to
health needs of individuals and (b) the public health investments and measures that are essential to the preservation and advancement of population
health.[15]

That the justification of these essential health-care provisions is based
on "the *development* and *preservation* of capacities that are essential to
normal range of human functioning" suggests that a comprehensive evaluation of the health-care system's performance should incorporate a normative life span perspective—a perspective that takes into account the
different health needs that arise at different stages of the complete human
life. As it happens, this is the approach to health system performance evaluation that has recently been incorporated by the AHRQ's annual National
Healthcare Quality Report series, which, beginning in 2013, includes an
evaluation of health-care services that improve health and quality of life
that are "often better characterized by stage over a lifespan rather than by
organ system" (AHRQ, 2014b, p. 95). From the standpoint of conceptualization and measurement, this divides health-care provisions between those
that target common diseases and health conditions (such as diabetes) and
those that focus on domains of clinical care over the life course (such as
adolescent health or palliative care in advanced age).

As can be seen in table 7.2, this is also the framework for the assessment
of health system performance as it applies to the full range of health-care
services (preventative, curative, rehabilitative, and adaptive) that make up
the substance of core health-care policy aim 3 (part A). As with the quality
of care measures discussed in the preceding section, rather than naming
the dozens of specific measures that apply to the full range of health services addressed in core health-care policy aim 3, it is assumed that the
specific measures that will be used (that themselves reflect the optimal
kinds of health services provided) will be those that yield the highest level

TABLE 7.2
Core Health-Care Policy Aims 3 and 4 and Health-Care System Performance Benchmarks

Core health-care policy aim	Health-care system performance measures	Target performance benchmarks
3a. Equitable distribution of preventative, curative, rehabilitative, and adaptive health-care services/ technologies specific to health needs		
Preventative	Common clinical conditions measures	$\mu benchmark$ $value = \mu c_1 = \mu c_2 = \ldots \mu c_i$
	Life span clinical care measures	$\mu benchmark$ $value = \mu c_1 = \mu c_2 = \ldots \mu c_i$
Curative	Common clinical conditions measures	$\mu benchmark$ $value = \mu c_1 = \mu c_2 = \ldots \mu c_i$
	Life span clinical care measures	$\mu benchmark$ $value = \mu c_1 = \mu c_2 = \ldots \mu c_i$
Rehabilitative	Common clinical conditions measures	$\mu benchmark$ $value = \mu c_1 = \mu c_2 = \ldots \mu c_i$
	Life span clinical care measures	$\mu benchmark$ $value = \mu c_1 = \mu c_2 = \ldots \mu c_i$
Adaptive	Common clinical conditions measures	$\mu benchmark$ $value = \mu c_1 = \mu c_2 = \ldots \mu c_i$
	Life span clinical care measures	$\mu benchmark$ $value = \mu c_1 = \mu c_2 = \ldots \mu c_i$
3b. Equitable distribution of public health investments and interventions	Distribution of public dollars in public health infrastructure/interventions (HI)	$HI \approx 0$
4. Compensatory entitlements and investments in health-care services and public health infrastructure/interventions for individuals, groups, and populations adversely affected by health disparities	Quality-adjusted life year (QALY) based on per capita compensatory investments	*QALY compensatory investment* (value subpopulation specific)

of net health benefits in accordance with the principle of allocative efficiency (Cylus & Smith, 2013). Also, as with the quality of care measures, target performance benchmark for the equitable distribution of the full range of health-care services will be expressed as $\mu benchmark\ value = \mu c_1 = \mu c_2 = \ldots$ μc_i, with the benchmark defined as the highest observed *health needs-adjusted* mean value on the health-care measure for any subgroup of the national population and μc representing the health needs-adjusted mean value on the health-care measure for subgroups of the population defined by age, income, race, ethnicity, sex, geographic location, or other categories that represent high risk for health-care disparities. The "highest observed value" benchmarking criterion, aside from being consistent with the current national benchmarking approach adopted by the AHRQ, reflects the assumption validated by decades of research on fundamental social cause theory that the benefits of innovations in health care are distributed in accordance with hierarchies of economic advantage and power (Phelan et al., 2004). Finally, the approach to the adjustment for health needs would be determined by the multivariate regression methods appropriate to the specific health-care measure and data sources (Hernandez-Quevedo & Papanicolas, 2013).

Consistent with the health system performance measures that pertain to the amelioration of health-care disparities, it assumed that with respect to the optimal delivery of the health-care services delineated in core health-care policy aim 3, on a broad array of measures, the health-care system will fall short of its benchmarks. These health system performance gaps will persist for two reasons. The first is that to the extent that the health-care system continues to function within embedded systems of oppression and injustice, the delivery of health care will continue to reflect those systems of oppression and injustice just as disparities in health will persist (Link & Phelan, 1995). At best, well-conceived health-care reform can only hope to reduce the effects of social stratification on health care.

The second reason that health system performance gaps will continue to persist is that both societal evolution and innovations in health care will create the necessity for new kinds of health system performance benchmarks and revisions to the existing ones. For this reason, as with the need to assess health system performance trends and progress benchmarks in the amelioration of health-care disparities, there will need to be performance trend tracking and progress benchmarking specific to the delivery of the health services identified in core health-care policy aim 3. Because the national investments in the specific array of preventative, curative, rehabilitative, and adaptive health-care services provided as a social right of citizenship must vary in response to the dynamic nature of population health risks and changing social priorities (for example, as with the investments in the AIDS epidemic that emerged in the 1980s), so too must the health system performance benchmarks and the markers of adequate health system performance improvement.

Assessing the Equitable Distribution of Public Health Investments
and Interventions

Public health investments refer to the public dollars that are distributed to the public health infrastructure at the national, state, and local community levels that (1) target the prevention of disease and disability and prevention and (2) are focused on the health of entire populations, rather than individuals (CDC, 2000). The components of public health infrastructure include a network of federal, state, and local health departments and laboratories that provide the essential public health services (such as monitor health risks and investigate/diagnose population health problems, enforce laws and regulations that protect the health of the public, mobilize community partnerships and actions to address local health problems, and inform and educate the public about important health issues); the local, state, and national public health data and information systems; and the public clinics and hospitals that comprise a large part of the nation's health-care safety net (Shi & Singh, 2001). Public health interventions refer to the subset of public health investments in population-based health interventions that target specific population health risks, such as diabetes prevention programs or population-based sexually transmitted disease prevention measures.

There are three fundamental premises to the equitable distribution of public health investments and interventions. The first is that governments are accountable for the general health of the national population and progress toward the achievement of optimal population health, just as they are responsible for a nation's economic stability and progress toward an optimal standard of material well-being (Karanikolos et al., 2013). The second is that a significant share of a national population's avoidable mortality (deaths that can be prevented) can be affected either negatively or positively by political decisions about the magnitude and distribution of population-based health interventions (Karanikolos et al., 2013). The third is that variations in the preventable death rates among the different segments of the national population reflect, in part, historic disequities in public health investments and the provision of population-based health interventions (CDC, 2010).

The effectiveness of the nation's health-care system in terms of the equity of its investments in public health infrastructure and interventions brings us back to the concept of *horizontal equity*, previously defined as the equal treatment of persons who are equal with respect to health needs (Hernandez-Quevedo & Papanicolas, 2013). In the context of realized primary care access discussed earlier in this chapter, *horizontal equity* meant that the utilization of primary health care would be observed to be equal across persons once individual differences in health-care needs were taken into account. In the context of public health investments, *horizontal equity* becomes defined as the equal treatment of communities and populations that are equal with respect to health needs, with equity observed as an equal distribution of public health dollars across populations and communities once aggregate within-population/community differences in health needs are taken into account. In that differences in the health needs of populations and communities are measured as variations in the rates of disease, disability, and death, the HI that was introduced at an earlier point in this chapter is advanced as a particularly useful measure of this aspect of a health system's performance (van Doorslaer et al., 2006).

To recap, the HI is an application of the Lorenz curve methodology for estimation of distributional inequities that adjusts the coefficient of distributional inequity for differences in health needs, with $HI \approx 0$ representing equity and a progression toward equity represented in a decrease in the absolute magnitude of HI toward 0 (Hernandez-Quevedo & Papanicolas, 2013). Conceptually, this could be visualized by reexamining figure 7.2, substituting on the Y-axis the cumulative proportion of public health dollars for the cumulative proportion of primary care episodes. For the X-axis, income could be the dimension of equity considered, as could communities and populations ranked by any number of other indicators. In keeping with this general approach, table 7.2 shows that the target performance benchmark for the distribution of public health investment dollars across populations and communities is therefore set to be $HI \approx 0$.

POLICY AIM 4: COMPENSATORY ENTITLEMENTS AND INVESTMENTS IN HEALTH-CARE SERVICES AND PUBLIC HEALTH INFRASTRUCTURE AND INTERVENTIONS FOR INDIVIDUALS, GROUPS, AND POPULATIONS ADVERSELY AFFECTED BY HEALTH DISPARITIES

As discussed in chapter 4, compensatory health service investments to individuals, groups, and populations adversely affected by health disparities pertain to "downstream" funds that are allocated to the facility, workforce, and technological components of the diagnosis and treatment of disease and disability, whereas compensatory public health infrastructure investments entail resources targeted toward "upstream" population health strategies that are intended to reduce disparities in disease risk and prevalence. Although (as discussed in chapter 4) the primary justification for such compensatory investments is the role that health plays as a functional requisite to fair equality of opportunity, compensatory health service investments are also justified by the general goal of equity in health outcomes.

To the extent that achievement of equity in health outcomes relies on equity in health care, there are two forms of equity in health care at play. The first is the previously described *horizontal equity* health-care provisions that are based on the moral principle of equal treatment of persons and groups that are equal with respect to health needs. The second form of equity, *vertical equity*, calls for unequal health-care investments on behalf of persons and groups that are unequal with respect to health and health-care needs—in particular, those segments of society carrying a disproportionate burden of disease and disability (Hernandez-Quevedo & Papanicolas, 2013). Vertical equity in health care is realized to the extent that compensatory investments in health care are proportionate to disparities in health, and this in turn serves as the criterion for the evaluation of the health-care system's performance in response to core health-care policy aim 4. But by what specific metric should the magnitude of these compensatory health-care investments be calibrated? For several reasons, it is suggested that the preferred metric should be based on the age-adjusted cost for the QALY.

Calibrating the Magnitude and Distribution of Compensatory Health-Care Investments

As discussed at an earlier point in the chapter, a QALY is a measure of life expectancy that takes into account both the quantity of life in number of years and the quality of life in different health states, with 1 representing a year in perfect health and 0 representing death. It is in essence the arithmetic product of a life year and a measure of life quality in functional health that ranges between 0 and 1.

Because the QALY captures both the quantity and quality of aspects of life years, it has long been favored and extensively researched as the standard metric for the cost-benefit analysis of national investments in health-care benefits, programs, and emergent health-care technologies. In the United States, the QALY has been extensively used for these purposes since the 1970s, when it was used to determine the gains in functional life years relative to expenditures for the kidney dialysis coverage of Medicare beneficiaries with end-stage renal disease (Neumann et al., 2014). As discussed earlier in this chapter, we have also seen that in the more recent work of Meltzer and Chung (2014), the QALY was selected as the criterion metric for the determination of the most optimal measures of health-care quality.

While the QALY measure of healthy life expectancy has been used extensively as a tool in the United States and elsewhere to guide public health-care investments, it has also been used as a population-based measure of health disparities that captures disparities in the years of life lived in optimal health (Howard et al., 2014; McCollister et al., 2012). For example, it has been shown that the racial disparity in *healthy* life expectancy between whites and African Americans is significantly larger than the disparity in *overall* life expectancy (Molla, 2013). It is this second feature of the QALY, the ability to capture the disparities in both the length and the quality of life, that makes the QALY a particularly useful metric for the calculation of compensatory investments in health care.

However, what is also needed is an estimated dollar value to attach to a QALY that can serve as the benchmark for compensatory health-care investments to those segments of the national population most affected by health disparities. In keeping with the principle of vertical equity, the magnitude of compensatory investments in health-care services would thus be calibrated in proportion to the gap in QALYs between the least and most advantaged groups in society.

One approach to setting the compensatory value of a QALY for the disadvantaged segments of the population would be to tie the compensatory value of the QALY to the prevailing monetary threshold for public fund (primarily Medicare) expenditures for expanded health-care benefits and new technologies, which by historic convention has been fixed at $50,000 per QALY (Neumann et al., 2014). That is, under the prevailing standards for extending Medicare coverage for new innovations in medical technology and treatments, up to $50,000 for each added QALY for a Medicare beneficiary is considered a justifiable social investment.[16] From an equity point of view, since no distinction should be made between the maximum social investment for an added QALY for a Medicare beneficiary and the QALY of a member of group that carries a disproportionate burden of morbidity and mortality, it would seem that magnitude of social investments in closing the QALY gap in health disparities should at least be proportionate to the social investments we as a society are willing to make to extend the QALY's for Medicare beneficiaries.

As intuitive as this approach might be from the standpoint of equity, the limited literature on an empirically based standard for the monetary value of a QALY suggests that the $50,000 benchmark actually falls far from historic health resource allocation decisions (Braithwaite et al., 2008; Hirth et al., 2000). The $50,000 benchmark also refers to a maximum expenditure threshold per QALY, as opposed to what should be a target average expenditure per QALY. The preferred standard of equity would actually be some form of an age-adjusted QALY benchmark. An example of this would be a QALY expenditure benchmark based on the age-adjusted worth in terms of human capital—that is, the productive capacity of one year of life in good health. By this criterion, Hirth et al. (2000) estimated that the benchmark for an age-adjusted QALY should be fixed at $36,544 (in 2014 dollars).[17] While this might seem to be an overly conservative figure, it reflects the average annual valuation of productivity over the entire length of life, including childhood and old age. If we used $36,544 as a hypothetical QALY expenditure benchmark, then the compensatory health-care investments over an individual lifetime that would be proportional to the disparity in QALYs would be calculated as follows:

$$(QALYs \text{ } reference \text{ } population - QALYs \text{ } comparison \text{ } population) \times \$36,544$$

As an empirical example, recent CDC data on functional life expectancy between African Americans and whites suggest that whites can expect the equivalent of sixty-seven QALYs over the complete lifetime while African Americans can expect only sixty-one QALYs over a complete lifetime, a difference of six QALYs (Molla, 2013). If the age-adjusted QALYs were valued at $36,544 (as suggested by Hirth et al., 2000), then the compensatory health-care investment over the lifetime of an African American would be $219,264 [(67 QALYs $white$ − 61 QALYs $African American$) × $36,544]. Spread over the expected full lifetime of an African American (seventy-nine years), this would require compensatory health-care investments of $2,775 ($219,264/79) annually per capita if in fact compensatory health-care investments were completely proportional to the value of an age-adjusted QALY as determined by its worth in human productive capacity. While this might seem to be an exorbitant investment, it is actually but 32 percent of the nation's $8,713 per-capita health expenditure rate (OECD, 2015). Still, it is both an unrealistic level of compensatory investment (both politically and fiscally) and also disproportionate to the contributions that health-care investments alone could make to closing the racial QALY gap. What is needed is a further adjustment to the compensatory worth of an age-adjusted QALY that takes into account the estimated contribution of health-care investments to the closing of QALY disparities.

For this, we draw from literature on the contribution of health care to the reduction of disparities in life expectancy, which uses the concept of amenable mortality (or avoidable mortality), meaning causes of premature mortality that can be affected by health-care policy interventions—whether through individual-level clinical health care or population-based public health programs. The most recent evidence suggests that 42 percent of the racial gap (African American vs. white) in life expectancy is attributable to causes of death that can be affected through more equitable access to health care and investments in targeted public health interventions (Ilo et al., 2014),[18] With this as an example of a general approach to an equity-based calibration of compensatory health-care investments, we would arrive at an annual per-capita compensatory health-care allocation for African Americans as follows:

$$(67 \text{ QALYs} white - 61 \text{ QALYs} African\ American) \times (\$36,544 age\text{-}adjusted$$
$$QALY\ value) \times (.42 amenable\ mortality\ adjustment)/79 African\ American$$
$$life\ expectancy = \$1,166$$

While this is arguably an equitable means of determining the magnitude and distribution of compensatory investments in health care for populations burdened by disparities in health, is it fiscally pragmatic and sustainable? Assuming the 2014 U.S. Census estimate of 42 million African Americans and then multiplying this by the above per-capita compensatory health-care investment of $1,166, this amounts to an annual allocation of $49 billion of compensatory health-care investments targeted to the reductions of health disparities for the African American population, or the equivalent of 1.7 percent of the $2.9 trillion total national health expenditures for the year 2013 (CMS, 2014b). It is a formidable reallocation of national health expenditures, but not when viewed in relationship to the historic racial disequities in access to health care. Also, the compensatory funds would decline over time in proportion to the reduction in the racial gap in QALYs.

In sum, the proposed approach to setting the target benchmark for compensatory investments in health-care services and public health infrastructure/interventions for the amelioration of health disparities would be to calibrate them in accordance with the magnitude and distribution of health disparities as measured by subpopulation differences in QALYs. It is also proposed that the allocation of annual compensatory investments could be based on the age-adjusted productive value of a QALY, weighted by effect of individual- and population-level health-care interventions on overall life expectancy. This would be represented in the following benchmarking equation:

$$
\begin{aligned}
&(\text{QALYs}reference\ population - \text{QALYs}comparison\ population) \times \\
&(\text{Age-adjusted QALY Value}) \times (\text{Amenable Mortality Adjustment})/ \\
&\text{LE}comparison\ population\ life\ expectancy = \text{QALY-based Target} \\
&\text{Benchmark for Annual Per-Capita Compensatory Investment} \\
&(QALY\ compensatory\ investment)
\end{aligned}
$$

Since the specific target value of compensatory health-care investments would vary greatly by the subpopulation affected by health-care disparities, the statistic representing the target performance benchmark determined by the above equation is shown in Table 7.2 as *QALY compensatory investment*. The components of *QALY compensatory investment* value estimation that would vary by subpopulation include the expected QALY value, the amenable mortality adjustment, and overall life expectancy. There are also a variety of different methods for determining the value of a QALY that would yield very different results and policy implications for the overall magnitude of equitable compensatory health-care investments (Hirth et al., 2000).

CONCLUDING REMARKS ON THE ASSESSMENT OF HEALTH-CARE SYSTEM PERFORMANCE

The general framework, dimensions of health-care system performance, proposed measures, and the target performance benchmarks proposed represent but a highly reduced synthesis of an extensive literature on health system performance that has been crafted to the particular health-care policy objectives advanced in earlier chapters of this book. There is nothing sacro-sanct about any particular health system performance measure proposed in this chapter or even the target benchmarks. Collectively, they are intended to provide the broad outlines of a coherent and plausible approach to the assessment of health system performance that is based on the normative principles embedded in the policy objectives of a fundamentally reformed and more inclusive health-care system. Perhaps the trickiest aspect of health system performance assessment is not in the selection of the dimensions of health system performance to evaluate, the best measures specific to each dimension, or even in the selection of target performance benchmarks that reflect the normatively defined optimal. It is more likely in the benchmarking of achievable progress toward end goals, which requires both scientific consensus and a sophisticated political appraisal of the possibilities and boundaries of social change.

Chapter Eight

SPECIAL ISSUES AND CONSIDERATIONS

This final chapter is about the social rights to health care for segments of the national population that fall outside of the general justifications for a right to health care, such as presented in chapter 3—that is, the justifications for a social right to health care based on the status of citizenship, the realization and preservation of the capacities essential to the exercise of political citizenship, and the requisites of fair equality of opportunity that John Rawls advanced as inherent to the meaning of democratic citizenship as well as the related rationales for T. H. Marshall's defense of social citizenship (Marshall & Bottomore, 1992; Rawls, 1971). Clearly, insomuch as undocumented immigrants are precluded from citizenship status and the possibility of political citizenship, either they have no claims to health-care rights or other justifications must exist that uphold some social citizenship rights to health care in absence of the de jure capacity to exercise political citizenship. It is also true that citizens who are at the more extreme range of disablement (whether from birth, trauma, or old age) and thus are de facto unable to exercise political citizenship rights require other justifications for social rights to health care. In addition, with respect to both the extremes of age and disabilities, there are also questions and enduring disagreements pertaining to the limits of health-care intervention (and ergo the rights to health care) in terms of beneficence, sustainability, and intergenerational equity. Then there are segments of the national population who may have rights to health care that go beyond those of the general citizenry, specifically military veterans and Native Americans. This chapter is therefore organized around three discussions: the social rights to health care for noncitizens, the boundaries to the social rights to health care for all citizens, and the special social rights to health care for some citizens.

THE SOCIAL RIGHTS TO HEALTH CARE FOR NONCITIZENS

The term *citizen* refers to a person who has been granted the status of U.S. citizen through right of birth within the territorial boundaries of the United States, is the child born to a U.S. citizen, or is a person in the process of becoming a naturalized citizen as specified by applicable federal law (The Immigration and Nationality Act, Public Law No. 82-414). The noncitizens are divided into three separate categories: nonimmigrant documented aliens, documented permanent residents, and undocumented immigrants. The first category of noncitizens (comprising tourists, foreign students, temporary workers, etc.) are visiting the United States for a specific purpose and are not assumed to have any claims to health care except via special contract (such as health-care coverage through temporary employment or student health-care benefits provided through an educational institution) or on humanitarian grounds. The second category, documented permanent residents (also known as *lawful permanent residents* or *permanent resident aliens*), refers to individuals who have been issued the so-called Green Cards—immigrant visas under the Immigration and Naturalization Act as permanent residents. Members of this group are on the path to becoming naturalized U.S. citizens or in all other respects have entered into the de facto realm of social citizenship through their decision and capacity to embrace American society as permanent residents. As with the Medicare social insurance fund for health care as it exists today, immigrants within this permanent resident category both pay into and are covered by the Tier I social insurance fund for health care. This leaves the undocumented immigrant category, which includes those who have not made a commitment to embrace American society as permanent residents (such as Mexican nationals who enter the United States for seasonal work and then prefer to return to their home communities in Mexico) and those who have made the decision to embrace American society as permanent residents but must live their lives "in the shadows" to avoid deportation.[1] From the standpoint of a social right to health care such as it has been argued in preceding chapters, the distinction between the decision to embrace American society as a permanent resident and the capacity to do so is crucial.

UNDOCUMENTED IMMIGRANTS, LABOR MARKETS, AND THE SOCIAL CONTRACT

The case for a social right to health care such as has been presented in this book has been built on a synthesis of the theories of John Rawls and T. H. Marshall on the requisites of political democracy and democratic citizenship. The problem now confronted is that neither lived long enough to adapt their theories of democratic citizenship, political democracy, and social rights to a globalized economy—each treated democratic societies as closed systems within which workers were presumed to possess the status and rights of citizenship. Neither Rawls nor Marshall anticipated the emergence of political democracies with a large share of the national population contributing to the collective well-being of society in the absence of a path to the status and rights of citizenship—in effect, nominally democratic societies predicated economically (if not even politically) on a permanent underclass of so-called *illegal* immigrants. As sociologist Kitty Calavita notes, "Illegal immigrants are the prototype of such marginality, confined as they are to the worst jobs and excluded from social membership not only by virtue of their status as immigrants but by their illegality" (Calavita, 2005, pp. 403–404).

The Emergence of the New Underclass

In broad strokes, the emergence of undocumented workers as the new underclass is in large part an artifact of two interrelated phenomena, one economic and the other political. Economically, as the global economic model shifted from a Henry Ford–style high-wage/high-productivity industrial manufacturing model to a "post-Fordist economic model espousing just-in-time production, downsized production units, and temporary and low-wage employment," the labor markets in modern democracies (including the United States) became bifurcated between high-skill/education and high-wage employment and low-wage jobs filled by poorly educated/unskilled indigenous workers and immigrant workers (Calavita, 2005, p. 416). In the United States, the proximity of a semi-permeable border with Mexico meant that as the availability of low-wage employment fluctuated both seasonably and in response to economic cycles, the migrant labor stream adapted accordingly (Massey et al., 1990).[2]

Although the availability of a low-wage labor pool from Mexico also functioned to weaken the collective bargaining power of low-wage indigenous American workers and undermined popular support for increasing the federal minimum wage in proportion to the pace of inflation, up until the mid-1980s, the largest share of the nation's undocumented workers considered themselves Mexican nationals rather than undocumented permanent residents aspiring to American citizenship (Massey et al., 2015). This changed in the early 1980s when President Ronald Reagan, following the long tradition in American politics of demonizing immigrants during times of social and economic insecurity, framed immigration from Central America and Mexico as a threat to national security (Massey, 2007). This charge, in combination with both a growing conviction among American workers that Mexican migrants were stealing their jobs and nativist xenophobia, culminated in the 1986 Immigration Reform and Control Act (IRCA)— legislation aimed at stemming the tide of illegal immigration through massive investments in border security, deportation of undocumented immigrants, and access to legal permanent resident status for migrants able to demonstrate facility in English and five years of residence. In a classic example of social policy with unintended consequences, IRCA's provisions largely destroyed the institutionalized pattern of circular cross-border labor migration that had functioned for decades. During the ten years that followed the 1986 passage of IRCA, the probability of an undocumented immigrant remaining in the United States as a permanent resident rose from 39 percent to 80 percent, thus solidifying a new underclass of Americans comprising undocumented previously migrant workers and their dependents (Massey, 2007).

Revisiting the Purposes of the Social Contract

As noted by Rawls, in the history of democratic thought, two contrasting visions of a society have been prominent. The first is a utilitarian one—that is, the idea of society as a social system organized so as to produce the most good summed over all of its members. The second, associated with political liberalism, is the idea of society as a fair system of cooperation between citizens regarded as free and equal (Rawls, 2001, p. 95). In an interesting and disturbing way, politically enfranchised Americans thus far have elected to tolerate, if not even embrace, a ruthlessly utilitarian version of society—that is, one that affirms the legitimacy of a system of collective prosperity that is sustained by an underclass of American workers who have no political rights and few social rights just as long as there is the public sense that the collective interest is advanced. While many may argue that undocumented workers by virtue of their illegal residency status are not legitimate members of society, their excluded status is an artifact of social policies such as IRCA and North American Free Trade Agreement (NAFTA) that were presumed to advance the collective good (in essence, policies argued to be "good for the country") and also the capacity of the politically enfranchised majority of Americans to exploit their powerlessness.[3] Functionally, undocumented workers and their dependents are not peripheral to American society but are deeply embedded in the social and economic fabric of the nation. While the presence of 11.3 million undocumented immigrants from Mexico and elsewhere is in large part a consequence of ill-conceived immigration policies, famines, territorial conflicts, and the unintended consequences of free trade agreements (Portes, 2006), most have become (in the language of Rawls's theory of justice) "fully cooperating members of society" in all senses of the term but those pertaining to formal citizenship status. As with previous generations of immigrants from throughout Europe, with few exceptions, they are here to work and build a better future for themselves and their children, and their presence is a net benefit both to the nation's gross domestic product (GDP) and the solvency of the nation's old-age entitlement programs (Alba, 2006; Hanson, 2007; Van de Water, 2008). With respect to their future and the national interest, there are but three policy choices.

The first policy choice, argued as legitimate and practical by some, combines aggressive deportation and employment enforcement measures, the latter prosaically referred to by the 2012 GOP presidential candidate Mitt Romney as "self-deportation" (Boroff & Planas, 2012). Even if the mass deportation (voluntary or otherwise) of millions of undocumented immigrants were feasible logistically (which no credible scholar of immigration policy suggests is true), the economic consequences themselves would be dramatic if not disastrous. By the year 2005, at which point the undocumented immigrant population and elsewhere was reaching its apex at 12.2 million, undocumented immigrants represented 24 percent of the workers in agriculture, 17 percent in the cleaning industry, 14 percent in the construction industry, and 12 percent in the food preparation industry (Hanson, 2007; Krogstad & Passel, 2015). Aside from the negative impacts on the nation's economic productivity, the payroll taxes deducted from the wages of undocumented workers also contribute to the solvency of the Social Security and Medicare trust funds (Van de Water, 2008). This leaves policy choices two and three, both of which are far more plausible.

The second policy choice would largely be a continuation of the current social policies toward undocumented immigrants, which in effect perpetuates their underclass status through expropriation of their low-wage labor while at the same time precluding their political citizenship and marginalizing their social citizenship. That is, the status quo social policy holds that undocumented workers should continue to labor in the absence of the social safety net available to other American workers in the form of such antipoverty provisions as unemployment insurance, Medicaid, Social Security Disability Insurance, and Temporary Assistance to Needy Families. The term *expropriation of labor* is used very deliberately here, in keeping with the idea that stratified societies are built upon the capacity of the dominant groups of a society to expropriate the resources produced by subordinate groups while preventing those subordinated from realizing the full value of their efforts in producing the resources (Massey, 2007). Undocumented workers, by virtue of their delegitimized status, labor without the minimum wage protections, employment benefits, or collective bargaining rights that are afforded other workers. In fact, undocumented workers are the perfect reincarnation of the nineteenth-century immigrant laborer in a twenty-first-century economy—they can be hired at the most meager of wages, mistreated at the workplace with impunity, and discarded at will. To complete this bleak picture, undocumented workers from Mexico have the propensity to return home when they are too sick or too old to work (Palloni & Arias, 2004), thus relieving local governments of their need to also re-create nineteenth-century poorhouses. The problem is, of course, that while enhancing the standard of living of the majority on the backs of a disenfranchised underclass may be consistent with a kind of ruthless utilitarianism or even the imagined social order of Aldous Huxley's *Brave New World*, it is inconsistent with the general idea of a just democratic society. It is also not a sustainable social policy over time or without long-term costs to the prosperity and political stability of the nation—a lesson that might have been learned from the African American experience.

This leads to the third social policy solution, which recognizes that the presence of the undocumented immigrant population exists as an *irreversible* unintended consequence of the immigration and economic policies of past decades, and that much is lost and nothing truly gained by their continued exclusion from the American social contract, particularly its social citizenship provisions.

Undocumented workers toil, produce, pay taxes, and endeavor to lawfully live out their lives as ordinary Americans in the penumbra of civil society, and despite political rhetoric to the contrary, the overwhelming evidence is that the far majority are here to stay irrespective of punitive immigration policies (Massey et al., 2015). Although the common belief is that the undocumented immigrant population continues to grow at an unrestrained pace, the reality is that since its highest level of 12.2 million in 2007, the size of the undocumented immigrant population has been stable since 2008 at about 11.3 million (Krogstad & Passel, 2015). Within that population, there are those who aspire to full citizenship, others who prefer the status of foreign nationals with legalized U.S. residency status, and a minority who would prefer a return to migratory labor patterns with legalized U.S. entry and exits (Massey et al., 2015). With all of this is mind, how might the social contract with undocumented workers and their dependents be framed in a manner that is both fair and rational?

The primary limitations of Rawls's version of the idealized social contract, from which the rights and obligations of citizenship in a liberal democracy are derived (Rawls, 1971, 2001), are twofold. First, the Rawlsian version of the social contract assumes that all three dimensions of citizenship (civil, political, and social) are intrinsic to the social contract in a democratic society and there is no particular category for "fully cooperating members of society" who do not possess citizenship status.

Second, Rawls's theory of justice argues that the primary rationale for basic social institutions (inclusive of the education system and the healthcare system) is that they are essential to the development of the moral powers of citizens and thus "become fully cooperating members of a society of free and equal citizens" (Rawls, 2001, p. 37). That is, the justification of social rights is largely predicated on the functional requisites of citizenship. Both problems can be resolved, but only if the definition of a democratic society as a fair system of cooperation can be expanded to include "fully cooperating members of society" who do not possess and do not necessarily aspire to formal citizenship status in the legal meaning of the term. That is, it is necessary to delink the formal status of citizen from the construct of "a fully cooperating member of society" and imagine a category for fully cooperating members of society who are not citizens yet are full participants in the nonpolitical rights and reciprocal obligations that are typically associated with citizenship. That is, they would engage in productive labor, obey laws and respect the rights of others, pay taxes, and enjoy both the benefits of mutual prosperity and the protections associated with civil and social citizenship. As it happens, that category exists under current immigration law as "documented permanent residents" (or permanent resident aliens) or holders of the much sought after "Green Card" (U.S. Citizenship and Immigration Services, 2015).

While the granting of permanent residency status to millions of undocumented immigrants is politically unfeasible in the foreseeable future, so (as discussed previously) is mass deportation. By extending social citizenship rights to undocumented immigrants (education, health care, and antipoverty safety net programs), we have the opportunity to at least make more permeable the boundaries of social class and quite possibly replicate the successful economic and social assimilation of Italian Americans of the prior century. As noted by Alba (2006), like the typical undocumented immigrants of today, the Italian immigrants of the early twentieth century were poor, uneducated (nearly half were illiterate), and a target of inflammatory political rhetoric and xenophobic contempt. Today, the descendants of these former undesirables are at parity with prior groups of European immigrants in the ranks of the most prestigious professions, including the professoriate, medicine, and law (Alba, 2006). On the other hand, through the current social policy of excluding undocumented workers and their dependents from social rights to health care and a minimal economic safety net, we increase the likelihood of their failed or even downward economic assimilation—to our collective detriment both in the present and in the inevitable (and unforgiving) future (Portes et al., 2009).

The Social Right to Health Care for Undocumented Immigrants

Two compelling arguments for a social right to health care for undocumented immigrants have now been made, each predicated on the assumption that the presence of 11.3 million undocumented immigrants (like the former unwelcome immigrants from seventeenth-century Europe) is an irreversible fact of history. The first argument is deontological—that despite their delegitimized citizenship status, in all other respects, undocumented immigrants in the language of Rawls's theory of justice exist as "fully co-operating members of society" and therefore should be afforded the social rights and protections that derive from the social contract extended to legitimized citizens. To do otherwise would be an anathema to a vision of constitutional democracy as a fair system of cooperation among free and equal persons (if not citizens). The second argument is consequentialist; in essence, there is a collective price to be paid by all Americans when any group in American society is perpetually relegated to the vicissitudes of underclass status and class boundaries are made impermeable.

On the basis of these arguments, the immediate policy response should be the elimination of the ACA's mandated exclusion of undocumented immigrants from purchasing health insurance from the federal- and state-level health insurance exchanges, having income-based subsidies for health insurance coverage, and enrolling in comprehensive Medicaid coverage. It should be noted that all of the ACA's social right provisions are extended to documented immigrants who have resided in the United States for more than five years, in keeping with the idea that noncitizens who have made a commitment to U.S. residency can and should be regarded as fully cooperating members of American society. With respect to the Tier I social insurance fund for health care that is advocated in this book as the preferred approach to a social right to health care, as discussed in chapter 7, the mechanism through which undocumented immigrants could readily participate is the Individual Taxpayer Identification Number (ITIN), which functions as an alternative to the Social Security Number (SSN) that undocumented immigrants do not possess.[4] This is proposed as an interim solution that makes it possible to advance the realization of universal health insurance coverage in the absence of immigration policy reforms that would legitimize the status of the millions of undocumented immigrants who have become irrevocably woven into the social and economic fabric of the nation—the latter, of course, is infinitely preferable and likely inevitable.

THE BOUNDARIES TO THE SOCIAL RIGHTS TO HEALTH CARE FOR ALL CITIZENS

Health care is a finite social resource. At the national level, even with the cost-efficiency provisions of the ACA fully implemented, health-care national expenditures are projected to increase by 6 percent annually between 2015 and 2023, representing 19.3 percent of the GDP by 2023 (CMS, 2014d). Health-care rationing is not just an inevitable aspect of our nation's future but also a legacy of our nation's past—the difference being that historically, health care has been de facto rationed on the basis of race, ethnicity, and social class (Etzioni, 1991; Starr, 1982). While *health-care rationing* is a politically explosive term that has been cynically employed by politicians to scare the public with images of indifferent and even predatory government bureaucrats deciding who lives and who dies (as in the so-called death panels rhetoric of the ACA's 2010 congressional opposition), in more objective terms, it means engaging in a deliberative process for the allocation of limited social resources in accordance with both social priorities and principles of social justice. In contrast to the perspective of health-care economists, which frames this allocative process as a problem of efficiency maximization given certain desired social outcomes, this book frames the allocative process as primarily a problem of distributive justice. So what should be the principles of distributive justice that guide this allocative process at the extremes of either human existence or health-care needs?

In his final restatement of his theory of distributive justice, made shortly before his death in 2002, Rawls (2001) advanced a justification of a social right to health care, which he described as "[a] basic level of health care for all" (p. 176) as part and parcel of "the general means necessary to underwrite fair equality of opportunity and our capacity to take advantage of our basic rights and liberties, and thus be normal and fully cooperating members of society over the complete life" (p. 174). Marshall's justification of a social right to health care, while complementary, was distinct in its emphasis on the role that health care plays in the substantive requisites of social equality and an acceptable minimum standard of living that cuts across the boundaries of social class (Marshall & Bottomore, 1992, p. 33). While both justifications are foundational to the preventative, curative, restorative, and adaptive health-care provisions that comprise the Tier I health insurance coverage (summarized in chapter 5 as limited entitlement social insurance for health care), they do not address the two fundamental distributive justice questions that any country that provides universal health-care coverage to its citizens must grapple with. The first is the boundaries of a social right to costly health care that does not contribute significantly to cure, the maximization of quality of life where death is inevitable and imminent, or the restoration of functional capacity commensurate with what most people would consider a minimal quality of life. The second concerns intergenerational equity, that is, the fair distribution of limited health-care resources over the complete human life course.

CONTEMPLATING THE BOUNDARIES TO A SOCIAL RIGHT
TO HEALTH CARE AT THE EXTREMES OF EXISTENCE

The question addressed here is as follows: What are the upper limits to our individual and collective expectations to health-care expenditures where there are no discernable or likely benefits to either the protection or restoration of a minimal quality of life? One way to think about this is that point where one no longer possesses the capacity to perceive, experience, and interact with one's physical and social environment in a cognitively sapient state. The typical medical diagnosis associated with this circumstance is the persistent vegetative state (PVS). Although the exact prevalence of this condition is unknown due to differences in clinical diagnosis, the mid-range estimate of the prevalence of PVS in the United States is 10.4 per 100,000 persons or, in population terms, about 33,000 patients nationwide (Donis & Kraftner, 2011). This is in stark contrast with the much lower PVS prevalence rates in Denmark and the Netherlands (respectively at .13/100,000 and .2/100,000), where the withdrawal of artificial nutrition and hydration in PVS and like cases is more widely accepted than in the United States (Donis & Kraftner, 2011). Leaving aside the tragic emotional consequences on the families and loved ones of PVS patients regarding whether or not life in a PVS condition is ended or prolonged, the costs of ongoing care for PVS patients are enormous, ranging from $246,000 annually for institutional care to $180,000 for in-home care.[5] Assuming the national prevalence rate of 10.4 per 100,000, this translates to a cost that ranges from $6 billion to $8 billion nationally depending on the mix of in-home versus institutionalized care. Using the more conservative figure of $6 billion, were the United States to have the PVS prevalence of Denmark (at .13/100,000), the dollars that could be shifted from PVS care to other health-care priorities (such as reductions in preventable infant mortality) would exceed $5.8 billion. While it might seem that we can never know the mental life of an individual in a persistent vegetative state or to rule out the possibility of miraculous recovery, in contemplating these metaphysical considerations, we should also acknowledge the reality of the social choice being made between funding a high incidence of ongoing PVS care and other health-care investments that are far more likely to yield measurable and meaningful years of life.

Another way to think about the boundaries of a social right to health care at the extremes of existence are medical interventions that are provided to prolong life in the absence of a clear therapeutic goal outside of prolonging life itself. There are many examples of this, but one that comes to mind (a real case) is the physician who continues to order bimonthly blood transfusions for treatment of a blood disorder in a nursing home patient with advanced Alzheimer's disease. We will call her M. Consistent with this tragic condition, M does not know who she is or where she is, does not recognize her family or even the staff involved in her daily care, requires full assistance for bathing and incontinence care, and is incapable of communicating a coherent thought. M is slowly dying of one disease that has no cure, and her life is only being prolonged through her physician's insistence that she should not be allowed to die of another treatable disease she happens to have. To add to the dilemma, the documentation regarding M's end-of-life preferences only speaks to her reluctance to accept "heroic intervention" that would prolong her life in an incapacitated condition— M's physician believes that biweekly blood transfusions fall under the category of ordinary and routine supportive therapy for her particular blood disorder diagnosis.

Were health-care resources unlimited, we might contemplate the circumstances of M's medically prolonged existence solely from the perspective of which course of action values the dignity and sanctity of life more—treating her for one chronic life-threatening condition while awaiting the final stages of her death from another untreatable one, or simply suspending all but comfort care while the inevitable takes its course. However, we are not free to be wholly oblivious and indifferent to the larger normative questions regarding M's tragic situation about the just and reasonable allocation of limited health-care resources—whether in the financial costs of prolonging her life (or some might say her death) or in the consumption of limited blood product supplies that are donated under the assumption that the medical community will be good stewards of their use. We are also not free to be oblivious to the reality that the revenue to her physician's nursing home practice is maximized to the extent that there is a higher caseload of nursing home residents. Although most of us would be inclined to give the physician's motivation the benefit of the doubt absent an established pattern of financial exploitation, there is a large literature that shows that clinical decisions in end-of-life care are not made independently of perverse financial incentives (Institute of Medicine, 2015). This shows up not just in individual cases but also in the regional variations in healthcare expenditures for end-of-life care (care during the last six months of life) that range from a low of $9,735 per Medicare beneficiary in Colorado to a high of $24,578 in Texas (Barnado et al., 2007).[6] Were older adults not entitled to social insurance for health care, it could be speculated that the variation in end-of-life expenditures would vary not so much by region as by income, race, ethnicity, and other correlates of private health insurance coverage.

Finally, we are not free to ignore a longstanding cultural dynamic in American medicine, which might be referred to as "the tyranny of the possible"—that is, the tendency to confuse the capacity to sustain life at the margins of functional existence and true prospects for meaningful recovery (often at the price of futile and unneeded suffering) with a concrete and transparent justification for doing so (Mohindra, 2007). There are two aspects to the tyranny of the possible.

The first has to do with the nature of remote probabilities in many incurable fatal diseases with a rapid progression to death, highlighted by Harvard Medical School professor and award-winning author Atul Gawande in *Being Mortal: Medicine and What Matters at the End* (2014). Using the case example of a scientist diagnosed with abdominal mesothelioma, a rare and lethal form of cancer typically associated with asbestos exposure with a median survival of only eight months postdiscovery, Gawande points out that the distribution of survival points was not clustered around the median of eight months but rather fanned out in both directions, with a very long tail representing the data points of rare cases of patients with abdominal mesothelioma who survived well beyond eight months.[7] Notwithstanding the reality that each of the cases that survived more than a few months beyond the median survival of eight months represented miniscule probabilities of extended survival that were near zero, they were *not* zero, thus representing the exceedingly small chance of having a few extra months of life or perhaps even a year or more. In the minds of many patients facing their imminent death from a terminal disease (and their families), *why should they not* pin their hopes on the "medical miracle" lottery ticket and opt for aggressive treatment at all costs? American physicians, notes Gawande, are extraordinarily reluctant to push patients toward a discussion of near-zero probabilities and the true costs (in their suffering and loss of quality of life) of their desperate quest for a medical lottery ticket win. Instead, physicians of gravely ill patients are more likely to buy into the quest themselves, because it allows them to do what they are trained to do—fight death with all means at their disposal. Poignantly and authentically, Gawande admits to his own emotional turmoil and complicity in gut-wrenching case examples from his own practice of aggressive and futile medical interventions in the face of the inevitable (pp. 165–173).

The second aspect of the "tyranny of the possible" is connected to but distinct from the hopes of patients and their loved ones in the face of imminent death from incurable diseases—that is, the availability of a wide range of cutting-edge and experimental medical interventions in drugs, radiation, and surgery that have some remote or unknown possibility of affecting the course of the disease. For example, in too many cases, patients barter what remains of the most precious aspects of their quality of life for their selection into Phase I clinical trials of new chemotherapies and experimental radiation treatments when the primary purpose of these trials is to calibrate the range of toxicity rather than to extend life (Gawande, 2014). Were these patients choosing to participate in Phase I clinical trials for altruistic motivations (as some no doubt do), from an ethical and humanitarian perspective, this would be sad but also noble and acceptable. But in too much of American medicine, it is neither; patients volunteer for early trial experimental treatments solely out of desperate hope without true knowledge about what they have bartered away—those precious last days and months of well-managed symptoms to embrace what has made their lives worth living. Those of us who are health-care practitioners become complicit in this aspect of the tyranny of the possible to the extent that we find ourselves unable or unwilling to convey to patients and their families in these tragic situations the truth as we know it. Only when we can muster the empathy, courage, and skills to confront and convey the difficult truths about the therapeutic trade-offs in fatal health conditions to our patients are the choices theirs and not our own.

Normative Expectations Versus "Death Panels"

Among the most cynical and perhaps effective tactics in the ongoing political debates over the public versus private financing of health care is the use of "death panel" imagery to represent the inevitable consequence of so-called government health care—represented in former Republican vice presidential candidate Sarah Palin's 2009 claim that Democrats would create a death panel of government bureaucrats who would decide whether elderly and disabled patients are "worthy of health care" (Ubel, 2013). The language and imagery evoked harken back to the community panels of the early 1960s (sometimes referred to as "God committees") that in fact determined which end-stage renal disease patients would be eligible for the limited local charity funds for the prohibitively expensive kidney dialysis. Ironically, it was the 1965 Medicare social insurance entitlements to health insurance coverage for the kidney dialysis care of patients with chronic kidney disease (irrespective of age) that eliminated the need for these local community panels (Buntin, 2009).

The alternative to a kind of bureaucratic process for the rational and hopefully just allocation of limited health-care resources and intrinsically the outer boundaries to a social right to health care is an ongoing public and political discourse, as well as deliberative process, that leads to an overlapping consensus on what should be the full range of expectations for health care at all stages of the human life course—a process and fundamental feature of democracy that Rawls (2001) describes as "public justification" (pp. 26–29).[8] Rawls introduced the idea of public justification as an alternative to the futility of finding a comprehensive doctrine that would reconcile all of the religious and philosophical perspectives that are represented in a pluralist society or, for that matter, could transcend the evolutionary progression of human societies.

Two examples of a version of a fruitful public discourse on the substance and boundaries to a social right to health care help shape a pluralist normative context for the design of health-care delivery systems, the allocation of limited health-care resources, and individual-level clinical decision making. The first dates back to the 1989 Health Services Act in the state of Oregon, otherwise known as the so-called Oregon Plan. To extend Medicaid health-care coverage to all Oregon residents who were not covered by Medicare or employment-based health insurance, the state legislature established a "Health Services Commission" to specify the scope of Medicaid entitlements through an objective and public process that incorporated both evidence of clinical efficacy and public values specific to health-care priorities. This process included forty-seven public forums held throughout the state on health-care values and priorities, as well as representative surveys of all segments of the state's population.

The outcome of this process was a prioritized list of 709 health conditions and related clinical interventions that was used by the State Health

Service commission to determine the range of health-care needs and services covered under Oregon Medicaid, contingent on the state's fiscal resources (Oberlander et al., 2001). Although the Oregon Plan has been heavily criticized as both draconian and unfair, in that its list of health-care priorities only applied to low-income Medicaid recipients, Oregonians have kept the process in place as a preferred alternative to (1) arbitrary bureaucratic decisions about which health services to either cover or not cover given the fiscal resources in any one year or (2) vested interests within the health-care industry that promote funding of the most profitable health-care interventions as opposed to those that optimize cost efficiency and clinical efficacy.

A second example, a less direct approach to shaping the normative guidelines for the just and efficacious allocation of limited health-care resources through public discourse, is the Institute of Medicine's process for the development of its groundbreaking *Dying in America: Improving Quality and Honoring Individual Preferences Near the End of Life* (2015). This report (which represents the collaborative work of prominent voices from academic and clinical medicine, bioethics, the nursing profession, social work, and the health insurance and hospital industry), in its exhaustive critique of the nation's deeply flawed approach to end-of-life health care and reframing of end-of-life health-care needs and priorities, seeks to advance normative change through education and the fostering of public and professional dialogue. It does not advance a comprehensive doctrine on end-of-life care so much as it invites and fosters deliberation over the social purposes of end-of-life care, the priorities of clinical practice, and what should be the reasonable and realizable substantive expectations of a social right to health care for all as the inevitability of death approaches.

CONTEMPLATING THE PROBLEM OF INTERGENERATIONAL EQUITY IN A SOCIAL RIGHT TO HEALTH CARE

Every modern democracy is grappling with the sustainability of a social right to comprehensive health care in the face of an aging population. In the United States, where national health-care expenditures are already two times those of the average of other developed democracies, the sustainability challenge is far more formidable. In addition, the United States also has a very high child poverty rate, which at one child in poverty out of every five is 60 percent in excess of the average child poverty rate for all other modern democracies (OECD, 2014b). This is in stark contrast with the poverty rates for older adults in the United States, which, at 9.5 percent of adults aged sixty-five and older, is slightly less than half that of the nation's child poverty rate (DeNavas-Walt & Proctor, 2014). This is so because the nation's older adults are the only segment of the population that benefits from the dual coverage of the country's only two social insurance programs (Medicare and Social Security's Old-Age and Survivors Insurance), whereas the safety net for the nation's children comprises means-tested programs that primarily target economic dependence rather than poverty.

From the standpoint of *intergenerational equity*—in essence, the idea that each generation possesses an equal share in the resources and rights that comprise the core benefits of society—this is an egregiously unjust state of affairs. While T. H. Marshall did not directly address this problem (except perhaps by implication), Rawls did so directly and extensively in his original full treatise, *A Theory of Justice* (1971), through two interconnected ideas: *just savings* and the *social minimum.*

Rawls describes the *just savings* principle as "an understanding between the generations to carry their fair share of the burden of realizing and preserving a just society" (p. 289). This means that each generation "must not only preserve the gains of culture and civilization, and maintain intact those just institutions that have been established, but must also put aside in each period of time a suitable amount of real capital accumulation" necessary to preserve and develop both economic infrastructure and the social resources that are crucial to the development of human capital (p. 285).[9] The societal resources that are set aside for future generations should be guided by a concern for the *social minimum*, that is, the minimum material security and human capital investments that are guaranteed to the least advantaged in society. In keeping with Rawls's "Difference Principle" (discussed in chapter 3), the social minimum "is to be set at that point which, taking wages into account, maximizes the expectations of the least advantaged" in terms of the resources needed for a minimum standard of well-being and fair equality of opportunity (p. 285).

Ideally, then, we should want to provide a social right to health care for older adults that strikes the proper balance between the health-care investments that optimize quality of life and "capacity preservation" at the extremes of old age, while retaining the resources for social investments in the development and protection of citizenship-relevant capacities in younger generations and a minimally decent standard of living through all stages of the life course. In our quest to accomplish this, we are confronted with two formidable health-care policy challenges, the first pertaining to the long-term solvency of the Medicare program entitlements and the second concerning the financing of long-term care services for older adults.

Medicare Trust Fund Solvency

When the Medicare program was established in 1965, it was predicated on an acute care paradigm, one that assumed that the health-care expenditures of older adults largely derived from short-term illnesses that would be characterized by recovery or death. It was also designed with the assumption that the post–age sixty-five life expectancy of Medicare would be limited to an average of no more than 15 years. Since 1965, in large part due to the beneficial impacts of the Medicare program on the health of the nation's older adults, the health-care paradigm for aging Americans has shifted from an acute transitory disease model to one predicated on the long-term management of multiple chronic diseases over a post–age sixty-five life expectancy that itself has grown by five years (NCHS, 2011). Moreover, the largest gains in post–age sixty-five life expectancy subsequent to the Medicare program's establishment have been among older adults aged eighty-five and older—that is, those older adults with the most extensive health-care needs (Crimmins et al., 1989).

There are two core problems with the Medicare program's long-term fiscal solvency. The first, but not necessarily the worst, problem is the well-documented aging of the population, particularly the size of the aging baby-boom cohorts of Medicare beneficiaries relative to younger generations of workers paying into the Medicare Hospital Insurance Trust Fund (CMS, 2014e). The second is the provider incentives and payment mechanisms of the Medicare program that have remained enmired in the old-age disease and mortality regime of fifty years ago, in significant part due to vested interests in the health-care industry (Boyd, 2010). Prior to the Medicare program reforms that were incorporated into the 2010 ACA legislation, the trustees for the Medicare Hospital Insurance Trust Fund had estimated that the assets of the fund would be totally depleted by 2017 (CMS, 2009), which would then require either a drastic reduction in Medicare hospital insurance benefits or significant ongoing and ever increasing Medicare program subsidies from general tax revenues. Under its current budgetary estimates, which assume that the ACA's Medicare program reforms are both implemented and fully effective as envisioned, the trustees for the Medicare Hospital Insurance Trust Fund project predict fiscal solvency through the year 2030 (CMS, 2014e).

Assuming that the Medicare Hospital Insurance Trust Fund will in fact retain its solvency through the year 2030 (which is a rather optimistic assumption given a dubious track record of large-scale social policy reforms), we must within the next decade find additional paths through which Medicare program expenditures can be reduced. Within the current structure of the Medicare program, there are four basic approaches for accomplishing this: (1) reducing the number of Medicare program beneficiaries through gradually raising the age of eligibility, (2) changing the Medicare program from a defined benefit to a defined contribution program (in essence, meaning Medicare beneficiaries would be given vouchers for the purchase of private health insurance plans), (3) reducing health-care utilization among Medicare beneficiaries through higher co-payments, and (4) finding ways to reduce even further Medicare program payments to providers.

The problem with the first strategy (aside from its political feasibility) is that by raising the age of eligibility, we would not only greatly increase the numbers of the nation's uninsured but also include among the uninsured a new group of older adults with very significant health problems. On the other hand, the voucher approach to reducing the growth in Medicare program expenditures, while favored by many conservatives, would quickly lead to the kinds of income disparities in the quality and accessibility of health care that have been a major feature of employment-based insurance. That is, higher-income Medicare beneficiaries would be able to supplement the Medicare voucher's health insurance purchasing power while lower-income Medicare beneficiaries (typically the poorer and sicker) would be relegated to low-cost/lower-quality health insurance plans (Marmor, 2012). The third alternative, raising the copayments among Medicare beneficiaries, invites exactly the kinds of income disparities in the quality and accessibility of health care as are produced by the voucher approach. Finally, with respect to the fourth alternative, while there might be some further marginal reductions in the payments to some classes of health-care providers that can be made without compromising health-care accessibility and quality for Medicare beneficiaries, provider payment reductions that are of sufficient magnitude to extend the fiscal solvency of Medicare would inevitably lead to reductions in the share of health-care providers willing to accept

Medicare patients—in particular, those with the most complex health problems and fewest resources (Orient, 2011).

Were the nation to adopt a social insurance plan for comprehensive health care along the lines that have been suggested in preceding chapters, the fiscal sustainability issues that currently threaten the social right to health care for the nation's older adults would be greatly mitigated if not even eliminated for the foreseeable future. So, too, would be the intergenerational disequities to a social right to health care that the Medicare program has represented over the past fifty years. This is so for three reasons.

First and foremost, eliminated are the antiquated provider payment structures, perverse incentives, and fragmented health-care delivery systems that have been promulgated and largely sustained over five decades under the traditional Medicare program. Second, through consolidating the tax contributions from Medicare, Medicaid, and the wage offsets represented in the premium contributions from employment-based insurance (as discussed in chapter 5) into a single social insurance trust fund, we will have created for the public interest enormous health-care purchasing power that can translate to better cost control and provider accountability. Third, and perhaps most crucially, are the health-care system delivery reforms (in particular the provider organization structures spelled out in chapter 6) that promote health care that is comprehensive and integrated through all stages of the life course. Much of this is not guaranteed by the transition to an age-inclusive social insurance fund for health care but would also be impossible to realize in the absence of a unified national fund for health care.

Even with this structural reform in place, large intergenerational justice problems remain that are consequent to the escalating long-term care needs of the aging generations. Since the 1970s, the public dollar expenditures on behalf of the long-term care needs of older adults have been in ever increasing conflict with needed social investments in such areas as public education, transportation infrastructure, and the economic safety net that are crucial to prospects for the generations that follow. So this becomes the next large intergenerational justice issue to be considered.

The Financing of Long-Term Care Services for Older Adults

Among the causes of the Medicare program's fiscal struggles are the long-term care needs of older adults who become "medicalized." That is, long-term needs are manifested in episodes of acute care that, while reimbursable under Medicare diagnostic criteria, remain unresolved and as such lead to ongoing Medicare program expenditures for problems that cannot be addressed within the acute care paradigm of patient care and health-care financing.[10] The much larger concern, though, pertains to the growth in state and federal Medicaid expenditures for the long-term care needs of older adults, which from 1995 through 2013 grew from $25 billion annually to $60 billion, and by the year 2023, the Congressional Budget Office projects long-term care Medicaid expenditures to reach $100 billion annually (CBO, 2013). While the aging of the national population is the primary cause of the projected growth in Medicaid expenditures, so also is the rise in the unit costs of long-term care services for older adults, particularly for those costs related to nursing home care (CBO, 2013).

As originally intended when signed into law in 1965, Medicaid was to function as the health-care safety net for the poor and those of limited means without health insurance. For working-age Americans and children, this remains largely true, even with the ACA's expansion of Medicaid eligibility to low-income households. Among older adults, however, Medicaid has long functioned as the financial safety net for middle-class households facing catastrophic expenditures for long-term care, particularly nursing home care. Among the 58 percent of nursing home residents who are enrolled in Medicaid for their nursing home care, about half entered as private patients, and many others qualified for Medicaid after transferring their assets (savings, real estate holdings, etc.) to meet the Medicaid means-based eligibility criteria in anticipation of a future need for nursing home care (Bassett, 2004; CBO, 2013).

Although long-term care insurance has long been promoted as the optimal solution for the risk of catastrophic nursing home and in-home care expenditures, only a small minority of older adults (11 percent as of 2010) carry long-term care insurance, and most older adults have no specific plans for their future long-term care needs (CBO, 2013). Also, those older adults at highest risk for nursing home care (low income and multiple functional impairments) are the least likely to carry private long-term care insurance (CBO, 2013). Because states in particular must grapple with the direct conflict between the ever increasing tax dollars required for Medicaid long-term care expenditures and the tax dollars needed for the public education, investments in economic infrastructure, and safety net programs for the poor and vulnerable, long-term care financing represents a significant intergenerational equity issue. To revisit the implications of Rawls's just savings principle (1971, p. 285), how do we finance a social right to an adequate scheme of long-term care services (within the boundaries of political feasibility) that strikes the proper balance between the optimization of quality of life and "capacity preservation" at the extremes of old age, while retaining the resources for social investments in the development and protection of citizenship-relevant capacities in younger generations and a minimally decent standard of living through all stages of the life course?

To respond to this question, it is useful to consider the relationship between what might be considered the reciprocity aspect of the just savings principle and the nature of social insurance. That is, as stated by Rawls (1971, p. 290), "In following the just savings principle, each generation makes a contribution to later generations and receives from its predecessors." This idea is embodied in both the Old-Age and Survivors Insurance (OASI) entitlements and the Medicare Hospital Insurance (HI) entitlements of the Social Security Act, in the sense that both old-age provisions are sustained by the revenues of payroll taxes paid by current generations as well as by the return on OASI and HI trust fund investments. Were we at the inception of the Medicare program in 1965, the perfect solution to the financing of long-term care needs would have been the addition of comprehensive long-term care services to the Medicare program, which could have been financed by a marginal increase in the Medicare payroll tax. Unfortunately, we are some fifty years past that point, and we must deal with the reality that any increase in the Medicare payroll tax sufficient to offset the projected long-term care expenditures for the baby-boom generation is both politically unfeasible and might also endanger the near-term prospects for economic growth. On the other hand, the present policy of taxing working-age households for the means-tested Medicaid subsidization of long-term health services for the generations of middle-class older adults who have elected not to purchase quite affordable private long-term insurance is unfair from an intergenerational equity standpoint. The current approach is also fiscally unsustainable as the baby-boom generation ages further into the years characterized by multiple long-term care needs and dwindling private resources with which to pay for long-term care services, and Medicaid long-term care expenditures cut ever more deeply into the public dollar resources needed for schools, economic infrastructure, and the social safety net for working-age families.

Given all this, is there an alternative long-term care policy strategy that recaptures the intergenerational reciprocity advantages of social insurance while making the financing of long-term care for the current generation of older adults more fair and fiscally sustainable? Conceptually and in actuarial terms, yes. In terms of political feasibility, only perhaps.

Conceptually, the optimal national policy strategy would first entail the addition of both institutional and community-based long-term care services to the Tier I social insurance trust fund for health care at a marginal increase in taxation, just as might have happened in 1965 had the pre-baby-boom generation (also known as "The Greatest Generation") had the knowledge of their risks for long-term care and its catastrophic costs. They did very well to accomplish the Medicare program, so there should be deep gratitude rather than criticism on this point of history. However, as a society, we now have infinitely better information about the realities of the true risks and costs of long-term care in advanced old age.

Also, the inclusion of long-term care financing in a unified social insurance trust fund for health care is both fiscally feasible and even desirable from the standpoint of cost management (Long & Marquis, 1994).

Again conceptually, the second part of the optimal national long-term strategy would be to increase the incentives of the current generations of middle- and upper-class older adults, those fifty-five and older, to invest in private-sector long-term care insurance, both as a way to protect their assets in savings and property and also as a means to increase the likelihood that they would be able to optimize their independence and quality of life through a flexible array of long-term care benefits. In effect, this would substantially reduce the utilization of Medicaid-funded long-term care services among older adults of means, thereby slowing the unsustainable growth in state and federal Medicaid expenditures. This is precisely the strategy of the Partnership for Long-Term Care (PLTC) program, which enables older adults who purchase private long-term care insurance to retain a larger share of their assets and qualify for Medicaid long-term care assistance at the point they have exhausted their private long-term care insurance benefits.

Initially pioneered by four states (California, Connecticut, Indiana, and New York) under the enabling legislation of the Deficit Reduction Act of 2005, as of 2015, the PLTC has expanded to forty states (CBO, 2013; PLTC, 2015). A crucial provision of the Deficit Reduction Act of 2005 also supports Partnership for Long-Term Care reciprocity between states, thus allowing policyholders who purchase a partnership policy in one state to move to another state and still qualify for the Medicaid eligibility benefits in their new state of residence (CBO, 2013). The problem is that only a small share of the nation's older adults participate in the Partnership for Long-Term Care program (substantially less than 10 percent by Congressional Budget Office estimates), which brings us back to the question of the political feasibility of long-term care financing reform.

From the standpoint of the politics of long-term care financing reform, the Partnership for Long-Term Care program (like the ill-fated Community Living Assistance Services and Supports [CLASS] provisions of the Affordable Care Act) serves as an object lesson of promising social policy in the absence of progressive political initiative and leadership—whether by Congress or via the bully pulpit of the presidency.[11] Largely due to an absence of political leadership in long-term care policy, the public and older adults in particular remain largely oblivious to their future likelihood of needing long-term care services and the potentially catastrophic costs entailed (CBO, 2013; The Urban Institute, 2001).

Moreover, the working-age adults who are at the cusp of entry into old age and retirement have few inducements to plan for and invest in their future long-term care needs because (1) the tax incentives for the purchase of long-term care insurance are relatively weak and limited to high-income earners and (2) Medicaid functions as the social safety net for catastrophic long-term expenditures for all but the most affluent share of older adult households (Baer & O'Brien, 2010; Bassett, 2004).

Ironically, finding a way to make the Partnership for Long-Term Care program actually work should be a fruitful area for bipartisan cooperation because it reduces the growth in public entitlement expenditures while retaining the integrity of the social safety net for catastrophic health-care expenditures. If liberals and conservatives could find a way to work together to promote the growth of the Partnership for Long-Term Care program as an alternative to traditional Medicaid financing of long-term care, the measures that should be pursued include (1) substantially increased tax credits at the state and federal level for long-term care insurance policy premiums of middle- and high-income earners, (2) direct and indirect subsidies for the long-term insurance premiums of lower-income earners, (3) closing the loopholes in state and federal Medicaid regulations that permit asset transfers for the purposes of qualifying for Medicaid among higher-income households, and (4) investing in a large-scale public education campaign to increase the public's awareness of the risks and catastrophic costs of long-term care, the advantages of carrying long-term care insurance as a way to sustain independence and quality of life in old age, and long-term care insurance as a means of preserving property and wealth for one's children.

The political feasibility of incorporating the marginal costs of both community-based and institutional long-term care services in the Tier I social insurance fund is not an insurmountable challenge, but only to the extent that (1) the growth in national health-care expenditures is reduced as anticipated by the health-care system delivery reforms proposed in chapter 6 (thus limiting the costs of social insurance for health care as a share of household income) and (2) there is a sea of change in the public awareness of escalating long-term care needs as a normal and inevitable aspect of the aging process.

THE SOCIAL RIGHT TO HEALTH CARE FOR THE PROFOUNDLY DISABLED

There are both easy and difficult questions pertaining to claims to health care that have no relevance to political citizenship, fair equality of opportunity, and social mobility, as in the case of persons having profound intellectual disabilities that cannot be ameliorated by investments in health care, as well as the health and mental health care for the severely and persistently mentally ill. In the final version of his theory of justice, Rawls conceded that while "we have a duty towards all human beings, however severely handicapped," there are unresolved questions concerning "the weight of these duties when they conflict with other basic claims" (Rawls, 2001, p. 176, n. 59). In other words, when it comes to making allocative decisions between the specialized and costly long-term care needs of the severely disabled and other socially crucial investments in basic education and health care, the principles of justice advanced by Rawls based on equality of status, equal basic rights and liberties, and fair equality of opportunity provide no clear answers.

However, health-care policy ethicist Norman Daniels suggests that for the disabled who fall below the minimum threshold of the normal range of functioning, the allocative priorities for health needs shift from the protection, maintenance, and restoration of normal functioning to meeting those health and related social needs of the severely disabled that optimize social inclusion and functioning *as close as possible* to the normal range—within the limits of reasonable resource constraints (Daniels, 2008, pp. 145–149). As stated by Daniels, "The right to health care can yield entitlements only to those needs we can reasonably meet" (p. 146).

As sensible as this seems, determining the boundaries of the reasonable in cases of severe disability is often exceedingly difficult and even morally and emotionally excruciating, as in the hypothetical case of a quadriplegic having ongoing public expenditures for daily in-home care assistance (to optimize her health and prospects for social inclusion) that exceed twice the median income of the typical household. By virtue of these public expenditures for daily care assistance, this individual is able to experience a greatly enhanced quality of life relative to institutional care, can more readily develop and use her intellectual gifts for productive work, and thereby would be likely to live longer as well. In parallel with the problem of intergenerational equity and the long-term care needs of older adults, when taken to population-level scale, there is a daunting deliberative conflict between her claims to the social resources needed to optimize her longevity and quality of life and the social resources needed to optimize fair equality of opportunity for the non–severely disabled.

What, then, should determine the threshold of the reasonable when it comes to the health needs of the severely disabled? Daniels (2008) suggests that the limiting considerations include not only the protection of fair equality of opportunity but also the extent to which all of the social institutions that are essential to fair equality of opportunity are themselves dependent on society's productive capacities (p. 146). That is, the share of social resources allocated to the special health needs of the severely disabled begin to exceed the threshold of the reasonable at the point that (1) the social resources that are essential to fair equality of opportunity are threatened and (2) the social investments that are essential to the nation's (or the states) productive capacities become undermined.[12] In practical application, these moral criteria for the determination of the boundaries of the reasonable in efforts to meet the special health needs of the severely disabled are useful only to the extent that they are applied to objective empirical evidence about the effects of alternative approaches to the allocation of limited social resources. Hopefully, in the processes of litigation and legislation that will ultimately define the parameters of the feasible in meeting the health needs of the most disabled among us, the moral consideration of empirical knowledge will triumph as the final arbitrator.

THE SPECIAL SOCIAL RIGHTS TO HEALTH CARE
FOR SOME CITIZENS

Neither Marshall nor Rawls contemplated the question of special social rights for some distinct classes or groups of citizens, apart from (1) the general justifications of social rights that might give some groups special rights related to special needs (such as the severely disabled discussed in the preceding section) or (2) the case of Rawls's Difference Principle, which legitimizes only those social and economic inequalities that are to the greatest benefit to the least advantaged of society.[13] Yet there are two groups in the United States that, for historical reasons, have long had special social rights to health care: Native Americans and military veterans. The question is whether, under the reformed health-care financing and delivery scheme advanced in the preceding chapters, these two groups should retain a right to health care that is substantively distinct from the general class of citizens. To explain why the response for both groups is yes, each case must be considered on its own merits.

American Indians and Alaska Natives

As of the 2010 decennial census, there were 2.9 million Americans identified as American Indian or Alaska Native (AIAN) alone and another 3.2 million Americans who identified as AIAN in combination with at least one other race (Norris et al., 2012). The special rights to health care for the AIAN population are derived from two principle justifications, the first being welfare rights and obligations to AIAN tribes that originate in treaties that were signed by the federal government in exchange for the expropriated aboriginal territories, beginning with the Treaty with the Delawares in 1778 and culminating with the Fort Laramie Treaty of 1868. These social right obligations were embodied in such treaty language as the "promise of all proper care and protection" in exchange for forcefully expropriated tribal land and natural resources and were further validated by the U.S. Supreme Court in its 1831 decision, *Cherokee Nation v. Georgia* (Warne & Frizzell, 2014, p. 263). However, throughout the nineteenth century and much of the twentieth century, the U.S. government sought in various ways to abrogate the social and human rights of AIANs that extended from treaty obligations, and it was not until the Snyder Act of 1921 that the federal government made any meaningful provision for the health care of indigenous Americans through funds for contracts with physicians to provide medical care on tribal reservations. Although the Indian Health Service (IHS) was established in 1955 in an effort to make a more significant effort toward the health needs of the AIAN population, the IHS has been chronically underfunded and poorly staffed relative to the health-care needs of the AIAN population, as well as geographically isolated from the urban AIAN population (Kunitz, 1996; Warne & Frizzell, 2014). It was not until the Indian Health Improvement Act of 1976 that Congress acknowledged the U.S. government's responsibility to maintain and improve the health of the AIAN population at a level commensurate with the health of the U.S. population as a whole and allocated investments in the IHS infrastructure toward that end goal (Warne & Frizzell, 2014).

The second justification for the special social rights to health care for the AIAN population is rooted in compensatory grounds, arising from the genocidal repercussions of the conquest of the indigenous territories of North America by the European ancestors and founders of the modern American republic that by 1900 had all but eradicated the indigenous peoples of the continent. Although the scholarly estimates of the pre-Columbian (1492) population in North America vary widely, ranging from as few as 2 million indigenous Americans to as many as 18 million, what is clear is that by 1900, the combined indigenous populations of the continental United States, Canada, and Greenland had dwindled to no more than 375,000 (Thornton, 1997). Notwithstanding the enduring controversy about the relative effects of the specific mechanisms of indigenous population decline that took place over the 400-year period of continental conquest (mass violence, disease, territorial displacement, and cultural genocide) and even the use of the term *genocide*, there is no question that all causes of the near eradication of the indigenous American population are entirely rooted in the coercive and deadly processes of colonialization that established the modern American republic (Thornton, 1997).

While the nation's AIAN population has rebounded over the past century from more progressive policies toward the rights and well-being of indigenous Americans to the 2.9 million count estimated in the 2010 U.S. Census, the compensatory justifications of the special health-care rights of the AIAN population continue to arise from the legacies of colonialization that are quite literally embodied in current AIAN health disparities.

American Indians and Alaska Natives have a life expectancy that is 4.2 years less than that for the U.S. population as a whole, and persons of primarily AIAN ancestry continue to die at dramatically higher rates from a range of preventable causes of death, including chronic liver disease and cirrhosis, diabetes mellitus, unintentional injuries, assault/homicide, intentional self-harm/suicide, and chronic lower respiratory diseases (IHS, 2015). Given these justifications for special entitlements to health care for AIANs, what should be the substantive response?

Although it might be argued that the special social rights to health care that belong to persons of AIAN ancestry can be addressed through the general health disparity amelioration provisions and evaluative processes discussed in chapters 6 and 7, two distinctive aspects of the AIAN health-care entitlements transcend the requirements of general health-care policy provisions. The first pertains to the prioritization of national investments in the reduction of health disparities, which should accord particular respect for the unique obligations to the health and well-being of AIAN tribes that are rooted in historical treaty rights and the magnitude of health disparities carried by the AIAN population.

The second distinctive aspect relates to the role that tribal sovereignty and tribal governance play in mediating the substantive specifics (or institutional arrangements) of the health-care rights for its AIAN members, as embodied in Presidential Executive Order 13175, which, since it was issued by President Bill Clinton in 2000, has required all federal agencies to consult directly with tribes on any actions that involve tribal resources and members or in any way might affect tribal interests.[14]

While it can be said the special social rights to health care for persons of AIAN ancestry are to a significant extent included in key provisions of the ACA that are specific to the AIAN population (such as the permanent reauthorization and expansion of the Indian Health Care Improvement Act, the special health insurance subsidies available to AIANs), in the final analysis, what is required is the full funding of health services to AIAN persons and communities commensurate with the expressly stated legislative intent of the Indian Health Care Improvement Act—that is, "to ensure the highest possible health status for Indians and urban Indians and to provide all resources necessary to effect that policy" (Warne & Frizzell, 2014, p. S265). If implemented in adequate funding allocations, this would be a significant and welcome departure from 200 years of federal policy history.

Military Veterans

As noted previously, neither Marshall nor Rawls addressed special social rights to health care for groups other than the severely disabled, and therefore both bypassed at least direct reference to special rights based on military service. Rawls, a combat veteran of World War II, as deeply as he must have felt about the nation's debt to its veterans, did not *directly* refer to any special considerations for military service in his original (1971) or restated (2001) theory of distributive justice. However, fundamental to his framing of a just society as "a fair system of social cooperation" are the two core ideas of equality and reciprocity,[15] the latter of which pertains directly to the justification of special social rights based on military service. Military service by definition entails the subordination of liberty rights to military order and discipline, the willingness to risk and even surrender life and limb on behalf of what is politically defined as the national interest, and the acceptance of numerous other sacrifices and hardships that are in the nature of life in the military, such as living in strange and unpleasant places isolated from one's country and kin, or spending months confined within a submarine deep below the surface of the world's oceans. Not surprisingly, over the nation's history, the likelihood of military service is lowest among families of high income, and during different periods in history, both race and class disadvantages have typically been associated with the likelihood of combat roles and fatalities (Coffey, 1998; Lutz, 2008).

In keeping with the idea of reciprocity for military service, since the Revolutionary War, the nation's government has assumed special obligations on behalf of its military veterans, particularly those who have suffered combat-related injuries during times of war. At various points in history and usually at the conclusion of major wars, Congress has extended and enlarged upon special provisions and compensations for military service, including homes for the aged and disabled veterans, veterans' pensions, survivors' benefits for dependents of veterans, special loan programs for homes and small businesses, and special entitlements to health care (Almgren, 2013). The most ambitious and well-known example of these compensatory actions by Congress is the Servicemen's Readjustment Act of 1944 (better known as the GI Bill), which included in its core provisions the educational stipend and home ownership loan programs that were pivotal to the creation of the great American middle class and the post–World War II suburbanization of the American landscape (Massey, 2007).

The Struggles of the Veterans Administration Health-Care System

The special social rights to health care for military veterans are provided through the nation's Veterans Administration (VA) health-care system, which encompasses 153 medical centers, 882 ambulatory care clinics, 136 nursing homes, forty-five residential rehabilitation programs for drug and alcohol dependence, and ninety-two comprehensive home-based care programs (Almgren, 2013). The care for veterans is provided through twenty-two regional networks that are financed primarily on a capitated-based global budgeting basis, on funds allocated biennially from Congress. Significantly from the standpoint of the de facto substantive rights to health care for veterans, although all veterans honorably discharged from military service are eligible to enroll in the VA health-care system, eligibility for care is determined by the year-by-year balance between utilization of care by veterans and congressional appropriations, as well as the individual veteran's standing in a system of prioritized eligibility. The only veterans who are automatically eligible for VA system care are those who have an established service-connected disability of at least 50 percent disablement and recently discharged veterans with a service-connected disability that is as yet unrated (Almgren, 2013).

Importantly, the VA system has also long served as the health-care safety net for low-income veterans without health insurance. In the year prior to the ACA being signed into law, low-income veterans without qualifying service-connected disabilities accounted for 28 percent of all VA health system enrollees (CBO, 2010). Although the ACA is expected to reduce the share of low-income veterans without health insurance, it is likely that the VA system will continue to serve as the health-care safety net for many thousands of low-income veterans well into the foreseeable future.

As the VA health system approaches the centennial of the 1917 War Risk Insurance Act that first established medical benefits for veterans, the special social rights to health care for veterans remain often unrealized and in constant jeopardy due to level of funding that is insufficient to contend with the aging of the veterans of long past wars (World War II, Korea, and Vietnam) and the casualties of more recent ones (Iraq 1991, Iraq 2003–2010, and Afghanistan 2001–2016).[16] In 2015, one year after former VA Secretary Eric Shinseki was forced to resign amid the scandal involving the falsification of records to hide the long wait times facing veterans seeking care, the number of veterans on wait lists to be treated for a wide range of health needs had increased by 50 percent (Wax-Thibodeaux, 2015). Despite a broad-based political consensus that it has met the health-care needs of those veterans returning from service in Iraq and Afghanistan, the VA system in many parts of the country is essentially broken, and it has remained woefully understaffed, underfunded, and politically embattled.

Toward the Full Realization of Special Social Rights to Health Care for Military Veterans

The VA health system's ongoing struggles are rooted in an enduring lack of political consensus as to which and what health-care needs of veterans fall within the boundaries of just reciprocity for military service. Veterans are reified in the campaign language of politicians, but in the hard-nosed budgetary negotiations in Congress, their specific health-care entitlements are rank-ordered and reduced to what is deemed fiscally feasible in light of other national priorities—ironically including the means with which to mount new wars. So the first fundamental question must be the following: Just what is owed to the nation's veterans for military service in keeping with principles of fair reciprocity?

At a minimum, it would seem to include full and complete compensation for the costs of military service borne by the veteran and his or her immediate family—in health terms, either full restoration of preservice healthy functioning or the complete fulfillment of adaptive health-care needs where full restoration of preservice health is not possible. However, this minimum compensatory standard does not get either a social reward for military service or compensation for the lost opportunity costs of military service, which may be met (as they have been at different points in the history of veterans' health care) through such special health-care entitlements as long-term care in old age, the elimination of health insurance copays for veterans, and health-care programs that target the optimization of quality of life for military veterans at all stages of the life course. The overall point is that the principles of fair reciprocity for military service and their related health-care entitlements should be developed in advance of congressional budgetary negotiations and not be a product of them.

Another large question pertains to whether veterans are best served by a separate health-care system from the health-care financing and delivery system advanced in the preceding chapters of this book. The most scathing critics of the VA health-care system see it as a bloated, inefficient, and entrenched bureaucracy staffed by well-compensated federal civil servants who are far more interested in protecting and advancing their careers than serving the nation's veterans.

Unfortunately, both the 2014 VA health-care system scandal that involved the falsification of waiting time records and the related narratives of veterans who felt abandoned and betrayed by the VA system added some credence to this line of criticism. In the most recent presidential election cycles, mainstream conservative presidential candidates Mitt Romney (2012) and Jeb Bush (2016) each called for the use of vouchers for the purchase of private health insurance as an alternative to health care in the VA system, although both stopped short of risking the ire of millions of veterans by calling for the complete dismantling of the VA health-care system (Epstein, 2015; McAuliff, 2012).

To many conservative politicians, the VA health-care system is a penultimate example of the waste and ineptitude that is intrinsic to government-run health care, irrespective of the high costs and poor quality of care that are widespread throughout private-sector medicine (Institute of Medicine, 2001). The VA health-care system's defenders (which include such venerated veterans' advocacy organizations as the American Legion and the Veterans of Foreign Wars) can point to the findings from an exhaustive 2004 RAND Corporation study published in the *Annals of Internal Medicine* that showed relative to private-sector medicine delivered to nonveterans, VA health care was superior in fourteen of fifteen categories of care and comparable in the one category that was the exception (Asch et al., 2004). Overall, the VA patients in the RAND study received about two-thirds of the care recommended by national standards, compared with about half for non-VA patients relying on the private-sector health-care system (RAND Corporation, 2005). It should be noted, though, that this study was conducted in the early years of the Iraq and Afghanistan wars, before the VA health-care system was challenged to absorb the tsunami of discharged veterans in need of health care that emerged in the latter years of the decade.

In a more recent and equally nonideological dispassionate analysis of policy alternatives for meeting the nation's special obligations toward its veterans, Stefos and Burgess (2014) have suggested that selective use of private health insurance subsidies, matched with care coordination, could induce Medicare-eligible veterans with less complex health-care needs to obtain their health care from private-sector Medicare providers, thus enabling the limited resources of the VA health-care system to be shifted to the care of veterans with more complex health-care needs. They note, for example, that from 2009 through 2011, the average annual VA health system expenditures for Medicare-eligible veterans amounted to $28.9 billion (Stefos & Burgess, 2014). These findings suggest some promise for an approach, in the context of a national single-payer system model with comprehensive basic benefits, for giving veterans the alternative of mainstream health care when and where they feel their health-care needs can be better met while retaining the integrity of the VA health-care system for the more complex and specialized needs of veterans. This is very different from the simple voucher approach that is advocated, at least in part, as an ideologically motivated Trojan horse for the dismantling of the VA health-care system.

CONCLUDING REMARKS: ANTICIPATING THE UNKNOWNS OF EVOLUTIONARY SOCIAL CHANGE

This final chapter has been about a few of the known special considerations and complexities that arise as the nation's health-care system evolves toward a more complete realization of a social right to comprehensive health care for all its citizens, as well as the extension of a social right to health care to many noncitizens based on principles of fairness, just compensation, and reciprocity. There are, of course, a range of special considerations and complexities that have been bypassed in the enduring trade-off between adequate coverage and unwieldy exposition or as a reflection of the author's biases and blind spots. Critics require fodder for critique, and this chapter (as with the book as a whole) may be overgenerous in that regard.

This acknowledged, even more special considerations and complexities to the model of evolutionary health-care reform envisioned in this book are unknown and perhaps even unknowable. Health-care policy scholars, like the prisoners in Plato's *Allegory of the Cave*, infer the shape and nature of the future in health care from bounded frames of reference. Also like Plato's prisoners, we confer and debate with each over the nature of a reality that (often unknown to us) is beyond our powers of perception and imagination. Trapped as we are within the limits of historical experience and our particular disciplinary and ideological perspectives, our best guess (inferred from historical experience) can only be that (1) unanticipated policy consequences and complexities are intrinsic to all fundamental institutional reforms, even the most desirable of them, and (2) while inevitable, they are not insurmountable. We also can know, with more certainty, that we should neither replicate nor build further upon the flawed social policy foundations of the past.

NOTES

1. STATEMENT OF THE PROBLEM: AMERICAN EXCEPTIONALISM IN HEALTH CARE AND THE EMERGENCE OF THE GREAT UNSUSTAINABLE COMPROMISE

1. This number includes both undocumented immigrants who are excluded from ACA coverage and other groups that, while technically eligible for means-tested health-care coverage, face significant barriers to enrollment (e.g., homeless persons and the seriously and persistently mentally ill). In this book, the term *Americans* encompasses all those who occupy a place in American society—those with citizenship status, legal resident aliens, and undocumented immigrants.

2. Between 1975 and 2014, the General Social Survey's (GSS) representative sample of American adults was asked every other year whether they believed it is the federal government's responsibility to help people pay for doctor and hospital bills when they are sick or that people should "take care of these things for themselves." Survey respondents were then asked to rate their beliefs on a five-point scale between these two extremes, with "5" representing a strong belief that helping people to pay for their health care when sick was a government responsibility and "1" representing the belief that it was the responsibility of the individual to pay for his or her health care, not the federal government. "3," the position in between these extremes, indicates the belief that paying for health care was the responsibility of *both* the government and the individual. Over the four decades that Americans were surveyed on this question, the average share of Americans placing themselves on the "3" to "5" response range (indicating a belief that the government has either a primary or at least a shared responsibility in ensuring that people have help in paying for needed health care) was 80 percent. In contrast, an average of only 17.1 percent of Americans surveyed over this forty-year period did not believe that helping people pay for their health care when sick was the responsibility of the federal government.

3. Harry S. Truman, *Special Message to Congress Recommending a Comprehensive Health Program*. November 19, 1945. Cited from Public Papers from the Presidents, Harry S. Truman 1945–1953. Harry S. Truman Library and Museum. http://www .trumanlibrary.org/publicpapers/index.php?pid=483&st=&st1=.

4. The Republican Party, fueled by renewed public confidence in the superiority of free-market capitalism and growing fears of postwar communist expansionism, gained fifty-five House seats and twelve Senate seats—enough to give them control of both houses of Congress for the first time since 1928.

5. The Sheppard-Towner Act, formally titled the "Congressional Act for the Promotion of the Welfare of and Hygiene of Maternity and Infancy," was the first federal program that included federally funded health care for preventative and primary health care to ordinary citizens. As such, it was vigorously opposed by the AMA, which, among other things, saw Sheppard-Towner as a threatening first step toward socialized medicine. Related to that concern were developments in American medicine that by the mid-1920s identified both maternal hygiene and well-baby care as potentially lucrative domains for medical free enterprise (Almgren et al., 2000).

6. In their analysis of Hill-Burton funds allocated between 1950 and 1973, Hochban et al. (1981) found that the per-capita amount of Hill-Burton funds distributed for hospital construction was 1.5 times higher in middle-income communities relative to low-income counties and slightly higher in wealthy counties ($23.59 per capita in wealthy counties versus $20.93 per capita in poor counties). This translated very directly to increasing rather than reducing disparities in the availability of hospital beds in poor communities relative to middle-income communities.

7. Both the Blue Cross and Blue Shield voluntary health insurance associations originated as artifacts of an innovation and diffusion process rather than as a result of a national health-care policy agenda that encouraged the development of voluntary health insurance. Blue Cross began as an innovative strategy to create a fund for the hospital care of school teachers at Baylor University Hospital in Texas in 1929, while the first Blue Shield plan was organized by the California Medical Association and its county medical societies in 1939. The late development of the Blue Shield insurance plans for physician services relative to that of hospital insurance is attributed to the entrenched resistance of the AMA to even the idea of voluntary health insurance until the real possibility of social insurance for health care became evident with the success of the Social Security Act of 1935.

8. Some of this decline can also be attributed to structural changes in the economy as well, particularly the decline in labor union representation and high-wage and benefit blue-collar employment in the wake of deindustrialization.

9. The "Harry and Louise" television ad series was designed to lead the viewer to a set of conclusions about the Clinton plan, through the depiction of a typical suburban couple having a conversation about their negative reactions to health-care reform's supposed detrimental impacts on their health-care choices and costs.

10. According to the Henry Kaiser Family Foundation (2012), in 2011, 61.5 percent of the nonelderly population was covered by a combination of employer-based and private non-group coverage health insurance. The U.S. Census Bureau (1975) historical estimates of health insurance coverage for the years 1939 to 1970 show that in 1953, the voluntary insurance coverage for the total national population (including those aged sixty-five and older) had reached the 61.5 percent mark.

11. According to the Henry Kaiser Family Foundation's March 2014 Health Tracking Poll, the public's 46 percent opposition to the ACA comprised objections against an expanded government role in the provision of health care, dislike of the ACA's so-called individual mandate, and concerns about both the cost of health insurance to individuals and the cost of health-care reform for the country.

2. THE EMERGENCE OF THE NEW ERA OF REFORM

1. This health-care reform typology does not include selective expansions of health-care entitlements under Medicare and Medicaid, such as the inclusion of the hospice care benefits under Medicare in 1982 and the Medicare Part D (drug benefit program) added in 2003.

2. The source of this quote of Johnson's, and the circumstances under which it occurred, is Pulitzer Prize–winning journalist Nick Kotz's (2005) definitive history of Johnson's successful effort to achieve the civil rights and voting rights legislation that transformed American society, *Judgement Days: Lyndon Baines Johnson, Martin Luther King Jr. and the Laws that Changed America.* This quote is taken in its entirety from page 16 of this book.

3. Nixon had, however, departed from the AMA at an early point in his political career when, in 1947, he supported voluntary *federal* health insurance as an alternative to compulsory social insurance (Quadagno, 2005).

4. Although the Health Insurance Affordability and Accountability Act (HIPAA) of 1996 is also a very major piece of policy legislation enacted during the Clinton administration that had the effect of extending access to employment-based insurance to workers who had lost or were at risk of losing their employment-based insurance, it is regarded here as primarily offsetting some of the unintended consequences of the 1974 Employment Retirement and Income Security Act on workers and their dependents with preexisting health conditions. HIPAA was not about expanding health insurance coverage so much as preventing its loss.

5. Jill Quadagno (2005, p. 136) notes that the AHA leadership supported PPS as an alternative to the strict cost controls under TEFRA. However, outside of Washington, D.C., the hospital administrators and board members that comprised the rank and file of the AHA had hardly heard of PPS or DRGs until they were forced in 1983–1984 to radically and rapidly transform the incentives of their medical staff and department heads.

6. As quoted from "President Bush Visits Cleveland, Ohio," The Office of the Press Secretary, The White House, July 10, 2007.

7. As originally signed into law, the ACA was intended to achieve health insurance coverage for 93 percent of the national population and almost all U.S. citizens. This estimate of the intended health insurance coverage effects of the ACA is taken from the CMS actuarial estimates provided to the U.S. Congress on April 22, 2010 (CMS, 2010), combined with U.S. Census projections for the U.S. population as of 2019 (U.S. Census Bureau, 2008), the point at which the ACA was projected to be fully implemented.

8. These criteria for successful social policy were originally summarized in a previous book: Almgren, *Health Care Politics, Policy and Services: A Social Justice Analysis* (2013). For a more complete analysis of the political prospects for the ACA's success as social policy, see pages 355–360.

9. The three U.S. Supreme Court cases that represented a broad-based effort to over-turn key provisions of the ACA were as follows: *The National Federation of Independent Business v. Sebelius, No. 11-393; U.S. Department of Health and Human Services v. Florida, No. 11-398;* and *Florida v. Department of Health and Human Services, No. 11-400.*

10. In a debacle that was politically costly to both the Obama administration and the midterm election prospects for the Democratic Party, during the first months of its operation, the federal health insurance exchange website repeatedly crashed, produced errors in enrollment registration and health insurance cost estimates, and altogether confirmed for a large share of the public the expectation that the ACA would be a bureaucratic disaster. At the state level, the health insurance exchange development efforts reflected the extremes of robust success (Washington) and catastrophic failure (Oregon).

3. THE THEORETICAL FOUNDATIONS FOR HEALTH CARE AS A SOCIAL RIGHT OF CITIZENSHIP

1. Daniels (2008, p. 42) uses the phrase "normal species functioning," by which he clearly means *Homo sapiens* or humans.

2. Stated in full, Rawls's second principle of justice reads as follows: "Social and economic inequalities are to satisfy two conditions: first, they are to be attached to offices and positions open to all under conditions of fair equality of opportunity; and second they are to be to the greatest benefit to the least-advantaged members of society" (Rawls, 2001, pp. 42–43).

3. Notably, this very powerful statement on a universal right to health care was embraced by the United States well over sixty years ago—and to date, the United States is the only signatory democracy of the United Nations Universal Declaration of Human Rights that has yet to achieve a universal right to health care for its citizens.

4. Olson (2012) actually provides a very thorough and much more extensive analysis of the moral foundations of a universal right to health care within Christian theology. Interested readers are referred to his book as cited in the list of references for this chapter.

5. As cited from Richard McBrien, "What the Church Teaches on Health Care Reform," *National Catholic Reporter,* October 5, 2009, http://ncronline.org/blogs/essays-theology/what-church-teaches-health-care-reform.

6. Callahan's famous book, *Setting Limits: Medical Goals in an Aging Society,* goes well beyond a simple utilitarian argument that age might serve as a fair and rational criterion for the limitations of entitlements to health care. In particular, he makes the case that age, as a universal criterion, is a far more just criterion for limiting health-care entitlements than such particularistic criteria as race and social class—as is the de facto case in the current structure of the U.S. health-care system. That acknowledged, three decades after his book was published, Daniel Callahan at age seventy-nine incurred $80,000 in Medicare costs for treatment of his heart condition (Baker, 2009).

7. Although Sen acknowledges Rawls and the contribution of liberal political philosophy to the development of his own social justice framework, he offers multiple criticisms of political liberalism and the epistemological traditions it represents. Chief

among them is the premise in Western political philosophy that optimal social justice can be advanced by reliance on so-called transcendental theories of justice based on abstract thought experiments, as opposed to real-world comparisons of alternative systems of social organization and social justice. His specific critique of Rawls and liberalism generally is its focus on the just distribution of the *means* that are presumed to advance human well-being as opposed to the *ends* realized.

8. Herbert Hart (1907–1992) was a legal philosopher and professor of jurisprudence at Oxford, while Sir Isaiah Berlin (1909–1997) was principally known as a political philosopher. Stuart Hampshire (1914–2004), a fellow at Oxford at the time that Rawls was there in 1952, is known for his work at bridging the one-time intellectual chasm between moral philosophy and politics. It therefore comes to no surprise that Rawls's *A Theory of Justice* is such a rich synthesis of thought from legal philosophy, political philosophy, and classic moral philosophy.

9. This question has been framed in language that simplifies and gets to the essence of Rawls's idea of the Original Position as the hypothetical basis of the just social contract, as refined in the final version of his theory of justice (Rawls, 2001, pp. 15–16).

10. Sir William Beveridge, former director of the London Stock Exchange, in response to a request from government to investigate alternative approaches to social security for British subjects, delivered his famous Beveridge Report (formally titled *The Social Insurance and Allied Services: Report by Sir William Beveridge Presented to the Parliament by Command of His Majesty, November, 1942*), which became the template for the modern British welfare state.

11. The residualist welfare state places emphasis on meager, means-tested, and selective provisions that are limited to failures of the labor market to meet essential human needs over universalistic human capital investment and safety net provisions.

12. As pointed out by Nancy Fraser and Linda Gordon (*Beyond Contract-versus-Charity, Toward Participation and Provision: On the Concept of Social Citizenship*, CSST Working Paper No. 76, University of Michigan, Ann Arbor, 1992), aside from the flaws and inconstancies in Marshall's historical sequence in the evolvement of the different dimensions of citizenship, political rights *may* but do not necessarily precede social rights. "Thus, although it is true in principle that political rights can be used to secure social rights, social security has proved necessary in practice for the full and effective exercise of political power. Historical struggles for either one have usually also involved the other" (p. 36).

13. In fact, as discussed at an earlier point in this chapter, Marshall does so in pointing out the clear connections between freedom of speech and the right to a basic education.

14. As argued by Boaz (1997), affordable health care is not an entitlement of citizenship but a matter of self-responsibility and market-based risk management through voluntary associations and contracts (meaning private health insurance).

4. A PRINCIPLED CRITIQUE OF THE ACA AND THE ACA IN AN EVOLUTIONARY PERSPECTIVE

1. Social epidemiologist Nancy Krieger (2002) refers to health disparities among marginalized individuals, groups, and populations as the biological "embodiment" of social stratification.

2. The health-care resources listed here are taken directly from Daniels's (2008) list of six health needs commensurate with the requirements of normal functioning (p. 42). Daniels refers directly to "preventative, curative, rehabilitative, and compensatory medical services (and devices)," although I substitute *adaptive* for *compensatory*. Public health investments and measures are implied from Daniels's list.

3. Rawls's full phrase is "normal and fully cooperating members of society," by which he means citizens as persons possessing the normal range of human capabilities. Here Rawls is not advocating that the disabled and other dependent persons be denied citizenship status, so much as he is laying the groundwork for the justification of social rights that are essential to the realization and preservation of the normal range of functioning that, in turn, is essential to fair equality of opportunity.

4. Under the original provisions of the ACA, the federal government would have the power to coerce states to expand Medicaid eligibility through the withholding of funds for already established Medicaid programs. Even liberal Justice Elaine Kagan viewed this as an unconstitutional overreach of federal power.

5. Health insurance, like all other forms of insurance, is based on creation of risk pools of the insured that include a critical mass of low-risk enrollees that is needed to offset the health insurance costs incurred by high-risk enrollees. Because the ACA intends to enroll formally uninsured adults badly in need of health care, it is critical to the fiscal viability of the ACA's approved insurance plans that healthy young adults enroll in insurance in large numbers, as opposed to paying a modest tax penalty and continuing to take their chances against the possibility of catastrophic health expenditures. Because also the ACA's tax penalties for failing to carry health insurance are relatively modest compared to the cost of even subsidized health insurance and the fear of "medical bankruptcy" is not prominent among the concerns of young adults, the ACA's health insurance enrollment assumptions are highly optimistic if not dubious.

6. Although there is no agreed-upon specific definition of a medical home, there is broad consensus on some essential elements: close and regular contact with a primary care provider who takes the lead referring the patient to specialists, integrated electronic health records, and active participation of the patient and the patient's family/support network in the patient's care (Cassidy, 2012).

7. As discussed at an earlier point in the chapter, as originally signed into law, the ACA funded the expansion of Medicaid coverage to millions of uninsured through a substantial ($17 billion) reduction in DSH program payments to financially at-risk safety net hospitals. It was assumed by the architects of the ACA that safety net hospitals that had formally relied on DSH payments to offset uncompensated care losses would experience reductions in uncompensated care losses as a larger share of the previously uninsured would be enrolled in Medicaid. However, subsequent to the 2012 U.S. Supreme Court ruling that the ACA could not coerce states into accepting federal funds for Medicaid coverage expansion, it appears that in many parts of the country, safety net hospitals will suffer drastic DSH reductions in the absence of offsetting Medicaid program expansion revenue.

8. This comes as no surprise, in that Sweden's health-care system is based on a universal social insurance plan and Sweden's national population is relatively homogeneous with respect to both race and socioeconomic status.

9. As originally signed into law, the ACA designated $15 billion over ten years for the Prevention and Public Health Fund section of the ACA, an amount that Congress reduced by $6.25 billion as a part of the 2012 Middle Class Tax Relief and Job Creation

Act. This reflects the vulnerability of the ACA to congressional obstructionism and political horse trading. In contrast to early twentieth-century marginalization of public health explained by Starr (1982), these reductions in the ACA's public health funding are not at the behest of the AMA but rather are a reflection of competing budget priorities and partisan politics.

10. The distinction between "upstream" and "downstream" investments in health care draws on a prevention science analogy that is common to both the public health and child welfare literatures. The idea is that treatment interventions are analogous to the "downstream" act of tossing a lifeline to a person drowning in a swift river, whereas prevention strategies are akin to "upstream" actions (such as putting up a fence or posting a warning sign) that make it less likely that people will be swept away by the river to begin with.

11. *The 2014 Annual Report of the Boards of Trustees of the Federal Hospital Insurance and Federal Supplementary Medical Insurance Trust Funds* predicts that the Hospital Insurance Trust Fund (Medicare Part A) will have a fund balance of zero by 2030, with expenditures exceeding revenue beginning in 2022.

5. A PRINCIPLED APPROACH TO RADICAL HEALTH-CARE FINANCE REFORM

1. Wendt's (2009) analysis included indicators for expenditures per capita, the percentage of total health expenditures covered by public funds, the health-care provider mix, the basis of entitlement to health care, and regulation of access to care.

2. While public health-care expenditures as a proportion of the GDP are slightly higher in the United States than the OECD average (6.6 percent vs. 8.3 percent), this comparison is distorted by the much higher costs of the U.S. health-care system as opposed to a stronger level of support of health care as a social right (OECD, 2014a).

3. The poverty measure employed is relative poverty among the zero to seventeen age group after taxes and transfers (OECD, 2014b), observed either in 2011 or the nearest corresponding year available.

4. Massey attributes Southern support for the Taft-Hartley Act as originating in the success of Northern-based unions in organizing black textile and service workers in the South, which Southern politicians feared would fuel demands for civil rights. They were probably correct but of course ultimately on the wrong side of history as well as political democracy.

5. As measured by generational earning elasticity—in essence, the extent to which a child's income at the end of the length of a generation can be predicted by his or her parent's income. See Corak (2013) for a full explanation of this and alternative measures of social mobility.

6. This quote is cited from David Strauss's incisive critique of the myth of simple equality of opportunity that is embedded in this mantra, which he refers to as the illusionary distinction between equality of opportunity and equality of result.

7. Aside from a concerted lobbying effort supplemented by a strategic media campaign, the health insurance industry had as its trump card the vote of Senator Joe Lieberman (I-CT), the recipient of $448,000 in campaign contributions from the health insurance industry (Public Campaign Action Fund, 2009). Lieberman's vote was essential to the defeat of a Republican Party filibuster aimed at defeating the ACA in the

final months of 2009, and Lieberman made it very clear that he would block the final vote on any health-care bill that included a government-run public health insurance option.

8. The $24 million amount only represents the major health insurance industry contributors, Blue Cross/Blue Shield Plans and AHIP (America's Health Insurance Plans). As to the size of the health insurance industry, CMS actuaries estimated that the private health insurance industry accounted for $917 billion of the nation's health-care expenditures.

9. The specific restrictions governing the use of private health insurance vary by province; some provinces (British Columbia, Alberta, Manitoba, Ontario, Québec, and Prince Edward Island) prohibit the use of private insurance for publicly funded health services, while others (like Nova Scotia) indirectly constrain the private insurance market by precluding physicians from charging higher fees for privately insured patients than those charged for publicly insured patients (Hurley & Guindon, 2008). Countries that have a high prevalence of a duplicative role of private health insurance, which provides an alternative to the long lines of underfunded and overburdened publicly financed health-care services, include Australia (53 percent of Australians carry duplicative private health insurance) and Ireland (48 percent) (OECD, 2013).

10. This survey was sponsored by the Associated Press and Yahoo, and conducted by Knowledge Networks from December 14 to 20, 2007. Survey results are based on a probability sample of 1,823 adults (1,523 registered voters), with a margin of error of ±2.3 for all adults and ±2.5 for registered voters (AP/YAHOO Poll, 2008). The questions pertaining to support for national health insurance were included among a range of questions inclusive of gun control, the Iraq War, presidential candidate preferences, the economy, and a number of controversial social issues.

11. The exact description of a single-payer insurance plan used in the multiple surveys cited by Blendon et al. (2006) is as follows: "A national health plan, financed by taxpayers, in which all Americans would get their insurance from a single government plan" (p. 639).

12. In response to another question about specific worries, 64 percent cited "facing unexpected medical expenses" as among their significant concerns (which exceeded worries about all other items listed, including job loss, the inability to pay bills, and the loss of savings and investments). See http://surveys.ap.org/data/KnowledgeNetworks /AP-Yahoo_2007-08_panel02.pdf (item EC5).

13. Data are from the March 2014 wave of the Kaiser Family Foundation Health Tracking Poll series, which are based on nationally representative samples of adults aged eighteen and older. In response to the survey question "What would you like to see Congress do with the health care law?" 10 percent chose the response "keep the law as it is," 49 percent chose the response "keep the law in place and work towards improvements," and only 29 percent chose the either "repeal and replace" or "repeal and not replace"; see the full citation in the list of references for further details.

14. Even with full implementation of the ACA's health-care cost control provisions, the Board of Trustees for Medicare Part A Trust Fund estimates that expenditures will exceed revenues and assets by 2030 (Board of Trustees Medicare Trust Fund, 2014).

15. While the final revision of the ACA did include a provision that allowed the federal government to create multistate insurance plans that negotiate premium prices and benefit coverage with private insurance carriers, this is not a public plan or a single-payer plan.

16. The AMA's position on health-care reform, which remains wedded to a prefer-ence for voluntary private health insurance (AMA, 2014), is at odds with the direction of health-care reform opinions of physicians who are increasingly in favor of a single-payer approach.

17. The California legislature had successfully passed single-payer legislation with the support of a powerful coalition that included the California Nurses Association, only to have it vetoed by moderate GOP Governor Arnold Schwarzenegger—the last time in 2008. Although the California legislature again came close to passing a single-payer bill sponsored by California state senate chair Mark Leno (D) in 2012, the political priority given to the implementation of the ACA ultimately sidelined the legislation (Gallagher, 2013).

6. A PRINCIPLED APPROACH TO ESSENTIAL HEALTH-CARE DELIVERY SYSTEM REFORMS

1. While the differences in care between the first and second tiers in the "soft" ver-sion of a two-tiered health-care financing scheme may correlate with social class, in-somuch as both the tastes for and the means to pay for more convenience and a broader array of services may be influenced by socioeconomic status, class itself does not wholly determine the likelihood of carrying private health insurance in addition to the pub-lic benefit plan. This is because the level of quality, accessibility, and scope of coverage provided by the first-tier public plan would need to be more than minimalist to pro-tect the level of population and individual health commensurate with the normal range of human functioning.

2. Based on the author's analysis of hospital ownership data compiled by the Kaiser Family Foundation (2005 data), and both income inequality data and legislative po-litical party control from the Economic Policy Institute (2001–2003 data), the correla-tion between state levels of income inequality and the proportion of hospitals under for-profit ownership, adjusted for political party control, was modestly strong and statistically significant ($r=.47$, $p<.001$, $N=50$).

3. While the basic structural wagon wheel metaphor is cited from Cutler and Mor-ton (2013), the remarks pertaining to the competitive advantages derived from com-munity hospital affiliation with academic medical centers are the author's as much as Cutler and Morton's, based on the author's career experiences with hospital mergers.

4. An accountable care organization (ACO) is a Medicare program provider struc-ture that integrates patient care management, patient care data management systems, clinical case management models, and "bundled" payment mechanisms across primary care, specialty care, acute hospital care, rehabilitation care, skilled nursing facility care, and home health care.

5. The definition of a local health-care market adopted here is the Hospital Referral Region (HRR), pioneered by the Dartmouth Atlas Project and defined as a regional health-care market for tertiary medical care that generally requires the services of a major referral center (Dartmouth Institute for Health Policy and Clinical Practice, 2012). There are 306 HRRs nationwide.

6. Briefly described, the voucher approach would change the Medicare program from a "defined benefit program" that provides either full or substantial insurance cover-age for an array of guaranteed benefits, independent of cost, to a "defined contribution"

program that provides Medicare beneficiaries with a "voucher" worth a certain set dollar value with which to buy health insurance coverage through the private health insurance market. While Congress would almost certainly set minimum standards for benefit coverage and consumer disclosure of risks and out-of-pocket expenditures, critics of the voucher approach argue that low-income Medicare beneficiaries would be driven to the low-end health insurance market and inferior providers, despite their having higher levels of chronic disease and stronger needs for readily accessible, high-quality health care. Medicare would thus become a health-care entitlement program that, far from alleviating the linkages between social class and the quality of health care, actually would promote differences in the quality and accessibility of health care by class. The "commodification" of health care, as used here, is drawn from Esping-Andersen's (1990) notion of the "commodification" of human needs, which speaks to the extent to which social welfare provisions to address human needs (such as health care) are treated as market commodities in exchange for labor rather than as a provision to citizens from the state or as a social right of citizenship. In fact, under a voucher approach, the minimum acceptable provisions for the health-care needs of the most vulnerable elderly become much closer to becoming largely defined by market forces rather than by the legislative functions of the state—as it has been under the "defined benefits" approach of the Medicare program since its inception in 1965.

7. The only example of federal global budgeting for health care is the Veterans Administration (VA) health-care system. The VA formulates its health-care budget by developing annual estimates of its expenditures for all services and programs as a part of the congressional budget appropriations process (GAO, 2009). However, the VA health-care budget accounts for less than 2 percent of national health-care expenditures.

8. Comparisons in beneficiary expenditures by geographic location control for differences in age, race, and sex.

9. In the context of health care, the term *benchmarking* refers to the process of comparing clinical practice or health system performance against an external standard through the use of objective metrics of performance (AHRQ, 2013, January). A "benchmark" refers to a given measure of performance, such as the average number of minutes of wait time in a clinical practice (a process measure) or the incidence of complications from a given surgical procedure such as a total knee replacement (an outcome measure).

10. While the congressional budgeting process is currently based on an annual budget, Congress continues to debate the pros and cons of a biannual budget. The advantages of a biannual budget for federal spending as a whole to many are debatable. However, it is argued here that the budgeting of health-care services requires the stability and predictability of biannual budgeting as well as an adequate window of time for the development of essential feedback data on the cost-efficient delivery of core services.

11. While the approach to the oversight and limiting of private health insurance expenditures on noncore health-care services advocated by Long and Marquis (1994) entails states' limiting of private health insurance premiums, as discussed earlier in this chapter, there are two significant problems with this. As demonstrated with implementation of the Medicaid expansion provision of the ACA, many states have a high level of political tolerance for disparities in access to health care, which would make it unlikely that such states would be likely to impose limits on the coverage of health insurance. The second problem is that the American public generally opposes direct price controls of commodities, whereas excise taxes on nonessential commodities are

more tolerated. It is for these two reasons that a federal excise tax on Tier II health insurance coverage as a part of the Biannual National Health Expenditure Global Budget is presented as the most feasible limiting mechanism on Tier II expenditures.

12. This is a state-level version adapted from Edward Lawlor's (2003) proposed approach to the reform of Medicare, based on *agency theory* in economics.

13. The issues pertaining to the social right to health care of undocumented workers and their dependents will be addressed in the final chapter of the book.

14. It should be acknowledged that this PCP labor force does not account for the effect of supplementing the PCP labor force through the actions of state legislatures to expand the scope of practice for other professionals trained to provide primary care, most notably nurse practitioners. However, even a very radical shift in the politics of professional licensure will leave a large gap in the PCP labor force.

15. Based on a poll conducted January 9 to 15, 2015, by GBA Strategies on behalf of the Progressive Change Institute, a nationally representative sample of likely 2016 voters showed support at 51 percent, with a substantial majority (71 percent) supporting the option to choose between a single-payer plan and private health insurance. The interview sample was 1,500 likely 2016 voters nationwide (Margin of Error [MOE] ±2.5 percent) with every policy question posed to a split sample of 750 voters (MOE ±3.6 percent) to compare messaging and policy variations.

7. ASSESSING HEALTH-CARE SYSTEM PERFORMANCE AGAINST THE FOUR CORE AIMS OF HEALTH-CARE POLICY

1. While 100 percent enrollment can be set as a policy benchmark, it is assumed that there will be a margin of error in enrollment estimation that overlaps with the very small fraction of the population of citizens and legal immigrants that eludes aggressive enrollment efforts.

2. The health expenditure estimates used were based on 2009 expenditure data, and the discretionary income estimates were based on 2010 data. Given the low rate of both health-care inflation and general inflation during the 2009–2010 period, they are treated as equivalent data years.

3. The 2012 MEPS data show that the percentage of adults who were unable to obtain or delayed necessary medical care because they were unable to afford it ranged from 59 percent for the near-poor to 51 percent for middle-income earners (AHRQ, 2012a).

4. This is an almost verbatim quote from Shi and Singh's (2001, p. 493) very pragmatic and comprehensive definition of health-care access, with only the term *optimally effective health* care being used in place of the original *effective* health care, with *optimal* meaning what is achievable given the interactions between individual health needs/behaviors and the possibilities and limitations of medical science at any given point in time.

5. The Medical Expenditure Panel Survey (MEPS) is a set of large-scale surveys of families and individuals, their medical providers (doctors, hospitals, pharmacies, etc.), and employers across the United States. The health-care access measures that are shown in figure 7.1 are from the household component of the MEPS survey, which is based on a nationally representative set of households that have participated in the National Center for Health Statistic's ongoing National Health Interview Survey. The

household-level health-care access measures are either equivalent or align very closely with the individual- and household-level health-care access measures used in the European Union Statistics on Income and Living Conditions (EU-SILC), the Commonwealth Fund International Health Policy Survey, and the European Social Survey (ESS). For comparison, see Hernandez-Quevedo and Papanicolas (2013, p. 205).

6. A medically underserved area is defined by the Health Resources and Services Administration (HRSA) as a geography area (a county or group of contiguous counties in rural areas or a census tract representing a distinctive neighborhood in metropolitan areas) that has an Index of Medical Underservice (IMU) score of < 62 on a scale where 0 means a completely underserved area and 100 represents a best-served area. The IMU is based on four variables: the ratio of primary medical care physicians per 1,000 persons, the infant mortality rate, the percentage of the population with incomes below the poverty level, and the percentage of the population age sixty-five or older. A medically underserved population is also based on the IMU scale, with the same variables being applied to a population within a geographic area with distinctive economic, cultural, or linguistic access barriers to primary medical care services (HRSA, 1995).

7. Adjusted odds ratios are discussed at length at a later point in the chapter under the topic of logistic regression techniques as a tool to assess health-care disparities. Suffice it to say that adjusted odds ratios represent the relative risk of an event occurring that is associated with a given characteristic, adjusted for the effects of selected confounding influences. In this example, the relative risk of an African American residing in a medically underserved area would be adjusted for socioeconomic status (SES) to capture the risk specifically associated with race apart from the confounding effects of SES.

8. The Lorenz curve, developed by statistician M. O. Lorenz in 1905, has long been used as a method for depicting and measuring the distribution and concentration of wealth and the spatial concentration of populations. Its primary derivative measure, the Gini coefficient, has been widely used in comparative analyses of income inequality (Shryock & Siegel, 1976).

9. For a complete explanation of the conceptualization and calculation of the Index of Horizontal Inequity (HI), see Hernandez-Quevedo and Papanicolas (2013, pp. 204–210).

10. As mentioned previously, this is consistent with the approach to optimal performance benchmarking used by The Commonwealth Fund Commission on a High Performance Health System in its *Path to a High Performance U.S. Health System: A 2020 Vision and the Policies to Pave the Way* (2009).

11. Many readers will see that the $\mu benchmark\ value = \mu c_1 = \mu c_2 = \ldots \mu c_i$ criterion for perfect equity is but a simple extension of the null hypothesis for an analysis of variance (ANOVA) test for a difference in means between groups (Blalock, 1979).

12. The AHRQ methodological criteria define the threshold for an observed difference between the reference group and the comparison group as a statistically significant difference ($p < .05$, two-tailed test) that is greater than an absolute value of 10 percent.

13. This is a modified version of the definition of *allocative efficiency* provided by Cylus and Smith (2013), which in its original form reads "the extent to which limited resources are directed towards producing the current mix of health care outputs in line with the preferences of payers who supply the necessary inputs" (p. 284). The payer in the version of allocative efficiency employed in this book is the public as represented in the aims of national health-care policy.

14. Quality-adjusted life years (QALYs) is the most commonly reported measure of health benefits that incorporates both the length and quality of life in terms of health status. Meltzer and Chung's selection of the thirteen National Health Care Quality Report measures they analyzed was based on the availability of information on costs, effectiveness (in QALYs), the denominator population, and current implementation rate.

15. As explained in chapter 4, these specific health-care provisions are taken from those either stated directly or logically implied by Norman Daniels in his insightful and comprehensive extension of John Rawls's theory of justice to just health care policy: *Just Health: Meeting Health Needs Fairly* (2008).

16. The $50,000 per QALY standard that is the current (2015) social policy convention is far short of what we as a society have actually been willing to allocate to increase QALYs. An empirical analysis of the actual national health-care expenditures for the health-care advancements that occurred between 1950 and 2003 suggests that the lower and upper bounds for the maximum allocation for a QALY have been between $121,000 and $329,000 in 2015 equivalent dollars (Braithwaite et al., 2008).

17. The age-adjusted value of a QALY in accordance with the human capital criterion that was estimated by Hirth et al. (2000) was actually $24,777 in 1997 dollars. The $36,444 amount reflects the inflation adjustment to 2014 dollars.

18. Through a comprehensive analysis of causes of death by race and sex among the U.S. population between 1980 and 2007 and an exhaustive review of the literature on medically amendable causes of death, Ilo et al. (2014) estimated that two years of the racial gap in life expectancy were attributable to causes of death that could be affected by health-care policy interventions. This is 42 percent of the overall racial gap in life expectancy as estimated for 2007.

8. SPECIAL ISSUES AND CONSIDERATIONS

1. In-depth research on the modern history of Mexican migrants to the United States suggests that between 1965 and 1985, most undocumented migrants (as much as 85 percent of the annual total of undocumented migrants from Mexico) entered the United States as temporary workers and then returned to Mexico. After the border enforcement provisions of the Immigration and Reform and Control Act of 1986 (Public Law 99-603) went into effect, the return migration of undocumented workers from Mexico plummeted to 20 percent, which transformed a large share of the undocumented population from temporary workers to permanent U.S. residents by default rather than actual preference (Massey et al., 2015).

2. Although the undocumented immigrant population includes immigrants from Asia, the Caribbean, Central and South America, Africa, the Middle East, Canada, and Europe, the largest share and the focus of the undocumented immigrant policy debates are the approximately 6 million undocumented immigrants from Mexico (Krogstad & Passel, 2015).

3. As previously discussed, the border enforcement provisions of the Immigration and Reform Control Act of 1986 actually disrupted migratory work patterns and transformed a large share of the undocumented population from temporary workers to permanent U.S. residents by default rather than actual preference. The North American Free Trade Agreement of 1994 (NAFTA) was disastrous for the peasant agricultural

economy and small manufacturing industry of Mexico, sending millions of displaced peasants and workers seeking a living north of the border (Massey et al., 2015; Portes, 2006).

4. As discussed in chapter 7, under the current IRS code (Section 6103), the ITIN permits undocumented immigrants to access child tax credit subsidies while prohibiting the IRS to share taxpayer information with Immigration and Customs Enforcement (ICE), which is a clear example of a social citizenship provision that the federal government is already extending to undocumented immigrants that stands in stark contrast to the ACA's exclusionary language.

5. The annual costs of PVS care are difficult to estimate, and the published estimates are quite dated. The estimates cited are from an authoritative study on the prevalence and costs of PVS published in the *New England Journal of Medicine* in 1994 (Multi-Society Task Force on PVS, 1994) and adjusted for inflation to the year 2015.

6. These expenditure estimates are adjusted for inflation to the year 2015.

7. Gawande's case example is based on the 1985 essay of paleontologist and writer Stephan Jay Gould, who had extended his life, through surgery and experimental treatments, by some twenty years beyond his median abdominal mesothelioma survival prognosis of merely eight months.

8. While Rawls (2001) emphasized the public justification process as the means through which the basic structure of society is agreed upon (the general structure of government, the basic rights of citizenship) as opposed to the finer-grained social and political issues, this is a matter of priorities. The public justification process is meant to extend to the most divisive controversies of society in general (p. 28), within which we would include the substance of and limits to a social right to health care.

9. The just savings principle and its specific requirements, as with other principles of justice, are derived from the "original position" thought experiment, where principles of justice emerge from the deliberations among a group of equal citizens charged with the task of determining the agreed-upon conditions for a just society (as a fair system of cooperation between equals). They do so under "a veil of ignorance" as to both their own social characteristics (such as gender, social class, race, and age and related advantages and disadvantages therein) and the characteristics of their society (such as wealthy vs. poor, industrialized vs. agrarian economy, etc.) Because those charged with the task of determining the optimal accumulation and intergenerational transfer of assets between generations do not know the age or the generation to which they belong, generational bias is removed from the rules that guide the amount of just savings each generation is obligated to contribute as their fair share (Rawls, 1971, pp. 287–288). As stated by Rawls (1971, p. 289), "They try to piece together a just savings schedule by balancing how much at each stage they would be willing to save for their immediate descendants against what they would feel entitled to claim of their immediate predecessors."

10. A prime example of this "medicalization" of long-term care needs is an older adult who has repeat episodes of emergency department care for falls and injuries in a home environment that is ill-suited to her escalating needs for both social support and functional assistance in the basic activities of daily living.

11. The Community Living Assistance Services and Supports (CLASS) provisions of the ACA established a quasi-voluntary social insurance trust fund for long-term care, financed through the monthly premiums of adults who were automatically enrolled by their employers with a voluntary opt-out option. After concluding that an

insufficient number of healthy working-age adults would remain enrolled in the CLASS social insurance trust fund to make it affordable, in 2011 the Obama administration abandoned its effort to implement the long-term care insurance provisions of the ACA.

12. For readers familiar with the *Olmstead v. L.C.* (527 U.S. 581, 1999) decision of the U.S. Supreme Court that affirmed the right of individuals with disabilities to live in their communities and required states to provide support services for the severely disabled in community settings, it should be evident that these criteria for the threshold of "reasonable efforts" in meeting the social and health needs of the disabled are much higher than the "fundamental alteration" standard applied in the groundbreaking *Olmstead v. L.C.* decision. See Williams (2000) for a more complete discussion of the limits of "reasonable efforts" by states in meeting the community integration requirements of the ADA.

13. As previously discussed in chapter 2, Rawls's Difference Principle reads as follows: "Social and economic inequalities are to satisfy two conditions: first, they are to be attached to offices and positions open to all under conditions of fair equality of opportunity; and they are to be to the greatest benefit to the least advantaged of society" (Rawls, 2001, pp. 42–43). Here Rawls was speaking of inequalities of social status, income, and wealth that derive from special talents and abilities that in the end enhance the lives of the least advantaged of society (such as the high salaries and social status possessed by technology innovators that make the poor better off in the United States than most places in the world).

14. Executive Order 1375 has been reconfirmed by every successive U.S. president since Bill Clinton, and its continued reconfirmation is assumed to be a given for the presidencies of the foreseeable future.

15. As stated by Rawls (2001, p. 96), "The idea of society as a fair system of social cooperation is quite naturally specified so as to include the ideas of equality and of reciprocity." Note that Rawls pairs the idea of reciprocity on par with equality as fundamental to his theory of a just society.

16. Although the U.S. forces ceased their official combat role in 2014, the timetable for the withdrawal of all U.S. troops but those needed for embassy staffing and an unspecified "security component" has been extended by the Obama administration to 2016 (Office of the White House Press Secretary, 2014).

REFERENCES

Ackermann, R., & Carroll, A. (2003). Support for National Health Insurance among U.S. Physicians: A National Survey. *Annals of Internal Medicine, 139*(10), 795–801.

Agency for Healthcare Research and Quality (AHRQ). (2012a). *Medical Expenditure Panel Survey, 2012: Table 4.2: Percent of Persons Unable or Delayed in Receiving Needed Medical Care, United States, 2012.* Rockville, MD: Agency for Healthcare Research and Quality.

———. (2012b). *Medical Expenditure Panel Survey, 2012: Table 2.2: People Who Have a Usual Primary Care Provider a, by Family Income b, United States, 2012.* Rockville, MD: Agency for Healthcare Research and Quality.

———. (2013). *The Practice Facilitation Handbook: Module 7 Measuring and Benchmarking Clinical Performance.* Retrieved May 19, 2015, from http://www.ahrq.gov/professionals/prevention-chronic-care/improve/system/pfhandbook/mod7.html

———. (2014a). *2013 National Health Care Disparities Report.* Retrieved April 6, 2015, from http://www.ahrq.gov/research/findings/nhqrdr/nhdr13/2013nhdr.pdf.

———. (2014b). *2013 National Healthcare Quality Report.* Rockville, MD: Agency for Healthcare Research and Quality.

———. (2015). *Defining the PCMH.* Retrieved May 7, 2015, from http://pcmh.ahrq.gov/page/defining-pcmh.

Alba, R. (2006, July 28). *Looking Beyond the Moment: American Immigration Seen from Historically and Internationally Comparative Perspectives.* Retrieved July 27, 2015, from http://borderbattles.ssrc.org/Alba/.

Alker, J., Mancini, T., & Heberlein, M. (2012, October). *Uninsured Children 2009–2011: Charting the Nation's Progress.* Retrieved April 18, 2014, from http://ccf.georgetown.edu/wp-content/uploads/2012/10/Uninsured-Children-2009-2011.pdf.

Al-Khayat, M. (2004). *Health Care as a Human Right in Islam.* Cairo, Egypt: World Health Organization, Regional Office for the Eastern Mediterranean.

Almgren, G. (2007). *Health Care Politics, Policy and Services: A Social Justice Analysis.* New York: Springer.

——. (2013). *Health Care Politics, Policy and Services: A Social Justice Analysis.* New York: Springer.

Almgren, G., & Ferguson, M. (1999). The Urban Ecology of Hospital Failure. *Journal of Sociology and Social Welfare*, 26(4), 5–26.

Almgren, G., Kemp, S., & Eisinger, A. (2000). The Legacy of Hull House and the Children's Bureau in the American Mortality Transition. *Social Service Review*, 74(1), 1–19.

Altman, D., & Levitt, L. (2002). The Sad History of Health Care Cost Containment as Told in One Chart. *Health Affairs*, W2, 83.

American Indian Health and Family Services. (2010). *Health Reform for American Indians and Alaska Natives.* Retrieved June 17, 2014, from http://www.aihfs.org/pdf /IHS-ACA-Fact_Sheet.pdf.

American Medical Association (AMA). (2014). *H-165.888 Evaluating Health System Reform Proposals.* Retrieved August 11, 2014, from https://ssl3.ama-assn.org/apps /ecomm/PolicyFinderForm.pl?site=www.ama-assn.org&uri=%2fresources%2fhtm l%2fPolicyFinder%2fpolicyfiles%2fHnE%2fH-165.888.HTM.

American Medical Student Association. (2008). *AMSA Single-Payer 101.* Retrieved August 9, 2014, from http://www.amsa.org/AMSA/Libraries/Initiative_Docs/Single Payer101.sflb.ashx.

American Public Health Association (APHA). (2009, November 11). *Policy Statement Database: Public Health's Critical Role in Health Reform in the United States.* Retrieved May 15, 2013, from http://www.apha.org/advocacy/policy/policysearch/default.htm ?id=1386.

——. (2012, June 28). *APHA Press Release: Landmark Health Reform Law Ruling a Major Public Health Victory, Provisions Still Require Support.* Retrieved July 11, 2014, from http://www.apha.org/about/news/pressreleases/2012/scotus+ruling.htm.

Andersen, R. M. (1968). *Behavioral Model of Families' Use of Health Services.* Chicago: Center for Health Administration Studies, University of Chicago.

——. (1995). Revisiting the Behavioral Model and Access to Medical Care: Does It Matter? *Journal of Health and Social Behavior*, 36, 1–10.

Anderson, G., & Hussey, P. (2004). *Special Issues with Single-Payer Health Insurance Systems: HNP Discussion Paper.* Retrieved August 5, 2014, from http://siteresources .worldbank.org/HEALTHNUTRITIONANDPOPULATION/Resources/28162 7-1095698140167/AndersonSpecialIssuesFinal.pdf.

AP/YAHOO Poll. (2008). *The Associated Press Yahoo Poll Wave 2 Conducted by Knowledge Networks.* Retrieved August 7, 2014, from http://surveys.ap.org/data /KnowledgeNetworks/AP-Yahoo_2007-08_panel02.pdf.

Arend, J., Tsang-Quinn, J., Levine, C., & Thomas, D. (2012). The Patient-Centered Medical Home: History, Components, and Review of the Evidence. *Mt. Sinai Journal of Medicine*, 79(4), 433–450.

Asch, S., McGlynn, E., Hogan, M., Hayward, R., Shekelle, P., Rubenstein, L., et al. (2004). Comparison of Quality of Care for Patients in the Veterans Health Administration and Patients in a National Sample. *Annals of Internal Medicine*, 141(12), 938–945.

Assistant Secretary for Planning and Evaluation (ASPE). (2014, March 23). *Health Insurance Marketplace: March Enrollment Report: For the Period: October 1, 2013–March 1, 2014.* Retrieved April 24, 2014, from http://aspe.hhs.gov/health/reports/2014/market placeenrollment/mar2014/ib_2014mar_enrollment.pdf.

Atkinson, G. (2009). *State Hospital Rate-Setting Revisited*. Retrieved May 20, 2014, from http://www.hscrc.state.md.us/documents/AboutUs/InTheNews/AtkinsonState HospRatesetting.pdf.

Auerbach, D., & Kellerman, A. (2011). A Decade of Health Care Cost Growth Has Wiped Out Income Gains for an Average US Family. *Health Affairs, 30*(9), 1–7.

Australian Institute of Health and Welfare. (2013). *Health Expenditures Australia 2011–2012*. Canberra: Australian Institute of Health and Welfare.

Baer, D., & O'Brien, E. (2010). *Federal and State Income Tax Incentives for Long-Term Care Insurance*. Washington, D.C.: AARP Public Policy Institute.

Baker, B. (2009, December 10). *Ethicist Callahan: 'Set Limits' on Health Care*. Retrieved May 17, 2013, from http://www.kaiserhealthnews.org/Checking-In-With/Daniel -Callahan-Limits-On-Health-Care.aspx.

Barnado, A., Herndon, M., Anthony, D., Galllagher, P., Skinner, J., Bynum, J., et al. (2007). Are Regional Variations in End-of-Life Care Intensity Expained by Patient Preferences? *Medical Care, 45*(5), 386–393.

Barton, D. (2005). The Politics of Racial Disparities: Desegregating the Hospitals in Jackson, Mississippi. *Milbank Quarterly, 83*(2), 247–269.

Bassett, W. (2004). *Medicaid's Nursing Home Coverage and Asset Transfers*. Washington, D.C.: The Federal Reserve Board of Governors.

Bazzoli, G., Lee, W., Hsieh, H., & Mobley, L. (2012). The Effects of Safety Net Hospital Closures and Conversions on Patient Travel Distance to Hospital Services. *Health Services Research, 47*(1), 129–150.

Berenson, J., Doty, M., Abrams, M., & Shih, A. (2012, May). *Issue Brief: Achieving Better Quality of Care for Low-Income Populations: The Role of Health Insurance and the Medical Home for Reducing Health Inequities*. Retrieved June 17, 2014, from http://www.ncqa.org/portals/0/Public%20Policy/Berenson_achieving_better _quality_care_low_in come_8.30.12.pdf.

Berggren, R. (2005). Unexpected Necessities—Inside Charity Hospital. *New England Journal of Medicine, 353*, 1550–1553.

Bergman, M. (2014, April 1). *Obamacare Enrollment Hits Its Target, but Mission Accomplished?* Retrieved April 24, 2014, from http://www.neontommy.com/news /2014/04/obamacare-enrollment-hits-its-target-mission-accomplished.

Berkowitz, E. (2008). Medicare and Medicaid: The Past as Prologue. *Health Care Financing Review, 29*(3), 81–93.

Blalock, H. M. (1979). *Social Statistics*. New York: McGraw-Hill.

Blendon, R., & Benson, J. (2001). Americans' Views on Health Policy: A Fifty-Year Historical Perspective. *Health Affairs, 20*(2), 33–46.

Blendon, R., Benson, J., & Weldon, K. (2014). *Public Perceptions of the Massachusetts Health Insurance Law: Boston Globe/Harvard School of Public Health Public Opinion Survey*. Retrieved August 5, 2014, from http://c.oobg.com/rw/Boston/2011-2020/2014 /06/16/BostonGlobe.com/Business/Graphics/healthlaw.pdf?p1=Article_Related.

Blendon, R., Brodie, M., Altman, D., & Benson, J. H. (2005). Voters and Health Care in the 2004 Election. *Health Affairs, W5*, 86–96.

Blendon, R., Brodie, M., Benson, J., Altman, D., & Buhr, T. (2006). Americans' Views of Health Care Costs, Access, and Quality. *Milbank Quarterly, 84*(4), 623–657.

Blendon, R., Martilla, J., Benson, J., Shelter, M., Connolly, F., & Kiley, T. (1994). The Belief and Values Shaping America's Health Care Reform Debate. *Health Affairs, 13*(1), 274–284.

Blendon, R. M., Benson, J., Shelter, M., Connally, E., & Kiley, T. (1994). The Beliefs and Values Shaping Today's Health Care Reform Debate. *Health Affairs*, 13(1), 274–284.

Blumberg, L., Long, S., Keenney, G., & Goin, D. (2013). *Factors Influencing Health Plan Choice Among the Marketplace Target Population on the Eve of Health Reform*. Retrieved July 29, 2014, from http://hrms.urban.org/briefs/hrms_decision _factors.html.

Blumenthal, P. (2010, February 12). *The Legacy of Billy Tauzin: The White House-PhRMA Deal*. Retrieved April 22, 2014, from https://sunlightfoundation.com/blog /2010/02/12/the-legacy-of-billy-tauzin-the-white-house-phrma-deal/.

Board of Trustees Medicare Hospital Insurance Trust Fund. (2014). *2014 Annual Report of the Board of Trustees of the Federal Hospital Insurance Trust Fund*. Retrieved August 8, 2014, from http://www.cms.gov/Research-Statistics-Data-and-Systems /Statistics-Trends-and-Reports/ReportsTrustFunds/Downloads/TR2014.pdf.

Boaz, D. (1997). *Libertarianism: A Primer*. New York: Free Press.

Bonilla-Silva, E., & Dietrich, D. (2011). The Sweet Enchantment of Color-Blind Racism in Obamerica. *The Annals of the American Academy of Political and Social Science*, 634(1), 190–206.

Boroff, D., & Planas, R. (2012, January 24). Mitt Romney Says He Favors 'Self-Deportation' When Asked About Immigration During GOP Debate. *New York Daily News*. Retrieved July 27, 2015, from http://www.nydailynews.com/news/election-2012/mitt -romney-favors-self-deportation-asked-immigration-gop-debate-article-1.1010812.

Boyd, C. (2010). Medicare: It's Time to Talk About Changing It. *Annals of Health Law*, 19(1), 78–84.

Braithwaite, R., Meltzer, D., King, J., Leslie, D., & Roberts, M. (2008). What Does the Value of Modern Medicine Say About the $50,000 per Quality-Adjusted Life-Year Decision Rule? *Medical Care*, 46(4), 349–356.

Bristow, W. (2011, April 7). *Enlightenment*. Retrieved May 14, 2013, from http://plato .stanford.edu/archives/sum2011/entries/enlightenment.

Brookings Institution. (2014, June 14). *"Keeping the Promise: Site of Service Medicare Payment Reforms"; Testimony on Energy and Commerce, Subcommittee on Health Submitted by Barbara Gage, PhD*. Retrieved August 1, 2014, from http://www.brookings .edu/~/media/research/files/testimony/2014/05/gage%20pac%20testimony%20%20 additional%20questions%20for%20the%20record%20final.pdf.

Brown, L. (1992). Political Evolution of Federal Health Care Regulation. *Health Affairs*, 11(4), 17–37.

Bullock, H. (2006). *Justifying Inequality: A Social Psychological Analysis of Beliefs About Poverty and the Poor*. Retrieved July 28, 2014, from http://www.npc.umich.edu /publications/workingpaper06/paper08/working_paper06-08.pdf.

Buntin, J. (2009, August 23). Dialysis Death Panels and the Health Care Debate. *Washington Post*. Retrieved July 30, 2015, from http://www.washingtonpost.com /wp-dyn/content/article/2009/08/21/AR2009082101776.html.

Burtless, G., & Milusheva, S. (2013). Effects of Employer-Sponsored Health Insurance Costs on Social Security Taxable Wages. *Social Security Bulletin*, 73(1), Chart 1.

Calavita, K. (2005). Law, Citizenship, and the Construction of (Some) Immigrant "Others." *Law and Social Inquiry*, 30(2), 401–420.

Callahan, D. (1987). *Setting Limits: Medical Goals in an Aging Society*. New York: Simon and Schuster.

Callahan, D., & Bradley, E. H. (2012). *Global Competitiveness: How Other Countries Win*. Garrison, NY: The Hastings Center.

Calvin, J., Roe, M., Chen, A., Mehta, R. H., Brogan, G. X. Jr., Delong, E. R., et al. (2006). Insurance Coverage and Care of Patients with Non-ST Segment Elevation Acute Coronary Syndrome. *Annals of Internal Medicine, 145*(10), 739–748.

Carrier, E., Dowling, M., & Berenson, R. (2012). Hospitals' Geographic Expansion in Quest of Well-Insured Patients: Will The Outcome Be Better Care, More Cost, or Both? *Health Affairs, 31*(4), 827–835.

Carrier, E., Yee, T., & Stark, L. (2011). *Matching Supply to Demand: Addressing the U.S. Primary Care Workforce Shortage: NIHCR Policy Analysis No. 7*. Retrieved May 21, 2015, from http://www.nihcr.org/PCP_Workforce.html.

Carroll, A., & Ackerman, R. (2008). Support for National Health Insurance Among Physicians 5 Years Later. *Annals of Internal Medicine, 148*(7), 565–566.

Casalino, L., Gillies, R., Shortell, S., Schmittdiel, J., Bodenheimer, T., Robinson, J., et al. (2003). External Incentives, Information Technology, and Organized Processes to Improve Health Care Quality for Patients with Chronic Diseases. *JAMA, 289*(4), 434–441.

Cassidy, A. (2012, September 14). Policy Brief: Patient Centered Medical Homes. *Health Affairs*, pp. 1–6.

CBS/*New York Times* Poll. (2009, February 1). *CBS/New York Times Poll*. Retrieved May 28, 2015, from http://www.cbsnews.com/htdocs/pdf/SunMo_poll_0209.pdf.

Center for Healthcare Research and Transformation (CHRT). (2012, September 17). *Affordable Care Act Funding: An Analysis of Grant Programs Under Health Care Reform*. Retrieved July 14, 2014, from http://www.chrt.org/publications/price-of-care/affordable-care-act-funding-an-analysis-of-grant-programs-under-health-care-reform/.

Center for Responsive Politics. (2014). *Industry Profile: 2013: Annual Lobbying on Insurance*. Retrieved July 29, 2014, from http://www.opensecrets.org/lobby/indusclient.php?id=f09&year=2013.

Centers for Disease Control and Prevention (CDC). (2000). *Public Health's Infrastructure: A Status Report: Report Prepared for the Appropriations Committee of the United States Senate*. Atlanta: U.S. Department of Health and Human Services, Centers for Disease Control.

——. (2010). *Establishing a Holistic Framework to Reduce Inequities in HIV, Viral Hepatitis, STDs, and Tuberculosis in the United States*. Atlanta: U.S. Department of Health and Human Services, Centers for Disease Control and Prevention.

——. (2013a). State-Specific Healthy Life Expectancy at Age 65 Years—United States, 2007–2009. Atlanta: CDC.

——. (2013b, August 20). *Epidemiology and Laboratory Capacity for Infectious Diseases*. Retrieved July 11, 2014, from http://www.cdc.gov/ncezid/dpei/epidemiology-laboratory-capacity.html.

Centers for Medicare and Medicaid Services (CMS). (2009). *2009 Annual Report of the Trustees of the Federal Hospital Insurance and Federal Supplementary Medical Insurance Funds*. Retrieved October 25, 2013, from https://www.cms.gov/Research-Statistics-Data-and-Systems/Statistics-Trends-and-Reports/ReportsTrustFunds/downloads/tr2009.pdf.

——. (2010). *Estimated Financial Effects of the "Patient Protection and Affordable Care Act," as Passed by the Senate on December 24, 2009*. Washington, D.C.: Office of Chief Actuary, Centers for Medicare and Medicaid Services.

——. (2014a). *Children's Health Insurance Program (CHIP)*. Retrieved May 15, 2014, from http://www.medicaid.gov/Medicaid-CHIP-Program-Information/By-Topics /Childrens-Health-Insurance-Program-CHIP/Childrens-Health-Insurance -Program-CHIP.html.

——. (2014b). *National Health Expenditure Data: Historical NHE, 2013*. Retrieved July 9, 2015, from http://www.cms.gov/Research-Statistics-Data-and-Systems/Statistics -Trends-and-Reports/NationalHealthExpendData/NHE-Fact-Sheet.html.

——. (2014c). *National Health Expenditures; Aggregate and Per Capita Amounts, Annual Percent Change and Percent Distribution: Selected Calendar Years 1960–2012*. Retrieved July 29, 2014, from http://www.cms.gov/Research-Statistics-Data-and -Systems/Statistics-Trends-and-Reports/NationalHealthExpendData/Downloads/ tables.pdf.

——. (2014d). *National Health Expenditure Projections: 2013–2023*. Retrieved July 29, 2015, from http://www.cms.gov/Research-Statistics-Data-and-Systems/Statistics -Trends-and-Reports/NationalHealthExpendData/Downloads/Proj2013.pdf.

——. (2014e). *2014 Annual Report of the Boards of Trustees of the Federal Hospital Insurance and Federal Supplementary Medical Insurance Trust Funds*. Retrieved August 4, 2015, from https://www.cms.gov/Research-Statistics-Data-and-Systems /Statistics-Trends-and-Reports/ReportsTrustFunds/Downloads/TR2014.pdf.

Christianson, J., Leatherman, S., & Sutherland, K. (2009). *Financial Incentives, Healthcare Providers and Quality Improvements: A Review of the Evidence*. London: The Health Foundation.

Chung, A., Gaynor, M., & Richards-Subik, S. (2012, December). *Subsidies and Structure: The Lasting Impact of the Hill-Burton Program on the Hospital Industry*. Retrieved April 5, 2014, from http://igpa.uillinois.edu/system/files/HBCrowdOutpaper _AEAs.pdf

Clark, L. J., Field, M. J., Koontz, T. L., & Koontz, V. L. (1980). The Impact of Hill-Burton: An Analysis of Hospital Bed and Physician Distribution in the United States: 1950– 1970. *Medical Care, 18*(5), 532–550.

Cockburn, A. (2004, September 6). *How Many Democrats Voted for Taft-Hartley?* Retrieved March 18, 2014, from http://www.counterpunch.org/2004/09/06/how-many -democrats-voted-for-taft-hartley/.

Coffey, D. (1998). *African Americans During the Vietnam War*. Retrieved August 11, 2015, from http://www.english.illinois.edu/maps/poets/s_z/stevens/africanamer .htm.

The Commonwealth Fund Commission on a High Performance Health System. (2009). *The Path to a High Performance U.S. Health System: A 2020 Vision and the Policies to Pave the Way*. New York: The Commonwealth Fund.

Congressional Budget Office (CBO). (1994). *The Tax Treatment of Employment-Based Health Insurance*. Retrieved March 15, 2016, from https://www.cbo.gov/sites/default /files/103rd-congress-1993-1994/reports/1994_03_taxtreatmentofinsurance.pdf.

——. (2010). *Potential Costs of Veterans' Healthcare*. Retrieved January 26, 2012, from https://www.cbo.gov/sites/default/files/111th-congress-2009-2010/reports/2010_10 _7_vahealthcare.pdf.

——. (2013). *Rising Demands for Long-Term Care Services and Supports for Older Adults*. Washington, D.C.: Congressional Budget Office.

——. (2014). *Updated Estimates of the Effects of the Affordable Care Act Coverage Provisions, April 2014*. Retrieved April 24, 2014, from https://www.cbo.gov/publication /45231.

295

REFERENCES

Congressional Research Service (CRS). (2010, March 30). *Indian Health Care Improvement Act Provisions in the Patient Protection and Affordable Care Act (P.L. 111–148)*. Retrieved July 14, 2014, from http://www.ncsl.org/documents/health/IndHlthCare.pdf.

——. (2011, December 16). *Discretionary Funding in the Patient Protection and Affordable Care Act*. Retrieved July 14, 2014, from http://www.ncsl.org/documents/health/DisFundingACA.pdf.

——. (2013, March 13). *Appropriations and Fund Transfers in the Patient Protection and Affordable Care Act (ACA)*. Retrieved July 14, 2014, from http://fas.org/sgp/crs/misc/R41301.pdf.

A Conversation with Uwe E. Reinhardt, PhD: Health Care Deserves More Respect. (2013, November). *Managed Care*. Retrieved July 21, 2014, from http://www.managedcaremag.com/archives/2013/11/conversation-uwe-e-reinhardt-phd-health-care-deserves-more-respect.

Corak, M. (2013). Income Inequality, Equality of Opportunity, and Intergenerational Mobility. *Journal of Economic Perspectives, 27*(3), 79–102.

Corbie-Smith, G., Flagg, E., Doyle, J., & O'Brien, M. (2002). Influence of Usual Source of Care on Differences by Race/Ethnicity in Receipt of Preventive Services. *Journal of General Internal Medicine, 17*(6), 458–464.

Council of Accountable Physician Practices. (2011). *What Is the Difference Between a Medical Home and an ACO*. Retrieved May 6, 2015, from http://www.accountablecarefacts.org/topten/what-is-the-difference-between-a-medical-home-and-an-aco-1.

Crimmins, E., Saito, Y., & Ingegneri, D. (1989). Changes in Life Expectancy and Disability-Free Life Expectancy in the United States. *Population and Development Review, 15*(2), 235–267.

Cromartie, J. (2013). *How Is Rural America Changing?* Washington, D.C.: Economic Research Service, United States Department of Agriculture.

Cubanski, J., Swoope, C., Damico, A., & Neuman, T. (2014). *How Much Is Enough, Medicare Spending Among Beneficiaries: A Chartbook*. Retrieved May 26, 2015, from http://files.kff.org/attachment/how-much-is-enough-out-of-pocket-spending-among-medicare-beneficiaries-a-chartbook-report.

Cunningham, P. (2011). *State Variation in Primary Care Supply: Implications for Health Reform Medicaid Expansions*. Retrieved January 28, 2015, from http://www.rwjf.org/content/dam/farm/reports/issue_briefs/2011/rwjf69759.

Currie, J. (2004). *The Take-Up of Social Benefits: IZA Discussion Paper No. 1103*. Retrieved June 3, 2015, from http://ftp.iza.org/dp1103.pdf.

Cutler, D., & Gruber, J. (2001, June). *Health Policy in the Clinton Era: Once Bitten, Twice Shy*. Retrieved May 13, 2014, from http://www.hks.harvard.edu/m-rcbg/Conferences/economic_policy/CUTLER-GRUBER.pdf.

Cutler, D., & Morton, F. (2013). Hospitals, Market Share, and Consolidation. *JAMA, 310*(18), 1964–1970.

Cylus, J., & Smith, P. (2013). Comparative Measures of Health System Efficiency. In I. Papanicolas & P. Smith (Eds.), *Health System Performance Comparison* (pp. 281–312). Berkshire, UK: Open University Press.

Daniels, N. (2008). *Just Health: Meeting Health Needs Fairly*. New York: Cambridge University Press.

Dartmouth Institute for Health Policy and Clinical Practice. (2012). *Total Medicare Reimbursements per Enrollee, by Adjustment Type*. Retrieved April 6, 2015, from http://www.dartmouthatlas.org/data/table.aspx?ind=225&ch=191&loc.

Dash, P., & Meredith, D. (2010). *When and How Provider Competition Can Improve Health Care Delivery.* Retrieved July 12, 2016, from http://www.mckinsey.com /industries/healthcare-systems-and-services/our-insights/when-and-how-provider -competition-can-improve-health-care-delivery.

Davis, K., & Stremikis, K. (2009, December 21). *The Costs of Failure: Economic Consequences of Failure to Enact Nixon, Carter, and Clinton Health Reforms.* Retrieved May 20, 2014, from http://www.commonwealthfund.org/publications/blog/the-costs -of-failure.

Davis, K., Schoen, C., & Squires, D. (2014). *Mirror, Mirror on the Wall, 2014 Update: How the U.S. Health Care System Compares Internationally.* New York: The Commonwealth Fund.

Decker, S. (2013). Two-Thirds of Primary Care Physicians Accepted New Medicaid Patients in 2011–12: A Baseline to Measure Future Acceptance Rates. *Health Affairs, 32*(7), 1183–1187.

Dehlendorf, C., Bryant, C., Huddleston, H., Jacoby, V., & Fujimoto, V. (2011). Health Disparities: Definitions and Measurements. *American Journal of Obstetrics and Gynecology, 202*(3), 212–213.

DeNavas-Walt, C., & Proctor, B. (2014). *Income and Poverty in the United States: 2013.* Washington, D.C.: U.S. Census Bureau, U.S. Government Printing Office.

DeNavas-Walt, C., Proctor, B., & Smith, J. (2013). *Income, Poverty, and Health Insurance in the United States, 2012.* Washington, D.C.: U.S. Census Bureau.

Dharmananda, S. (2004). *Unani Medicine, with Reference to Hamdard of Pakistan and India.* Retrieved May 16, 2013, from http://www.itmonline.org/arts/unani.htm.

Dilandardo, J. (2011). Workforce Issues Related to Physical and Behavioral Healthcare Integration: Specifically Substance Abuse Disorders and Primary Care: A Framework. In *Workforce Issues: Integrating Substance Use Services into Primary Care* (pp. 1–39). Washington, D.C.: Substance Abuse and Mental Health Services Administration.

Dimick, J., Sarrazin, M., & Berkmeyer, J. (2013). Black Patients More Likely Than Whites to Undergo Surgery at Low-Quality Hospitals in Segregated Regions. *Health Affairs, 32*(6), 1046–1053.

Donis, J., & Kraftner, B. (2011). The Prevalence of Patients in a Vegetative State and Minimally Conscious State in Austria. *Brian Injury, 25*(11), 1101–1107.

Doty, M., Collins, S., Rustgi, S., & Kriss, J. (2008, August). *Issue Brief: Seeing Red: The Growing Burden of Medical Bills and Debt Faced by U.S. Families.* Retrieved April 22, 2014, from http://www.commonwealthfund.org/usr_doc/doty_seeingred _1164_ib.pdf?section=4039.

Dranove, D., & Millenson, M. (2006). Medical Bankruptcy: Myth Versus Fact. *Health Affairs, 25*(2), w74–w83.

Edwords, F. (2008). *What Is Humanism?* Retrieved May 13, 2013, from http://www .americanhumanist.org/humanism/What_is_Humanism.

Epstein, R. (2015, April 8). Jeb Bush Calls for Privatizing Elements of Veterans Health Care. *Wall Street Journal.* Retrieved August 13, 2015, from http://blogs.wsj.com /washwire/2015/04/08/jeb-bush-calls-for-privatizing-veterans-health-care/.

Esping-Andersen, G. (1990). *The Three Worlds of Welfare Capitalism.* Cambridge, UK: Polity Press.

Etzioni, A. (1991). Health Care Rationing: A Critical Evaluation. *Health Affairs, 10*(2), 88–95.

297

REFERENCES

Evans, R. (1990). Tensions, Compression and Shear: Directions, Stressors and Out-
comes in Health Care Cost Control. *Journal of Health Care Politics, Policy and Law*,
15(1), 105–128.
Experian Simmons. (2011). *The 2011 Discretionary Spending Report*. New York: Experian
Information Solutions, Inc.
Fisher, E., Goodman, D., Skinner, J., & Bronner, K. (2009). *Health Care Spending,
Quality and Outcomes: More Is Not Always Better*. Retrieved April 6, 2015, from
http://www.dartmouthatlas.org/downloads/reports/Spending_Brief_022709
.pdf.
Fleming, J. (1971). Letter to the Editor in Response to Berstein B, AJPH 60:1690–1700,
Sept., 1970. *American Journal of Public Health*, 61(1), 5–6.
Foley, M. (2008). *A Mixed Public-Private System for 2020: A Paper Commissioned by Aus-
tralian Health and Hospitals Reform Commission*. Retrieved April 28, 2015, from
http://www.health.gov.au/internet/nhhrc/publishing.nsf/Content/16F7A93
D8F578DB4CA2574D 7001830E9/$File/A%20Mixed%20Public-Private%20System%20
for%202020%20%28M%20Foley%29.pdf.
Freburger, J., Holmes, G., Ku, L., Cutchin, M., Heatwole-Shank, K., & Edwards, L.
(2011). Disparities in Postacute Rehabilitation Care for Stroke: An Analysis of the
State Inpatient Databases. *Archives of Physical Medicine and Rehabilitation*, 92(8),
1220–1229.
Freedman, S., Lin, H., & Simon, K. (2014, May). *Public Health Insurance Expansions
and Hospital Technology Adoption*. Retrieved June 17, 2014, from http://www.nber
.org/papers/w20159.
Friedman, G. (2013). *Funding HR 676: The Expanded and Improved Medicare for All Act*.
Retrieved August 5, 2014, from http://www.pnhp.org/sites/default/files/Funding%20
HR%20676_Friedman_7.31.13.pdf.
Fronstin, P., Salisbury, D., & VanDerhei, J. (2012, October). Savings Needed for Health
Expenses for People Eligible for Medicare: Some Rare Good News. *Employee Ben-
efit Research Institute Notes*, 33(10), 2–7.
Fuchs, V. (1986). *The Health Economy*. Cambridge, MA: Harvard University Press.
Fuchs, V., & Emmanuel, E. (2005). Health Care Reform: Why? What? When? *Health
Affairs*, 24(6), 1399–1414.
Gabel, J., & Ermann, D. (1985). Preferred Provider Organizations: Performance, Prob-
lems and Promises. *Health Affairs*, 4(1), 24–40.
Galewitz, P. (2011, October 21). *Nixon's HMOs Hold Lessons for Obama's ACOs*. Re-
trieved May 20, 2014, from http://capsules.kaiserhealthnews.org/index.php/2011
/10/nixons-hmos-hold-lessons-for-obamas-acos/.
Gallagher, T. (2013, May 2). California's Disappearing Health Care Reform. *Salon*.
Gallup Poll. (2014). *Health Care System*. Retrieved August 8, 2014, from http://www
.gallup.com/poll/4708/healthcare-system.aspx#1.
Galvin, R., & McGlynn, E. (2003). Using Performance Measurement to Drive Improve-
ment. *Medical Care*, 41(1, Suppl), I-48–I-60.
Garfinkel, I., Rainwater, L., & Smeeding, T. (2010). *Wealth and Welfare States: Is Amer-
ica a Laggard or a Leader?* New York: Oxford University Press.
Garrison, L., & Wilensky, G. (1986). Cost Containment and Incentives for Technology.
Health Affairs, 5(2), 46–58.
Gawande, A. (2014). *Being Mortal: Medicine and What Matters at the End*. New York:
Henry Holt.

GBA Strategies. (2015). *Progressive Change Institute Poll of Likely 2016 Voters*. Retrieved May 26, 2015, from https://s3.amazonaws.com/s3.boldprogressives.org/images/Big _Ideas-Polling_PDF-1.pdf.

Giddens, A. (2009). *Sociology*. Cambridge, UK: Polity Press.

Gilens, M. (2000). *Why Americans Hate Welfare: Race, Media, and Antipoverty Policy*. Chicago: University of Chicago Press.

Glied, S. (2009). Single Payer as a Financing Mechanism. *Journal of Health Politics, Policy and Law*, 34(4), 593–615.

Goldsteen, R., Goldsteen, K., Swan, J., & Clemena, W. (2001). Harry and Louise and Health Care Reform: Romancing Public Opinion. *Journal of Health Policy, Politics and Law*, 26(6), 1235–1352.

Goodman, D. C., Brownlee, S., Chiang-Hua, C., & Fisher, E. S. (2010). *Regional Variation in Primary Care and the Quality of Care Among Medicare Beneficiaries*. Retrieved March 31, 2015, from http://www.dartmouthatlas.org/downloads/reports /Primary_care_report_090910.pdf.

Gould, E. (2012, February 23). *A Decade of Declines in Employer-Sponsored Health Insurance Coverage*. Washington, D.C.: Economic Policy Institute.

Government Accountability Office (GAO). (2009, March 12). *Testimony Before the Subcommittee on Military Construction, Veterans Affairs, and Related Agencies, Committee on Appropriations, House of Representatives: VA Health Care: Challenges in Budget Formulation and Execution*. Retrieved April 13, 2015, from http://www.gao .gov/assets/130/121858.pdf.

——. (2011, June 30). *Medicaid and CHIP: Most Physicians Serve Covered Children but Have Difficulty Referring Them for Specialty Care*. Retrieved June 17, 2014, from http://www.gao.gov/products/GAO-11-624.

Gray, G. (2013). *Health Policy in Australia*. Retrieved November 18, 2013, from http:// apo.org.au/commentary/health-policy-australia.

Gruber, J. (2009, Winter). The Case for a Two-Tiered Health System. *Pathways*, pp. 10–13.

——. (2011). *The Impacts of the Affordable Care Act: How Reasonable are the Projections*. Working Paper Series (National Bureau of Economic Research), Working Paper No. 17168. Retrieved August 5, 2014, from http://www.nber.org/papers/w17168.

Hanson, G. H. (2007). *The Economic Logic of Illegal Immigration*. New York: Council on Foreign Relations.

Harris, J. (2010). *Citizenship in Britain and Europe: Some Missing Links in T. H. Marshall's Theory of Rights*. Retrieved May 24, 2013, from http://hdl.net/10419/43703.

Harrop, F. (2014, January 14). Single-Payer Is Not Dead. *RealClearPolitics*. Retrieved May 28, 2014, from http://www.realclearpolitics.com/articles/2014/01/14/single-payer _is_not_dead_121220.html.

Harvard School of Public Health. (2012, August 15). *Mexico Achieves Universal Health Coverage, Enrolls 52.6 Million People in Less Than a Decade*. Retrieved July 24, 2014, from http://www.hsph.harvard.edu/news/features/mexico-universal-health/.

Hatt, L., Thorton, R., Magnoni, B., & Islam, M. (2009). *Extending Social Insurance to Informal Sector Workers in Nicaragua via Microfinance Institutions: Results from a Randomized Evaluation*. Bethesda, MD: Private Sector Partnerships Abt Associates Inc.

Health Resources and Services Administration (HRSA). (1995). *Medically Underserved Areas/Populations: Guidelines for MUA and MUP Designation*. Retrieved June 16, 2015, from http://www.hrsa.gov/shortage/mua/.

———. (2013). *The Affordable Care Act and Health Centers*. Retrieved July 11, 2014, from http://bphc.hrsa.gov/about/healthcenterfactsheet.pdf.

———. (2015). *Shortage Designation: Health Professional Shortage Areas & Medically Underserved Areas/Populations*. Retrieved February 9, 2015, from http://www.hrsa.gov/shortage/.

HealthyPeople 2020. (2015). *Access to Health Services*. Retrieved June 16, 2015, from http://www.healthypeople.gov/2020/topics-objectives/topic/Access-to-Health-Services.

Helms, R. (2008). *Tax Policy and the History of the Health Insurance Industry*. Retrieved April 6, 2014, from http://www.taxpolicycenter.org/tpccontent/healthconference_helms.pdf.

Hendrickson, L., & Reinhart, S. (2010). *Global Budgeting: Promoting Flexible Funding to Support Long-Term Care Choices*. Retrieved April 12, 2015, from http://www.cshp.rutgers.edu/Downloads/4710.pdf.

Henry Kaiser Family Foundation. (2012). *Health Insurance Coverage of the Nonelderly Population, 2011*. Retrieved April 18, 2014, from http://kff.org/slideshow/health-insurance-coverage-in-america-2011/.

———. (2014a). *Kaiser Health Tracking Poll: March 2014*. Retrieved April 29, 2014, from http://kff.org/health-reform/poll-finding/kaiser-health-tracking-poll-march-2014/.

———. (2014b, May 1). *Medicare Advantage Fact Sheet*. Retrieved May 21, 2014, from http://kff.org/medicare/fact-sheet/medicare-advantage-fact-sheet/.

———. (2014c). *Health Reform Implementation Timeline*. Retrieved April 23, 2014, from http://kff.org/interactive/implementation-timeline/.

———. (2014d, April). *The Coverage Gap: Uninsured Poor Adults in States That Do Not Expand Medicaid*. Retrieved April 23, 2014, from http://kff.org/health-reform/issue-brief/the-coverage-gap-uninsured-poor-adults-in-states-that-do-not-expand-medicaid/.

———. (2014e). *State Decisions for Creating Health Insurance Marketplaces, 2014*. Retrieved April 24, 2014, from http://kff.org/health-reform/state-indicator/health-insurance-exchanges/.

Hernandez, S. (2000). Horizontal and Vertical Healthcare Integration: Lessons Learned from the United States. *HealthcarePapers, 1*(2), 59–65.

Hernandez-Quevedo, C., & Papanicolas I. (2013). Conceptualizing and Comparing Equity Across Nations. In I. Papanicolas & P. Smith (Eds.), *Health System Performance Comparison* (pp. 183–222). Berkshire, UK: Open University Press.

Hessler, K., & Buchanan, A. (2002). Specifying the Content of the Human Right to Health Care. In R. Rhodes, M. Battin, & A. Silver (Eds.), *Medicine and Social Justice*. New York: Oxford University Press.

Hill, I., Courtot, B., & Sullivan, J. (2005, May). *Ebbing and Flowing: Some Gains, Some Losses as SCHIP Responds to State Budget Pressure*. Retrieved April 18, 2014, from http://www.urban.org/uploadedpdf/311166_a-68.pdf.

The Hill-Burton Act, 1946–1980: Asynchrony in the Delivery of Health Care to the Poor. (1979). *Maryland Law Review, 39*(2), 316–375.

Hirschman, C. (2005). Immigration and the American Century. *Demography, 42*(4), 595–620.

Hirth, R., Chernew, M., Miller, E., Fendrick, M., & Weissert, W. (2000). Willingness to Pay for a Quality-Adjusted Life Year: In Search of a Standard. *Medical Decision Making, 20*(3), 332–342.

Hochban, J., Ellenbogan, B., Benson, J., & Olson, R. M. (1981). The Hill-Burton Program and Changes in Health Delivery. *Inquiry*, *18*(1), 61–69.

Horwitz, J. (2005). Making Profits and Providing Care: Comparing Nonprofit, For-Profit, and Government Hospitals. *Health Affairs*, *24*(3), 790–801.

Howard, G., Peace, F., & Howard, V. (2014). The Contributions of Selected Diseases in Disparities in Death Rates and Years of Life Lost for Racial and Ethnic Minorities in the United States, 1999–2010. *Preventing Chronic Disease*, *11*, 1–18.

Hsiao, W. C. (2011). State-Based Single-Payer Health Care—A Solution for the United States? *New England Journal of Medicine*, *364*, 1188–1190.

Hurley, J., & Guindon, E. (2008). *CHEPA Working Paper Series 08-04: Private Health Insurance in Canada*. Retrieved August 14, 2014, from http://chepa.org/docs/working-papers/chepa-wp-08-04-.pdf.

Hussey, P., & Anderson, G. (2003). A Comparison of Single- and Multi-Payer Health Insurance Systems and Options for Reform. *Journal of Health Politics, Policy and Law*, *66*(3), 215–228.

IBISWorld. (2015). *Nursing Care Facilities in the US: Market Research Report*. Retrieved May 22, 2015, from http://www.ibisworld.com/industry/default.aspx?indid=1594.

Ilo, I., Beltran-Sanchez, H., & Macinko, J. (2014). The Contribution of Health Care and Other Interventions to Black-White Disparities in Life Expectancy, 1980–2007. *Population Research and Policy Review*, *33*(1) 97–126.

Indian Health Service (IHS). (2015, January). *Fact Sheet: Indian Health Disparities*. Retrieved August 11, 2015, from http://www.ihs.gov/newsroom/includes/themes/newihstheme/display_objects/documents/factsheets/Disparities.pdf.

Institute of Medicine. (2000). *America's Health Care Safety Net: Intact but Endangered*. Washington, D.C.: National Academy of Sciences.

——. (2001). *Crossing the Quality Chasm: A New Health System for the 21st Century*. Washington, D.C.: National Academies Press.

——. (2002). *Unequal Treatment: Confronting Racial and Ethnic Disparities in Health Care*. Washington, D.C.: National Academies Press.

——. (2015). *Dying in America: Improving Quality and Honoring Individual Preferences Near the End of Life*. Washington, D.C.: National Academies Press.

Irvine, B., Ferguson, S., & Cackett, B. (2005). *Background Briefing: The Canadian Health Care System*. Retrieved November 18, 2013, from http://www.civitas.org.uk/pdf/Canada.pdf.

Jaffe, E. (2005). *Clinton Health Care Reform: The Squandering of Public Support*. Retrieved April 10, 2014, from http://cas.illinoisstate.edu/pol/downloads/icsps_papers/2006/Jaffe2005.pdf.

Jansson, B. S. (1988). *The Reluctant Welfare State*. Belmont, CA: Wadsworth.

Kaiser Commission on Medicaid and the Uninsured. (2013a, November). *How Do Medicaid Disproportionate Share Hospital (DSH) Payments Change Under the ACA?* Retrieved June 17, 2014, from http://kaiserfamilyfoundation.files.wordpress.com/2013/11/8513-how-do-medicaid-dsh-payments-change-under-the-aca.pdf.

——. (2013b, August). *What Is Medicaid's Impact on Access to Care, Health Outcomes and Quality of Care: Setting the Record Straight on the Evidence*. Retrieved June 17, 2014, from https://kaiserfamilyfoundation.files.wordpress.com/2013/08/8467-what-is-medicaids-impact-on-access-to-care1.pdf.

Kaiser Family Foundation. (2014, April 24). *A Closer Look at the Impact of State Decisions Not to Expand Medicaid on Coverage for Uninsured Adults*. Retrieved June 17,

2014, from http://kff.org/medicaid/fact-sheet/a-closer-look-at-the-impact-of-state-decisions-not-to-expand-medicaid-on-coverage-for-uninsured-adults/.

———. (2015). *Status of State Action on the Medicaid Expansion Decision*. Retrieved April 3, 2015, from http://kff.org/health-reform/state-indicator/state-activity-around-expanding-medicaid-under-the-affordable-care-act/#note-3.

Kaiser Family Foundation Health Tracking Poll. (2014). *Kaiser Family Foundation Tracking Poll: March 2014*. Retrieved August 7, 2014, from http://kff.org/health-reform/poll-finding/kaiser-health-tracking-poll-march-2014/.

Kaiser Family Foundation State Health Facts. (2013). *Hospital Beds per 1,000 Population by Ownership Type*. Retrieved April 3, 2015, from http://kff.org/other/state-indicator/beds-by-ownership/.

Kaiser Health Tracking Poll. (2009, September). *Kaiser Health Tracking Poll: Public Opinion on Health Care Issues*. Retrieved August 8, 2014, from http://kaiserfamily foundation.files.wordpress.com/2013/01/7990.pdf.

Kane, R., Kane, R., & Ladd, R. (1998). *The Heart of Long-Term Care*. New York: Oxford University Press.

Karanikolos, M., Khoshaba, E., Nolte, E., & McKee, M. (2013). Comparing Population Health. In I. Papanicolas & P. Smith (Eds.), *Health System Performance Comparison* (pp. 127–156). Berkshire, UK: Open University Press.

Kenney, G., & Pelletier, J. (2009). *Setting Income Thresholds in Medicaid/SCHIP: Which Children Should Be Eligible?* Retrieved May 15, 2014, from http://www.urban.org/UploadedPDF/411817_setting_income_thresholds.pdf.

Klein, E. (2014, January 16). Is the U.S. Too Corrupt for Single-Payer Health Care? *Washington Post*. Retrieved July 22, 2014, from http://www.washingtonpost.com/blogs/wonkblog/wp/2014/01/16/is-the-u-s-too-corrupt-for-single-payer-health-care/.

Klein, J. (2003). *For All These Rights: Business, Labor, and the Shaping of America's Public-Private Welfare State*. Princeton, NJ: Princeton University Press.

———. (2005). *For All These Rights: Business, Labor, and the Shaping of America's Private Welfare State*. Princeton, NJ: Princeton University Press.

Kotz, N. (2005). *Judgment Days: Lyndon Baines Johnson, Martin Luther King Junior, and the Laws That Changed America*. New York: Houghton Mifflin.

Krieger, N. (2002). A Glossary for Social Epidemiology. *Epidemiology Bulletin*, 23(1) 7–11.

———. (2005). Embodiment: A Conceptual Glossary for Epidemiology. *Journal of Epidemiology and Community Health*, 59(5), 350–355.

Krogstad, J., & Passel, J. (2015). *5 Facts About Illegal Immigration in the U.S.* Washington, D.C.: Pew Research Center.

Kunitz, S. (1996). The History and Politics of US Health Care Policy for American Indians and Alaska Natives. *American Journal of Public Health*, 86(10), 1464–1473.

Landefeld, J., Moulton, B., Platt, J., & Villones, S. (2010). *Survey of Current Business: GDP and Beyond: Measuring Economic Progress and Sustainability*. Washington, D.C.: Bureau of Economic Analysis, U.S. Department of Commerce.

Lawlor, E. (2003). *Redesigning the Medicare Contract: Politics, Markets, and Agency*. Chicago: University of Chicago Press.

Levitt, L., Gary, C., & Damico, A. (2013, December 17). *The Numbers Behind "Young Invincibles" and the Affordable Care Act*. Retrieved April 24, 2014, from http://kff.org/health-reform/perspective/the-numbers-behind-young-invincibles-and-the-affordable-care-act/.

Lieberman, R. (2001). *Shifting the Color Line: Race and the American Welfare State.* Cambridge, MA: Harvard University Press.

Lieberman, S., & Bertko, J. (2011). Building Regulatory and Operational Flexibility into Accountable Care Organizations and "Shared Savings." *Health Affairs, 30*(1), 23–31.

Link, B., & Phelan, J. (1995). Social Conditions as Fundamental Causes of Disease. *Journal of Health and Social Behavior* (special issue), 80–94.

———. (1996). Understanding Sociodemographic Differences in Health—The Role of Fundamental Causes. *American Journal of Public Health, 86*(4), 471–473.

Long, S., & Marquis, M. (1994, July). *Toward a Global Budget for the U.S. Health System: Implementation Issues and Information Needs.* Retrieved April 13, 2015, from http://www.rand.org/pubs/issue_papers/IP143/index2.html.

Lutz, A. (2008). Who Joins the Military? A Look at Race, Class and Immigration Status. *Journal of Political and Military Sociology, 36*(2), 167–188.

Madison, J. (1788a). The Alleged Danger From the Powers of the Union to the State Governments Considered. *The Federalist Paper No. 45.* Retrieved April 24, 2015, from http://www.constitution.org/fed/federa45.htm.

———. (1788b). The Conformity of the Plan to Republican Principles. *The Federalist Papers No. 39.* Retrieved July 12, 2016, from http://www.constitution.org/fed/federa39.htm.

Makuc, D., Halund, B., Ingram, D., Kleinman, J., and Feldman, J. (1991). Health Service Areas for the United States. *Vital and Health Statistics, 112*(Series 2), 1–102.

Mankiw, N. G. (2009, June 27). The Pitfalls of the Public Option. *New York Times,* p. BU5.

Marmor, T. (2000). *The Politics of Medicare* (2nd ed.). Hawthorne, NY: Aldine de Gruyter.

———. (2012). *Why Turning Medicare into Vouchers Will Not Work.* Retrieved August 4, 2015, from http://www.scholarsstrategynetwork.org/sites/default/files/ssn_basic_facts_marmor_on_medicare.pdf.

Marshall, T., & Bottomore, T. (1992). *Citizenship and Social Class.* London: Pluto Press.

Marx, K. (1938). *Critique of the Gotha Programme, by Karl Marx; with Appendices by Marx, Engles, and Lenin; A Revised Translation.* New York: International Publishers.

Massey, D. (2007). *Categorically Unequal: The American Stratification System.* New York: The Russell Sage Foundation.

———. (2009). Globalization and Inequality: Explaining American Exceptionalism. *European Economic Review, 25*(1), 9–23.

Massey, D., Alarcon, R., & Duran, J. (1990). *Return to Aztlan: The Social Process of International Migration from Western Mexico.* Berkeley: University of California Press.

Massey, D., Durand, J., & Pren, K. (2015). Border Enforcement and Return by Documented and Undocumented Mexicans. *Journal of Ethnic and Migration Studies, 41*(7), 1015–1040.

McAuliff, M. (2012, January 11). Mitt Romney: Maybe Veterans' Health Care Should Be Privatized. *Huffington Post.* Retrieved August 13, 2015, from http://www.huffingtonpost.com/2011/11/11/mitt-romney-veterans-health-care-privatization_n_1089061.html.

McCollister, K., Zheng, D., Fernandez, C., Lee, D., Lam, B., Arheart, K., et al. (2012). Racial Disparities in Quality-Adjusted Life-Years Associated with Diabetes and Visual Impairment. *Diabetes Care, 35*(8), 1692–1694.

303

REFERENCES

McDonough, J. (2015). The Demise of Vermont's Single-Payer Plan. *New England Journal of Medicine, 372*, 1584–1585.

McGlynn, E. (1997). Six Challenges in Measuring the Quality of Health Care. *Health Affairs, 16*(3), 7–21.

McQuire, T., Newhouse, J., & Sinaiko, A. (2011). An Economic History of Medicare Part C. *Milbank Quarterly, 89*(2), 289–332.

Mechanic, D. (2004). The Rise and Fall of Managed Care. *Journal of Health and Social Behavior, 45*(Suppl), 76–86.

Mehrotra, A., Damberg, C., Sorbero, M., & Teleki, S. (2009, January/February). Pay for Performance in the Hospital Setting: What Is the State of the Evidence? *American Journal of Medical Quality*, pp. 19–28.

Meltzer, D., & Chung, J. (2014). The Population Value of Quality Indicator Reporting: A Framework for Prioritizing Health Care Performance Measures. *Health Affairs, 33*(1), 132–139.

Miniño, A. (2011, July). *NCHS Data Brief No. 64: Death in the United States, 2009.* Hyattsville, MD: National Center for Health Statistics.

Mioreno-Serra, R., Thomson, S., & Xu, K. (2013). Measuring and Comparing Financial Protection. In I. Papanicolas & P. Smith (Eds.), *Health System Performance Comparison: An Agenda for Policy Information and Research* (pp. 223–254). Berkshire, UK: Open University Press, McGraw-Hill.

Mogulescu, M. (2010, March 16). NY Times Reporter Confirms Obama Made Deal to Kill Public Option. *Huffington Post.* Retrieved April 22, 2014, from http://www.huffington post.com/miles-mogulescu/ny-times-reporter-confirm_b_500999.html.

Mohindra, R. (2007). Medical Futility: A Conceptual Model. *Journal of Medical Ethics, 33*(2), 71–75.

Molla, M. (2013). Expected Years of Life Free of Chronic Condition–Induced Activity Limitations—United States, 1999–2008. *Morbidity and Mortality Weekly Report (MMWR), 62*, 87–92.

Monheit, A., & Vistnes, J. (2005). The Demand for Dependent Health Insurance: How Important Is the Cost of Family Coverage? *Journal of Health Economics, 24*(6), 1108–1131.

Morone, J. (2010). Presidents and Health Reform: From Franklin D. Roosevelt to Barack Obama. *Health Affairs, 29*(6), 1096–1100.

Multi-Society Task Force on PVS. (1994). Medical Aspects of the Persistent Vegetative State. *New England Journal of Medicine, 330*, 1572–1579.

Nakano-Glenn, E. (2002). *Unequal Freedom: How Race and Gender Shaped American Citizenship and Labor.* Cambridge, MA: Harvard University Press.

——. (2010). *Forced to Care: Coercion and Caregiving in America.* Cambridge, MA: Harvard University Press.

Nathan, R. (2005). Federalism and Health Policy: Medicaid as an Appropriate and Feasible Base on Which to Build Basic Health Care Coverage. *Heath Affairs, 24*(6), 1458–1466.

National Association of City and County Health Officials (NACCHO). (2012). *Public Health and Prevention Provisions of the Affordable Care Act.* Retrieved July 9, 2014, from http://www.naccho.org/advocacy/upload/PH-and-Prevention-Provisions-in -the-ACA-Revised.pdf.

National Association of Social Workers (NASW). (2011, December 29). *NASW Policy Statements: Health Care Policy.* Retrieved May 15, 2013, from https://www.social

workers.org/pressroom/swMonth/2012/toolkit/standards/Health%20Care%20P
olicy.pdf.

National Association of Urban Hospitals. (2012, September). *The Potential Impact of the Affordable Care Act on Urban Safety-Net Hospitals.* Retrieved July 1, 2014, from http://www.nauh.org/research/raw/98.html.

National Center for Health Statistics (NCHS). (2011). *Life Expectancy at Birth, at Age 65, and at Age 75, by Sex, Race, and Hispanic Origin: United States, Selected Years.* Retrieved August 4, 2015, from http://www.cdc.gov/nchs/data/hus/2011/022.pdf.

National Center for Health Workforce Analysis. (2014). *The Future of the Nursing Workforce: National- and State-Level Projections, 2012–2025.* Retrieved May 21, 2015, from http://bhw.hrsa.gov/healthworkforce/supplydemand/nursing/workforceprojections/nursingprojections.pdf.

National Committee on Vital and Health Statistics. (2001). *Information for Health: A Strategy for Building the National Health Information Infrastructure.* Retrieved May 5, 2015, from http://aspe.hhs.gov/sp/nhii/Documents/nhiilayo.pdf.

National Immigration Law Center. (2014). *The Individual Taxpayer Identification Number (ITIN): A Powerful Tool for Immigrant Taxpayers.* Retrieved June 4, 2015, from http://www.nilc.org/itinfaq.html#fn8.

National Opinion Research Center. (2006). *General Social Science Survey Codebook.* Retrieved April 13, 2006, from http://webapp.icpst.umich.edu/GSS.

———. (2016). *GSS Data Explorer: Should Govt Help Pay for Medical Care?* Retrieved March 15, 2016, from https://gssdataexplorer.norc.org/variables/846/vshow.

Needlenan, J., & Ko, M. (2012). The Declining Public Hospital Sector. In M. Hall & S. Rosenbaum (Eds.), *The Health Care Safety-Net in a Post Reform World* (pp. 200–213). New Brunswick, NJ: Rutgers University Press.

Neumann, P., Cohen, J., & Weinstein, M. (2014). Updating Cost Effectiveness—The Curious Resilience of the $50,000-per-QALY Threshold. *New England Journal of Medicine, 371*(9), 796–797.

Newhouse, J. (1993). An Iconoclastic View of Health Care Cost Containment. *Health Affairs, 12*(Suppl), 152–171.

A New Prescription for the Poor: America Is Developing a Two-Tier Health System, One for Those with Private Insurance, the Other for the Less Well-Off. (2011, October 8). *The Economist.* Retrieved August 1, 2014, from http://www.economist.com/node/21531491.

Nixon, R. (1972, March 2). *Special Message to Congress on Health Care.* Retrieved May 8, 2014, from http://www.presidency.ucsb.edu/ws/?pid=3757.

———. (1974, January 30). *Address on the State of the Union Delivered Before a Joint Session of the Congress, January 30, 1974.* Retrieved May 8, 2014, from http://www.presidency.ucsb.edu/ws/?pid=4327.

Noah, T. (2009, October 22). Did Lieberman Just Kill the Public Option? *Slate.*

Norris, T., Vines, P., & Hoeffel, E. (2012). *The American Indian and Alaska Native Population: 2010.* Suitland, MD: U.S. Census Bureau.

Nussbaum, M. (2000). *Women and Human Development.* New York: Cambridge University Press.

Oberlander, J., Marmor, T., & Jacobs, L. (2001). Rationing Medical Care: Rhetoric and Reality in the Oregon Health Plan. *Canadian Medical Association Journal, 165*(11), 1583–1587.

Office of the Press Secretary. (2014). *Remarks by the President on the Affordable Care Act, April 1, 2014.* Retrieved April 24, 2014, from http://www.whitehouse.gov/the -press-office/2014/04/01/remarks-president-affordable-care-act.

Office of the White House Press Secretary. (2014, May 27). *Statement by the President on Afghanistan.* Retrieved August 11, 2015, from https://www.whitehouse.gov/the -press-office/2014/05/27/statement-president-afghanistan.

Olson, C. (1995, March). Health Insurance Coverage Among Male Workers. *Monthly Labor Review,* 55–61.

Olson, P. (2012). *Moral Arguments for Universal Health Care.* Bloomington, IN: AuthorHouse.

Organization for Economic Cooperation and Development (OECD). (2011). *Health at a Glance 2011: OECD Indicators.* Paris: Organization for Economic Co-operation and Development.

——. (2012). *Health at a Glance 2011.* Retrieved October 25, 2013, from http://www.oecd-ilibrary.org/docserver/download/8111101ec053.pdf?expires=1382732057&id=id &accname=guest&checksum=70170CA03527B8EF4ABB4F2863DA6117.

——. (2013a). *Health at a Glance, 2013.* Retrieved July 18, 2014, from http://www.oecd .org/els/health-systems/Health-at-a- Glance-2013.pdf.

——. (2013b). *OECD Health Statistics 2013: Health Insurance Coverage for a Core Set of Services, 2011.* Retrieved June 17, 2014, from http://www.oecd.org/els/health-systems /Health-at-a-Glance-2013-Chart-set.pdf.

——. (2013c). *OECD Health Data 2013.* Retrieved October 23, 2013, from http://www .oecd.org/els/health-systems/oecdhealthdata2013-frequentlyrequesteddata .htm.

——. (2013d). *Most Frequently Requested Health Data, 2013.* Retrieved April 5, 2014, from http://www.oecd.org/els/health-systems/oecdhealthdata2013-frequently requesteddata.htm.

——. (2014a). *Health at a Glance, 2013.* Retrieved April 28, 2015, from http://www.oecd .org/els/health-systems/Health-at-a-Glance-2013.pdf.

——. (2014b, January 5). *Table CO2.2A Poverty Rates for Children and Households with Children.* Retrieved August 3, 2015, from http://www.oecd.org/els/family/CO2_2 _ChildPoverty_Jan2014.pdf.

——. (2014c). *Society at a Glance, 2014.* Retrieved July 23, 2014, from http://www.oecd -ilibrary.org/sites/soc_glance-2014-en/05/04/g5-07.html?contentType=&itemId =%2fcontent%2fchapter%2fsoc_glance-2014-20-en&mimeType=text%2fhtml&conta inerItemId=%2fcontent%2fserial%2f19991290&accessItemI ds=%2fcontent%2fbook%2 fsoc_glance-2014-e.

——. (2014d). *Income Distribution and Poverty.* Retrieved July 24, 2014, from http:// stats.oecd.org/Index.aspx?DataSetCode=IDD.

——. (2015). *Health Expenditures and Financing by OECD Country.* Retrieved July 9, 2015, from http://stats.oecd.org/index.aspx?DataSetCode=HEALTH_STAT.

Orient, J. (2011). Disenrollment from Medicare: A Fourth Option. *Journal of American Physicians and Surgeons, 16*(4), 104–109.

Page, S. (2005). *An Essay on the Existence and Causes of Path Dependence.* Retrieved April 5, 2014, from http://vserver1.cscs.lsa.umich.edu/~spage/pathdepend.pdf.

Palloni, A., & Arias, E. (2004). Paradox Lost: Explaining the Hispanic Adult Mortality Advantage. *Demography, 41*(3), 385–415.

Partnership for Long-Term Care (PLTC). (2015). *The Partnership for Long Term Care.* Retrieved August 6, 2015, from http://www.partnershipforlongtermcare.com/index .html.

PBS. (2000). "Interview with Uwe Reinhart." *The Healthcare Crisis: Who's at Risk.* Retrieved July 14, 2014, from http://www.pbs.org/healthcarecrisis/Exprts_intrvw /u_reinhardt.htm.

Peffer, R. G. (1990). *Marxism, Morality, and Social Justice.* Princeton, NJ: Princeton University Press.

Perry, S., & Foster, J. (2010, May). *Health Reform: Help for Native Americans and Alaska Natives.* Retrieved June 10, 2014, from http://research.policyarchive.org/95677.pdf.

Pew Research Center. (2013, May 23). *Chapter 3. Inequality and Economic Mobility.* Retrieved July 28, 2014, from http://www.pewglobal.org/2013/05/23/chapter-3-inequality -and-economic-mobility/.

Phelan, J., Link, B., Diex-Roux, A., Kawachi, I., & Levin, B. (2004). "Fundamental Social Causes of Social Inequalities in Mortality: A Test of the Theory. *Journal of Health and Social Behavior, 45*(3), 265–285.

Physicians for a National Health Program (PNHP). (2013). *PNHP Mission Statement.* Retrieved May 15, 2013, from http://www.pnhp.org/about/pnhp-mission-statement.

Politifact.com. (2012, October 1). *Chamber of Commerce Says Health Care "Public Option" Idea Was "Wildly Unpopular."* Retrieved August 9, 2014, from http://www .politifact.com/wisconsin/statements/2012/oct/01/us-chamber-commerce /chamber-commerce-says-health-care-public-option-id/.

Portes, A. (2006, July 31). *NAFTA and Mexican Immigration.* Retrieved July 27, 2015, from http://borderbattles.ssrc.org/Portes/.

Portes, A., Fernández-Kelly, P., & Haller, W. (2009). The Adaptation of the Immigrant Second Generation in America: Theoretical Overview and Recent Evidence. *Journal of Ethnic and Migration Studies, 35*(7), 1077–1104.

Pressman, J., & Wildavsky, A. (1984). *Implementation.* Oakland: University of California Press.

Public Campaign Action Fund. (2009). *Joe Lieberman and the Health Care Industry.* Retrieved July 29, 2014, from http://www.insurancepuppets.com/puppets/joelieberman.

Putnam, H. (2005). John Rawls. *Proceedings of the American Philosophical Society, 149*(1), 114–117.

Quadagno, J. (2004). Why the United States Has No Health Insurance: Stakeholder Mobilization Against the Welfare State. *Journal of Health and Social Behavior, 45* (Suppl.), 25–44.

——. (2005). *One Nation Uninsured.* New York: Oxford University Press.

RAND Corporation. (2005). *Improving Quality of Care: How the VA Outpaces Other Systems in Delivering Patient Care.* Retrieved August 13, 2015, from http://www .rand.org/content/dam/rand/pubs/research_briefs/2005/RAND_RB9100.pdf.

Rangrass, G., Ghaferi, A., & Dimick, J. (2013). Explaining Racial Disparities in Outcomes After Cardiac Surgery: The Role of Hospital Quality. *JAMA, 149*(3), 223–227.

Rawls, J. (1957). Justice as Fairness. *Journal of Philosophy, 54*(22), 653–662.

——. (1971). *A Theory of Justice.* Cambridge, MA: Belknap Press of Harvard University Press.

——. (2001). *Justice as Fairness: A Restatement.* Cambridge, MA: Harvard University Press.

307

REFERENCES

Raykar, N., Mandogo, M., Nagengast, E., Coffran, M., Hanks, J., Meara, J., and Tracci, M. (2014, March 1). *Medicaid Expansion Likely to Affect the Delivery of Surgical Care*. Retrieved June 17, 2014, from http://bulletin.facs.org/2014/03/medicaid-expansion-likely-to-affect-the-delivery-of-surgical-care/.

Redish, A., Sarra, J., & Schabas, M. (2006). *Growing Old Gracefully: An Investigation into the Growing Number of Bankrupt Canadians over Age 55*. Retrieved June 8, 2015, from https://www.ic.gc.ca/eic/site/bsf-osb.nsf/vwapj/Redish-Sarra-Schabas-2006-ENG.pdf/$FILE/Redish-Sarra-Schabas-2006-ENG.pdf.

Reid, D., & Wong, D. (2011, July). *Short Paper No. 9: The ACA and Health Disparities*. Retrieved July 14, 2014, from http://www.healthlaw.org/publications/aca-health-disparities#.U8QvbEB23To.

Reinhart, U. (2013, December 20). The Economics of Being Kinder and Gentler in Health Care. *New York Times*.

Religious Action Center of Reform (RAC). (2013). *Jewish Values and Health Care*. Retrieved May 15, 2013, from http://rac.org/Articles/index.cfm?id=1825.

Rescher, N. (1966). *Distributive Justice: A Constructive Critique of the Utilitarian Theory of Distribution*. New York: Bobbs-Merrill.

Rittenhouse, D., Shortell, S., & Fisher, E. (2009). Primary Care and Accountable Care—Two Essential Elements of Delivery-System Reform. *New England Journal of Medicine, 361*, 2301–2303.

Robbins, G., & Robbins, A. (1994, May). *Forecasting the Effects of the Clinton Plan*. Retrieved May 13, 2014, from http://www.ncpa.org/pdfs/st185.pdf.

Robert Wood Johnson Foundation. (2011, December). *Issue Brief: How Does the Affordable Care Act Address Racial and Ethnic Disparities in Health Care?* Retrieved June 17, 2014, from http://www.rwjf.org/content/dam/farm/reports/issue_briefs/2011/rwjf71997.

Robeyns, I. (2011). *The Capability Approach*. Retrieved from http://plato.stanford.edu/entries/capability-approach.

Robinson, J. (2008). Value-Based Purchasing for Medical Devices. *Health Affairs, 27*(6), 1523–1531.

Rodwin, V. G., & Sandier, S. (2008). *Health Care Under French National Health Insurance*. Retrieved November 15, 2013, from http://www.nyu.edu/projects/rodwin/french.html.

Roemer, M. (1961). Bed Supply and Hospital Utilization: A Natural Experiment. *Hospitals, 35*, 36–42.

Rogowski, J., Freedman, V., Wickstrom, S., Adams, J., & Escarce, J. (2008). Socioeconomic Disparities in Medical Provider Visits Among Medicare Managed Care Enrollees. *Inquiry, 45*(1), 112–129.

Rosenbach, M. (2007). *Increasing Children's Coverage and Access: A Decade of SCHIP Lessons* (Issue Brief No. 4, pp. 1–5). Washington, D.C.: Mathematica Policy Research Inc.

Rosenberg, C. (1987). *The Care of Strangers: The Rise of America's Hospital System*. New York: Basic Books.

Ross, D. (1991). *The Origins of American Social Science*. Cambridge, UK: Cambridge University Press.

Roy, A. (2013, August 10). Sen. Harry Reid: Obamacare 'Absolutely' A Step Toward a Single-Payer System. *Forbes*. Retrieved August 7, 2014, from http://www.forbes.com/sites/theapothecary/2013/08/10/sen-harry-reid-obamacare-absolutely-a-step-toward-a-single-payer-system/.

Scanlon, W. (2006). The Future of Medicare Hospital Payment. *Health Affairs, 25*(1), 70–80.

Schram, S., Soss, J., Fording, R., & Houser, L. (2009). Deciding to Discipline: Race, Choice, and Punishment at the Frontlines of Welfare Reform. *American Sociological Review, 74*(3), 398–422.

Schroeder, S. (2011). Personal Reflections on the High Cost of American Medical Care. *Archives of Internal Medicine, 171*(8), 722–727.

Scofea, L. (1994, March). The Development and Growth of Employer Provided Health Insurance. *Monthly Labor Review*, pp. 3–10.

Scott, F., Berger, M., & Black, D. (1989). Effects of the Tax Treatment of Fringe Benefits on Labor Market Segmentation. *Industrial and Labor Relations Review, 42*(2), 216–229.

Seifert, R., & Rukavina, M. (2006). Bankruptcy Is the Tip of a Medical-Debt Iceberg. *Health Affairs, 25*, w89–w92.

Sen, A. (2009). *The Idea of Justice*. Cambridge, MA: Belknap Press of the Harvard University Press.

Serwer, A. (2009, August 21). The De-Facto Segregation of Health Care. *American Prospect*. Retrieved July 24, 2014, from http://prospect.org/article/de-facto-segregation -health-care-o.

Shi, L. (2012). *The Impact of Primary Care: A Focused Review*. Retrieved January 28, 2015, from http://www.ncbi.nlm.nih.gov/pmc/articles/PMC3820251/.

Shi, L., & Singh, D. (2001). *Delivering Health Care in America* (2nd ed.). Gaithersburg, MD: Aspen Publishers.

Shi, L., & Stevens, G. (2005). Vulnerability and Unmet Health Care Needs: The Influence of Multiple Risk Factors. *Journal of General Internal Medicine, 20*(2), 148–154.

Shklar, J. (1991). *American Citizenship: The Quest for Inclusion*. Cambridge, MA: Harvard University Press.

Shojania, K., McDonald, W., Wachter, R., & Owens, D. (2007). *Closing the Quality Gap: A Critical Analysis of Quality Improvement—Volume 7, Care Coordination*. Rockville, MD: Agency for Healthcare Research and Quality.

Shryock, H., & Siegel, J. (1976). *The Methods and Materials of Demography*. New York: Academic Press.

Silverman, E., Skinner, J., & Fisher, E. (1999). The Association Between For-Profit Hospital Ownership and Increased Medicare Spending. *New England Journal of Medicine, 341*, 420–426.

Skocpol, T. (1992). *Protecting Soldiers and Mothers: The Political Origins of Social Policy in the United States*. Cambridge, MA: Harvard University Press.

——. (2010). The Political Challenges That May Undermine Health Care Reform. *Health Affairs, 29*(7), 1288–1292.

Slusky, R. (2011). *Report to the Legislature on Payment Reform*. Montpelier: State of Vermont, Agency of Human Services, Department of Vermont Health Access.

Social Security Administration. (2014a). Chapter 4: The Fourth Round—1957 to 1965. *Social Security History*. Retrieved April 10, 2014, from http://www.ssa.gov/history /corningchap4.html.

——. (2014b). *History of SSA During the Johnson Administration, 1963–1968*. Retrieved May 20, 2014, from http://www.ssa.gov/history/ssa/lbjmedicare4.html.

Soss, J., Schram, S., Vartanian, T., & O'Brien, E. (2001). Setting the Terms of Relief: Explaining State Policy Choices in the Devolution Revolution. *American Journal of Political Science, 45*, 378–395.

South Dakota Department of Public Health (SDDPH). (2012). *South Dakota Department of Public Health: Health Profiles by County*. Retrieved July 11, 2014, from http:// doh.sd.gov/statistics/2010Vital/HealthStatusByCounty.pdf.

Starr, P. (1982). *The Social Transformation of American Medicine*. New York: Basic Books.

——. (1995). What Happened to Health Care Reform. *American Prospect, 20*, 20–31.

State of Vermont. (2014, January 16). *Health Care Reform Timeline: Vermont Health Care Reform Population Grid*. Retrieved August 9, 2014, from http://hcr.vermont .gov/sites/hcr/files/2014/HCR%20Population%20Grid%20HHC%20011614.pdf.

Stefos, T., & Burgess, J. (2014, October 2). Establishing Vouchers for Veteran Health Care. *Health Affairs*. Retrieved August 13, 2015, from http://healthaffairs.org/blog /2014/10/02/establishing-vouchers-for-veteran-health-care/.

Strauss, D. (1992). The Illusionary Distinction Between Equality of Opportunity and Equality of Result. *William and Mary Law Review, 34*(1), 171–188.

Stuber, J., & Kronebusch, K. (2004). Stigma and Other Determinants of Participation in TANF and Medicaid. *Journal of Policy Analysis and Management, 23*(3), 509–530.

Sullivan, S., Watkins, J., Sweet, B., & Ramsey, S. (2009). Health Technology Assessment in Health-Care Decisions in the U.S. *International Society for Pharmacoeconomics and Outcomes Research, 12*(2), S39–S44.

Sussman, T., Blendon, R. J., & Campbell, A. L. (2009). Will Americans Support the Individual Mandate? *Health Affairs, 28*(3), w501–w509.

Talbott, W. (2010). *Human Rights and Human Well-Being*. New York: Oxford University Press.

Taylor, T. (2001). Threats to the Health Care Safety Net. *Academic Emergency Medicine, 8*(11), 1080–1087.

Teaching American History. (2012). *Progressive Party Platform of 1912*. Retrieved May 5, 1914, from http://teachingamericanhistory.org/library/document/progressive -platform-of-1912/.

Thornton, R. (1997). Aboriginal North American Population and Rates of Decline, c.a. A.D. 1500–1900. *Current Anthropology, 38*(2), 310–314.

Thorpe, K., Florence, C., & Seiber, E. (2000). Hospital Conversions, Margins, and the Provision of Uncompensated Care. *Health Affairs, 19*(6), 187–194.

Treasury Inspector General for Tax Administration. (2011). *Individuals Who Are Not Authorized to Work in the United States Were Paid $4.2 Billion in Refundable Credits*. Retrieved June 4, 2015, from http://www.treasury.gov/tigta/auditreports /2011reports/201141061fr.pdf.

Ubel, P. (2013, January 9). Why It Is So Difficult to Kill the Death Panel Myth. *Forbes*. Retrieved July 30, 2015, from http://www.forbes.com/sites/peterubel/2013/01/09 /why-it-is-so-difficult-to-kill-the-death-panel-myth/.

Ungar, R. (2012, February 23). Single-Payer Health Care Is Coming to America—Are We Ready? *Forbes*, pp. 1–3.

United Nations. (1948). *The Universal Declaration of Human Rights*. Retrieved May 13, 2013, from https://www.un.org/en/documents/udhr/index.shtml#a26

United States Senate Committee on Indian Affairs, 111th Congress. (2010). *In Critical Condition: The Urgent Need to Reform Indian Health Service's Aberdeen Area. Hearing Before the United States Senate Committee on Indian Affairs, September 28, 2011, 111th Congress*. Retrieved May 23, 2015, from http://www.indian.senate.gov/hearing

/oversight-hearing-titled-critical-condition-urgent-need-reform-indian-health
-services.

University of Delaware. (2012). Healthcare Law Gender Gap: New U.S. Poll Shows
Women Favor Mandate More Than Men. *Science Daily*. Retrieved August 7, 2014,
from http://www.sciencedaily.com/releases/2012/06/120626140953.htm.

The Urban Institute. (2001). *Long-Term Care: Consumers, Providers and Financing:
A Chartbook*. Washington, D.C.: The Urban Institute.

U.S. Census Bureau. (1975). *Historical Census of the United States: Colonial Times to
1970: Series B 401–412*. Retrieved April 7, 2014, from http://www2.census.gov/prod2
/statcomp/documents/CT1970p1-03.pdf.

———. (2008). *Projections of the Population and Components of Change for the United
States: 2010 to 2050*. Retrieved March 20, 2012, from http://www.census.gov/
population/www/projections/summarytables.html.

———. (2013). *2012 National Population Projections: Summary Tables: Table 1 Projections of
the Population and Components of Change for the United States: 2015 to 2060 (Middle
Series)*. Washington, D.C.: U.S. Census Bureau. U.S. Department of Commerce.

———. (2015). *Urban, Urbanized Area, Urban Cluster, and Rural Population, 2010
and 2000: United States*. Retrieved May 20, 2015, from http://www.census.gov/geo/
reference/ua/urban-rural-2010.html.

U.S. Citizenship and Immigration Services. (2015). *Lawful Permanent Resident (LPR)*.
Retrieved July 28, 2015, from http://www.uscis.gov/tools/glossary/lawful-permanent
-resident-lpr.

Van de Water, P. N. (2008). *Immigration and Social Security*. Washington, D.C.: Center
on Budget and Policy Priorities.

———. (2009). *2009 Trustees' Report Underscores Urgency of Health Reform, Medicare
Changes*. Retrieved April 29, 2014, from http://www.cbpp.org/cms/?fa=view&id
=2818.

Van Doorslaer, E., Clarke, P., Savage, E., & Hall, J. (2008). Horizontal Inequities in
Australia's Mixed Public/Private Health Care System. *Health Policy, 86*, 97–108.

Van Doorslaer, E., Masseria, C., & Koolman, X. (2006). Inequalities in Access to Medical Care by Income in Developed Countries. *Canadian Medical Association Journal,
174*(2), 177–183.

Venkatapuram, S. (2011). *Health Justice*. Cambridge, UK: Polity Press.

Warne, D., & Frizzell, L. (2014). American Indian Health Policy: Historical Trends
and Contemporary Issues. *American Journal of Public Health, 104*(Suppl 3),
S263–S267.

Warner, J. H. (2013). The Doctor in Early Cold War America. *Lancet, 381*(9876),
1452–1453.

Wax-Thibodeaux, E. (2015, June 23). One Year After VA Scandal, the Number of Veterans Waiting for Care Is Up 50 Percent. *Washington Post*. Retrieved August 12, 2015,
from http://www.washingtonpost.com/blogs/federal-eye/wp/2015/06/23/one-year
-after-va-scandal-the-number-of-veterans-waiting-for-care-is-up-50-percent/.

Weisbrod, B. (1991). The Health Care Quadrilemma: An Essay on Technological Change,
Insurance, Quality of Care, and Cost Containment. *Journal of Economic Literature, 29*(2), 523–552.

Wendt, C. (2009). Mapping European Healthcare Systems: A Comparative Analysis of
Financing, Service Provision, and Access to Healthcare. *Journal of European Social
Policy, 19*(5), 432–445.

White, C., & Reschovsky, J. (2012). *Great Recession Accelerated Long-Term Decline of Employer Health Coverage* (NIHCR Research Brief No. 8, pp. 1–6). Washington, D.C.: National Institute for Health Care Reform.

White, J. (2009). Gap and Parallel Insurance in Health Care Systems with Mandatory Contributions to a Single Funding Pool for Core Medical and Hospital Benefits for All Citizens in Any Geographic Area. *Journal of Health Politics, Policy and Law,* *34*(4), 543–583.

Williams, D., & Jackson, P. (2005). Social Sources of Racial Disparities in Health. *Health Affairs, 24*(2), 325–334.

Williams, L. (2000). Long Term Care After Olmstead v. L.C.: Will the Potential of the ADA's Integration Mandate Be Achieved? *Journal of Contemporary Health Law and Policy, 17*(1), 205–239.

World Economic Forum. (2012). *The Global Competitiveness Report 2012–20013.* Geneva, Switzerland: World Economic Forum.

Xu, K. (2002). Usual Source of Care in Preventive Service Use: A Regular Doctor Versus a Regular Site. *Health Services Research, 37*(6), 1509–1529.

INDEX

324

INDEX

INDEX

low-budget restricted access type health system: in Wendt's three-system typology, 134

low-income patients: disparities in usual source of care and, 163; quality of care disparities and, 163–164; unmet health needs disparities and, 164

low-wage caregiving labor force: budgetary challenges and, 191

low-wage employment, 239

LPNs. *See* licensed practical nurses

Luxembourg: health service provision-oriented type health system in, 133

managed care, 198; Medicare beneficiaries and, 51; rise and fall of, 28–29

Managed Care, 134, 140

managed competition: Clinton's Health Security Act and, 43

Mansuri Hospital (Cairo), 70

Marquis, M., 171, 179, 188, 192, 193

Marshall, Alfred, 79

Marshall, T. H., 35, 61, 62, 237, 239, 253, 263, 266; account of evolution of democratic citizenship, 80–82, 277n12; *Citizenship and Social Class*, 62, 63, 76, 77, 78, 82, 85, 92, 93; citizenship conceptualized by, 112; contrasting epistemologies of Rawls and, 74–76; on democratic citizenship, 111; evolution of democratic citizenship in Great Britain and, 79–80; fusion of Rawls and, on universal health care as requisite to democratic citizenship, 98–101; historical, personal, and intellectual context for, 74–76; justification of social right to health care by, 246; nature of democratic citizenship and, 93, 94–95; nature of democratic society and, 93–94; remarkable convergences in theories of John Rawls and, 74; social rights and exercise of civil and political citizenship and, 93, 96; social rights as requisites to citizenship status and, 93, 95–96; social rights as requisite to

collective sense of social equality and, 93, 97–98; social rights as requisite to permeable class structure and, 93, 97; theory of citizenship, 62, 63; theory of democratic citizenship in historical context, 76–79

Marx, Karl, 72, 73

Maryland: single-payer movement in, 200

Massachusetts Commonwealth Care plan, 27, 150

mass deportation of undocumented workers: potential economic consequences of, 241–242

Massey, D., 138

material security: citizenship status and, 102, 108

material social rights: Marshall on democratic citizenship and, 83

McCarthy era: national health insurance and rhetoric of, 7, 10

McCarthyism: "creeping communism" rhetoric of, 78

McDonough, John, 158

means-based social entitlements: stigma of, 33, 34, 58, 119

means-tested programs: low take-up rates and, 204; undocumented workers excluded from, 205

measurement of health-care equity: criterion for perfect equity, 220, 284n11; target performance benchmark for equitable distribution of health-care services and, 227–228; total amelioration of disparities in quality of care, 225

Medicaid, 26, 48, 70, 146, 158, 192, 193, 256, 260; ACA and state expansion of, 54, 55; ACA's amelioration of disparities in health-care access and, 117–118; American Medical Association and, 19–21; Clinton administration and preservation of, 44; Clinton's Health Security Act and, 42–43; cost-control aspects of ACA and, 31; creation of, 32, 40; expenditures for long-term care needs, growth in, 257; health-care

socioeconomic status (SES): global
budgeting approach and, 172
"soft" global budgeting process, 171
"soft" two-tiered health-care system:
characteristics of, 159–160, 281n1;
defined, 145; equitable vision of
health-care financing and, 144;
evolvement of, prospects for, 149–157;
explanations and caveats, 148–149;
OECD member nations and, 146;
reconciling core health-care policy
aims with, 145–149; Tier I (limited
entitlement social insurance trust
fund for basic care), 147; Tier II
(unsubsidized voluntary private
health insurance market), 147–148
Spain: low-budget restricted access type
health system in, 134
spatial mismatches: health-care facilities
and, 192
specialty hospitals, 191
SSN. *See* Social Security Number
Stalinism, 73, 77
Starr, Paul, 8, 20, 26, 37; analysis of
American medical profession by, 7–8;
on professional sovereignty, 9; *Social
Transformation of American
Medicine*, 7, 123, 199; three-layer cake
metaphor of, 22
State Children's Health Initiative
Program (SCHIP), 27; creation of, 44,
45; two significant achievements
represented by, 45
State Health Care Plan Authority—Tier I
health care: administrative
oversight functions, categories, 176,
182; biannual state plan for delivery
of Tier I core health-care services,
176, 180–182; research and
development, 176, 182
states: ACA's Medicaid expansion
provision and, 33, 54, 55, 113–114, 116,
117; ADA community integration
requirements, and limits of
"reasonable efforts" by, 287n12; global
budgeting approach, federalism, and,
175; global budgeting structure for
Tier I core services and, 177–178;

hospital resource disparities in,
161–162; numbers of PCPs relative to
population size in, 161; Partnership
for Long-Term Care reciprocity
between, 259–260; race and public
assistance in, 137; single-payer
movement and, 156–157
status equality: citizenship status and,
102, 108
Stefos, T., 269
stigma: of means-based social
entitlements, 33, 34, 58; Medicaid
coverage and, 117, 119
stratified societies: expropriation of
labor and, 242
Strauss, David: on equality of
opportunity *vs.* equality of result, 139,
279n6
structural budget: biannual global
budget for Tier I health-care services
and, 188
subsidized employment-based health
insurance: emergence of, 17–18; as
penultimate impediment to social
insurance for health care, 18
Substance Abuse and Mental Health
Services Administration (SAMHSA),
190, 221
suburbanization of American landscape:
post-World War II, 266
successful social policy: criteria for, 55
supplemental private health insurance
coverage, 133
supplementary health insurance: Tier II,
taxation triggers of, 173; two-tiered
global budgeting approach and,
172
Supreme Court: cases related to
overturning key provisions of ACA,
276n9
sustainability: limits of health-care
intervention in terms of, 237; political
dimension to, 197–198; Tier I
health-care services and, 197–198
Sweden, 62, 195; equity in health-care
system of, 122, 278n8; total health
expenditures uncovered by public
health insurance in, 132; universal